ULTRASOUND IN MEDICINE

Volume 2

A Continuation Order Plan is available for this series. A continuation order will bring delivery of each new volume immediately upon publication. Volumes are billed only upon actual shipment. For further information please contact the publisher.

ULTRASOUND IN MEDICINE

Volume 2

Proceedings of the 20th Annual Meeting of the
American Institute of Ultrasound in Medicine

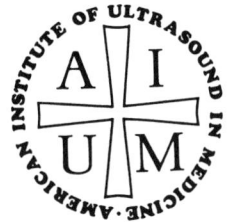

Edited by
Denis White
Department of Medicine
Queens University
Ontario, Canada

and

Ralph Barnes
Bowman Gray School of Medicine
Wake Forest University
Winston-Salem, North Carolina

PLENUM PRESS • NEW YORK AND LONDON

Library of Congress Catalog Card Number 74-32484
ISBN 0-306-34202-2

©1976 American Institute of Ultrasound in Medicine
and Plenum Press, New York
A Division of Plenum Publishing Corporation
227 West 17th Street, New York, N.Y. 10011

United Kingdom edition published by Plenum Press, London
A Division of Plenum Publishing Company, Ltd.
Davis House (4th Floor), 8 Scrubs Lane, Harlesden, London, NW10 6SE, England

All rights reserved

No part of this book may be reproduced, stored in a retrieval system, or transmitted, in any form or by any means, electronic, mechanical, photocopying, microfilming, recording, or otherwise, without written permission from the Publisher

Printed in the United States of America

AMERICAN INSTITUTE OF ULTRASOUND IN MEDICINE

PRESIDENT
William M. McKinney, M.D.

VICE PRESIDENT
Barry B. Goldberg, M.D.

SECRETARY
Richard L. Popp, M.D.

TREASURER
Horace E. Thompson, M.D.

PRESIDENT ELECT
Ross E. Brown, M.D.

PAST PRESIDENT
Gilbert Baum, M.D.

EXECUTIVE BOARD
Ralph Barnes, Ph.D.
Ernest N. Carlsen, M.D.
Kenneth R. Erikson, Ph.D.
Harvey Feigenbaum, M.D.
Barbara B. Gosink, M.D.
Joseph H. Holmes, M.D.
Professor Elizabeth Kelly Fry
Padmakar P. Lele, M.D.
George R. Leopold, M.D.
Richard A. Meyer, M.D.
Wesley L. Nyborg, Ph.D.
Renate Soulen, M.D.
Shirley Staiano, B.S.
Robert C. Waag, Ph.D.
Michael A. Wainstock, M.D.
Fred Winsberg, M.D.
Marvin C. Ziskin, M.D.

EXECUTIVE SECRETARY
Donna LaMaster

Preface

The use of ultrasound for various diagnostic techniques in medicine continues to increase in popularity and complexity. It seems possible that the prediction of the National Science Foundation that ultrasonic techniques may be used as frequently as X-ray techniques by the end of the decade may indeed be fulfilled. The annual scientific meeting of the American Institute of Ultrasound in Medicine is the only meeting held regularly on the North American continent and devoted solely to the diagnostic use of ultrasound. Under these circumstances it is not surprising to find that both the attendance at these meetings and the number of papers submitted for presentation, are increasing markedly each year. The papers presented at these meetings probably reflect the "state-of-the-Art" reasonably accurately. The Proceedings of these annual meetings are therefore a valuable record of the current state of ultrasonic diagnostic techniques in the U.S.A. Even though it is not possible to print in extenso every paper presented at the meeting, an attempt has been made with this volume, by increasing the length of the papers printed in abstract form, to enable the reader to obtain an overall view of current developments and research on this continent in all fields of ultrasonic medical diagnostic technology. Speed of publication is essential if this volume is to contain current information. The strike by Canadian postal workers seriously impeded the collection of the material printed and the editors apologise to any authors whose manuscripts were trapped by the strike.

This year an attempt was also made to increase the scientific value of these Proceedings by selection of the papers presented at the meeting.

The first part of this volume is devoted to papers describing the diagnostic potentialities of ultrasonic techniques in various medical fields. The Time-Motion display is unique to medical imaging with ultrasound and has been responsible for the plethora of papers describing the dynamic properties of the heart in health and disease. The restriction of this technique due to its one dimensional spatial display is now being overcome by the development of real-time imaging in two spatial dimensions which also, of course, is advantageous in other bodily regions. The development moreover of various new methods of signal processing, all included under the catch-all title of "grey-scale displays", is also opening up a new chapter in ultrasonic imaging in which differences in the parenchymatous structure of organs can be imaged to show the presence of localised or diffuse disease processes. Doppler shift measurements also can be made especially successfully with ultrasonic energy and the rapid development of more sophisticated Doppler techniques is resulting in the same advances in the measurement of blood flow that occurred in cardiology after the development of the time-motion display.

The development of ultrasonic diagnostic techniques depends upon the ingenuity of the bio-medical engineers so that, for many readers the section of these volumes describing New Techniques is the most interesting and rewarding. The present volume contains papers developing the technique described in the first volume whereby more information is extracted from the reflected pulse than the amplitude of its envelope. Moreover, as might be expected, increasing use is being made of computers in processing the received signals into more informative images.

A new section has been added this year describing the interactions of ultrasonic energy with tissue. It is these interactions which will determine the information that can be obtained from the body by means of ultrasound. They will moreover determine the nature of any therapeutic effects ultrasound may have, other than the non-specific heating of tissues long used in physical medicine departments.

Once again, the assistance of Mrs. Joan Carson is gratefully acknowledged. It was invaluable in the final preparation of the material printed.

D.N. White

Contents

CARDIOLOGY

Echocardiography of the Inter-Atrial Septum..................1
  N.C. Nanda, R. Gramiak, P. Viles,
  J. Manning and C.M. Gross

Echocardiographic Recognition of Intra-Atrial
    Baffle Dysfunction..13
  N.C. Nanda, R. Gramiak, S. Stewart and
  J. Manning

Usefulness of Echocardiographic Peak Velocity
    of Circumferential Fibre Shortening.....................21
  D.R. Boughner, J. Nolan and P. Rechnitzer

Myocardial Contractility in Normal and Post
    Infarction Subjects at Rest and During
    Isometric Exercise......................................31
  J.P. Nolan, D.A. Cunningham and
  D.R. Boughner

Echocardiographic Observations on Systolic
    Closure of the Aortic Valve in
    Mitral Incompetence.....................................37
  P.A.N. Chandraratna and A. Rashid

Hypertension in Adolescents - An Ultrasound
    Study...49
  W.P. Laird and D.E. Fixler

*Articles marked with asterisks are short communications

Two-Dimensional Echocardiographic Assessment of Normal Mitral Leaflet Motion*..................55
J. Kisslo, G. Friedman, M. Johnson and O.T. vonRamm

Quantitative Echocardiography: A Study of Champion Childhood Athletes*.........................57
H.D. Allen, N. Schy, J. Wood, S.J. Goldberg, D.J. Sahn and R. Wojcik

The Echocardiographic Spectrum of Mitral Valve (MV) Motion in Children With and Without Mitral Valve Prolapse (MVP)*...............59
D.J. Sahn, J. Wood, H.D. Allen, W. Peoples and S.J. Goldberg

Cross-Sectional Echocardiographic Assessment of Severity of Aortic Stenosis in Children*..61
A.E. Weyman, H. Feigenbaum, R.A. Hurwitz, D.A. Girod, J.C. Dillon and J. Stewart

Echocardiographic Observations Regarding Pulmonary Valve Motion in Children With Pulmonary Vascular Obstructive Disease*...63
S.J. Goldberg, H.D. Allen and D.J. Sahn

Echocardiographic Features of Common Ventricle*...65
J.B. Seward, A.J. Tajik, D.J. Hagler and D.G. Ritter

Detection of Intracardiac Right to Left Shunting by Echocardiography*........................67
L.M. Valdes-Cruz, D.R. Pieroni, J.M. Roland and P.J. Varghese

The Utility and Validity of Suprasternal Notch (SSN) Echocardiography in Congenital Heart Disease (CHD)*..................................69
D.J. Sahn, H.D. Allen, S.J. Goldberg, T. Ovitt and B.B. Goldberg

Correlation of Diagnostic Echographic Features of Mitral Stenosis with Findings at Catheterization and Surgery*........................71
J.H. Horgan, V.E. Kemp, W.E. Holland, R.R. Lower L. Bosher, R. Centor and A. Goodman

CONTENTS

The Effect of Transducer Placement on the
    Echocardiographic Pattern of Mitral
    Valve Prolapse*...73
  W. Markiewicz, J. Stoner, S. Hunt, E. London
  and R. Popp

Cross-Sectional Echocardiography in Evaluation
    of Patients with Discrete Subvalvular
    Aortic Stenosis*..74
  A.E. Weyman, H. Feigenbaum, J.D. Dillon and
  S. Chang

The Comparative Utilities of Real Time Cross-
    Sectional Echocardiographic Imaging
    Systems in Complex Congenital Heart Disease*..........75
  D.J. Sahn, W.L. Henry, H.D. Allen, J.M. Griffith
  and S.J. Goldberg

Spectrum of Echocardiographic Findings in Bacterial
    Endocarditis*...77
  P. Roy, A.J. Tajik, E.R. Giuliani,
  T.T. Schattenberg, G.T. Gau and R.L. Frye

Echocardiographic Features of Straddling
    Tricuspid Valve*...79
  J.B. Seward and A.J. Tajik

Detection of Congenital Ventricular Diverticulum
    by Cross Sectional Echocardiography*...................81
  E.S. Williams, A.E. Weyman, C.M. Estevez and
  H. Feigenbaum

Evaluation of Left Ventricular Apical Aneurysms
    by Cross Sectional Echocardiography*...................83
  A.E. Weyman, H. Feigenbaum, J.C. Dillon and
  S. Chang

Echocardiography in Patients with Marfan's
    Syndrome and Their Asymptomatic Relatives*..............84
  M.N. Payvandi, R.E. Kerber and F.M. Abboud

Echocardiography in Wolff-Parkinson-White
    Syndrome*...85
  M.S. Chandra, R.E. Kerber, D.D. Brown,
  D.C. Funk and F.M. Abboud

Echocardiographic Indocyanine Green (ICG) Dye
    Flow Patterns in Patients with Truncus
    Arteriosus (TA), Tetralogy of Fallot (TF),
    and Pulmonary Atresia with Ventricular
    Septal Defect (PA)*..87
  A.J. Tajik, J.L. Assad-Morell, J.B. Seward,
  D.J. Hagler, E.R. Giuliani and D.G. Ritter

Quantification and Prognosis of Acute Myocardial
    Infarction: Comparison of Echocardiographic
    and Catheterization Indices*.............................89
  A. DeMaria, J. Angel, E. Amsterdam and D. Mason

Right Ventricular Compression: A Reliable Echo-
    cardiographic Sign of Cardiac Tamponade*................91
  N.B. Schiller and E. Botvinick

Pre- and Postoperative Echographic Investigation
    of Left Ventricular Function in Aortic
    Stenosis (AS)*...93
  R.A. Meyer, J. Korfhagen, G.L. Johnson and
  S. Kaplan

Left Ventricular Volume Determinations of Canine
    Models*..95
  O.T. von Ramm, D.R. Cannon and J.A. Kisslo

Role of Echocardiography in the Assessment of
    Left Ventricular Function in Patients with
    Coronary Artery Disease*.................................97
  P. Chandraratna, A. Rashid, A. Tolentino,
  F. Hildner, A. Fester and B.B. Littman

Effects of Sodium Nitroprusside on Left Ventricular
    Size and Performance in Myocardial Infarction
    Determined by Ultrasound*................................99
  J. Angel, A. DeMaria, E. Amsterdam, A. Neumann,
  R. Miller and D. Mason

Echocardiographic and Ultrasono-Tomographic Study
    of the Left Ventricular Dynamics in LBBB*...............101
  J. Fujii, H. Watanabe, T. Watanabe, N. Takahashi,
  A. Ohta and K. Kato

The Effect of Phasic Respiration and Atrial Systole
    on the Echocardiographic Determination of
    Left Ventricular Function*..............................103
  J.I. Brenner and R.A. Waugh

CONTENTS

Echocardiographic (ECHO) Method of Scintillation Probe Placement for Radiocardiographic Assessment (RCG) of Left Ventricular Ejection Fraction (LVEF)*.....................105
   N. Kallos, A.R. Ghahramani, M. Groch, A. Miale, Jr. and S. Gottlieb

Medium for External Acoustic Transmission*.....................107
   H.D. Allen, S.J. Goldberg, D.J. Sahn, W.L. Henry and J.M. Griffith

ABDOMINAL

Differential Diagnosis of Echo-Free Renal Masses..............109
   W.M. Green, D.L. King and W.J. Casarella

Ultrasound Diagnosis in Renal Transplants.....................119
   T.G. Lee and J.M. Anderson

Ultrasound Diagnosis of Lymphoceles Following Renal Transplantation.....................................131
   A. Ben-Ora and N. Sander

Role of Ultrasound in the Diagnosis and Therapy of Perirenal Fluid Collections Following Renal Transplantation.....................................145
   D.G. Spigos and V. Capek

Aortosonography - The Diagnostic Method of Choice..157
   B.B. Goldberg

Radiation Therapy Planning Using Ultrasound...................165
   S. Porrath and L.T. Avallone

Accuracy of Grey-Scale Ultrasonic Examination of the Liver*..173
   K.J.W. Taylor, J.P. Glees, I.A. Smith and D.A. Carpenter

Correlative Studies Between Multi-Plane Tomographic Nuclear Imaging and Grey Scale Ultrasound in Extra and Intrahepatic Abnormalities*....................175
   W.F. Sample, J.B. Po, N.D. Poe, L.S. Graham and L.R. Bennett

Ultrasonic Evaluation of the Common Bile Duct*................177
   G.S. Perlmutter and B.B. Goldberg

Normal and Abnormal Pancreatic Echography*.....................179
   D.B. Rosenberg, K. Haber and W.M. Asher

Grey Scale Ultrasonography in the Differential
      Diagnosis of Chronic Splenomegaly*.......................182
   K.J.W. Taylor

Solid Renal Lesions: Ultrasonic and Angio-
      graphic Correlation*.....................................183
   N.F. Maklad, V.P. Chuang, B.D. Doust and
   J.E. Curran

The Place of B-scan Ultrasound in the
      Examination of Kidneys not seen on
      Intravenous Pyelography*.................................185
   R.C. Sanders

Long-Term Results of Ultrasonically Guided
      Percutaneous Aspiration of Renal Cysts*..................187
   Fl. Jensen, J.K. Kristensen, and H.H. Holm

Ultrasonic Imaging of the Abdominal Aorta
      with Real-Time Multielement Systems*.....................188
   S.H. Abowitt, E.B. Diethrich, V.E. Friedewald,Jr.,
   F. Ibrahim and B.J. Phillips

Normal Upper Abdominal Vasculature - A Study
      Correlating Contact B Scanning with
      Arteriography and Gross Anatomy*.........................189
   M.L. Skolnick and D.R. Royal

Prostatic Scanning with Gray Scale Ultrasound*.................191
   J.B. Po, W.F. Sample, L. Marks and R. Glenny

Measurement of Size and Weight of Prostate by
      Means of Transrectal Ultrasonotomography*................193
   H. Watanabe

Abdominal Ultrasound and Computerized Axial
      Radiographic Tomography*.................................195
   L. Gonzalez, J. Haaga and R.J. Alfidi

Use of Simethicone in Abdominal Echotomography*................197
   H.W. Pepper and J. Keene

CONTENTS

OBSTETRICS AND GYNECOLOGY

Real-Time Scanning in the Management of
  Early Pregnancy Complications.........................199
  D. Ziehm, L. Findleton and J. Ellis

Real-Time Gray-Scale B-Scan Ultrasound
  Recording of Human Fetal Breathing
  Movements In Utero....................................203
  C.W. Hohler and H.E. Fox

Detection of Fetal Heart Beats Using the
  TM-Mode...207
  S. Asokan and D. Premsagar

Use of Grey Scale Sonography in the Morpholo-
  gical Diagnosis of Selected Gynecologic
  Tumors..213
  A.C. Fleischer, M.D. Brown and P.L. Wilds

Application of the Multiple Head Transducer
  Scanning Device in Early Pregnancy*...................219
  L. Findleton, D. Ziehm and J. Ellis

Role of Ultrasound in the Detection and Management of Intrauterine Growth Retardation
  and Associated Placental Abnormalities*...............221
  H.R. Giles, C.F. Anderson, D.B. Rosenberg
  and C.D. Christian

Fetal and Neonatal Heart Size Correlation by
  Ultrasonic Imaging*...................................223
  F. Ibrahim, B.J. Phillips, S.H. Abowitt,
  V.E. Friedewald, S.A. Kinard and M.K. Laughead

Diagnostic Ultrasound for Detection of Intra-
  uterine Growth Retardation*...........................225
  J.T. Queenan, S.F. Kubarych, L.N. Cook,
  G.D. Anderson and L. Griffin

Ultrasonic Evaluation of Pelvic Masses in
  Pregnancy*..227
  A.A. Bezjian and M.M. Carretero

Aminocentesis under Ultrasound Guidance with
  Aspiration Transducer*................................229
  P. Barriga, G. Sarto and J. Cassidy

Ultrasonically Guided Fetal Injection of
    Vitamin-K (phytomenadione)*..............................231
  Fl. Jensen, B. Jacobsen, J.F. Larsen and
  J.F. Pedersen

Grey Scale Patterns in Pelvic Inflammatory
    Disease*..233
  W.F. Sample and J.B. Po

Use of B-Scan and Gray Scale Imaging in the
    Diagnosis of Benign Cystic Teratoma*......................235
  C.F. Anderson, H.R. Giles, D. Rosenberg
  and M.W. Heine

Ultrasonic Identification of the Position of
    Contraceptive Device in Utero and its
    Relation to Subsequent Performance*.......................237
  T. Chow and B. Wittmann

NEUROLOGY

Ultrasound for Identification of Brain Damage
    in Infants and Young Children.............................239
  R.F. Heimburger, F.J. Fry, T.D. Franklin,Jr.,
  R.C. Eggleton and E. Gresham

Ultrasound Scanning of Excised Brains to
    Localize Pathology*.......................................251
  R.F. Heimburger, F.J. Fry, T.D. Franklin,Jr.,
  R.C. Eggleton and J. Muller

Lateral Ventricular Measurement During Infancy*...............253
  M.S. Tenner, G. Wodraska and C. Montesinos

OPHTHALMOLOGY

Power Spectral Resonance Analysis in the
    Evaluation of Vitreous Pathology*.........................255
  M.E. Smith, L.A. Franzen, F.L. Lizzi
  and D.J. Coleman

Ultrasonographic Diagnosis of Tumors of the
    Anterior Choroid and Ciliary Body*........................257
  L.A. Franzen, M.E. Smith, D.J. Coleman
  and R.L. Jack

The Ultrasonographic Characteristics of
    Orbital Dermoid Cysts*..................................259
  G.K. Sterns and D.J. Coleman

Posterior Ocular Curvature by B Scan
    Ultrasonography*..261
  W.E. Cappaert, E.W. Purnell and K.E. Frank

Ultrasonic Findings in Diabetic Vitreo-
    retinopathy*..263
  K.E. Frank, E.W. Purnell and W.E. Cappaert

OTHER ORGANS

Evaluation of Solitary Cold Thyroid Nodules
    by Echography and Thermography*.........................265
  G.C. Coggs, O.H. Clark, F.S. Greenspan
  and L. Goldman

A Large Aperture Real-Time Equipment for
    Imaging the Carotid Artery*.............................267
  A.K. Nigam and C.P. Olinger

Ultrasound in Orthopedic Diagnosis*..........................269
  V. Mayer

Patellar Tracking by Ultrasound*.............................271
  V. Mayer, A. Wardell and J.L. Marshall

DOPPLER

Calibration of a Doppler Blood Flowmeter
    for Measurements Independent of Flow
    Angle, Velocity Profile, and Lumen
    Shape...273
  C. Hottinger, L. Gerzberg and J.D. Meindl

Resolution Performance of Pulsed Ultrasound
    Doppler Blood Flowmeters................................277
  J.M. Griffith and W.R. Brody

The Doppler Ultrasonic Cerebrovascular
    Examination: Improved Accuracy by
    Refinement of Technique.................................281
  H.E. Russell, R.J. Burger and R.W. Barnes

Common Carotid Flow During Graded Stenosis
    and Occlusion of the Internal Carotid
    Artery..285
  R.R. Gonzalez, Jr. and H.R. Müller

Aortic Velocity Patterns Using Transcutaneous
    Doppler Ultrasound....................................297
  J.A. Persaud and D.R. Boughner

The Use of Pulsed Doppler Ultrasound to Identify
    Arterial Flow Abnormalities...........................309
  W.R. Felix, Jr., B. Sigel, R. Gibson, J. Williams
  A. Edelstein and J. Justin

Cardiac Blood Flow Detection*.................................317
  D.W. Baker, R.E. Daigle, V. Simmons and R. Olson

A Real-Time High-Resolution Ultrasonic
    Arterial Imaging System*..............................319
  J.C. Taenzer, S.D. Ramsey, J.F. Holzemer,
  J. Suarez and P.S. Green

Preclinical Evaluation of the SRI Real-Time
    Arterial Imaging System*..............................321
  J.W. Marich, P.S. Green, T.C. Evans and C.E. Harrison

Noninvasive Detection of the Atherosclerotic
    Plaque: The Carotid Bifurcation*......................324
  M.P. Spencer, J.W. Li, E.C. Brockenbrough and
  J.M. Reid

Velocity Maps in the Canine Aorta*............................325
  C.W. Miller, F.D. McLeod and R.C. Nealeigh

Measurement of Hemodynamic Properties in the
    Abdominal Aorta and Iliac Artery via an
    Intravenous Catheter-Tip Probe*.......................327
  R.C. Nealeigh, C.W. Miller and F.D. McLeod

Transcutaneous Assessment of Forearm Reactive Hyperemia
    by Doppler Ultrasonography: Correlation with
    Venous Occlusion Plethysmography*.....................329
  R.W. Barnes, P.G. Miller and E.V. Miller

NEW TECHNIQUES

OCTOSON - A New Rapid General Purpose Echoscope..............333
  G. Kossoff, D.A. Carpenter, D.E. Robinson
  G. Radovanovich and W.J. Garrett

CONTENTS

The OCTOSON in Use..341
   W.J. Garrett, G. Kossoff, D.A. Carpenter
   and G. Radovanovich

An Analog Echocardiogram for Estimating
     Ventricular Stroke Volume.............................351
   M.L. Petrovick, G.S. Malindzak Jr. and E.D. Haak, Jr.

A New Three-Dimensional Random Scanner for
     Ultrasonic/Computer Graphic Imaging
     of the Heart..363
   D.L. King, S.J. Al-Banna and D.R. Larach

Real-Time B-Mode Echo-Encephalography........................373
   S.W. Smith, D.J. Phillips, O.T. von Ramm
   and F.L. Thurstone

Versatile Echoscanner 383
   J.B. Williams and T.B. Smith

Ultrasound Transaxial Tomography by Recon-
     struction...391
   P.L. Carson, T.V. Oughton and W.R. Hendee

Raylography, A Pulse Echo Technique with
     Future Biomedical Applications........................401
   I. Beretsky, G. Farrell and B. Lichtenstein

Medium Characterization by the Application of
     a Deconvolution Technique in an Acoustic
     Pulse Echo System -- Raylography......................411
   B. Lichtenstein, I. Beretsky, G. Farrell
   and A. Winder

Ultrasonic Spectral Investigations for
     Tissue Characterization...............................427
   F.L. Lizzi and M.A. Laviola

Effect of Drugs on Mouse Embryo Hearts in
     Organ Culture Visualized by Acoustic
     Microscopy..441
   R.C. Eggleton, L.W. Kessler, F.S. Vinson
   and G.B. Boder

Field Evaluation of the AIUM Standard 100 mm
     Test Object...445
   K.R. Erikson, P.L. Carson and H.F. Stewart

Technical Considerations of Ultrasonic Photography: Choosing the Right Film and Photographic paper for Your Present Ultrasound Camera System..................................453
   H.W. Pepper and S. Arnon

A New Mechanical Real Time Ultrasonic Scanner*..459
   H.H. Holm, J.K. Kristensen, J.F. Pedersen, S. Hancke, A. Northeved and F. Jensen

Abdominal Scanning with a Rotating Transducer*..461
   J.K. Kristensen, Fl. Jensen and H.H. Holm

THAUMASCAN: Improved Image Quality and Clinical Usefulness*...................................463
   O.T. von Ramm and F.L. Thurstone

Real-Time Ultrasound Abdominal Imaging*......................465
   M.L. Johnson, O.T. von Ramm, J.A. Kisslo and F.L. Thurstone

Continuous Contact B Abdominal Scanning with Photographic Recording from a Non-Storage Oscilloscope on 70 MM Film*............................467
   M.L. Skolnick

High Resolution Ultrasound Mammography*......................469
   G. Baum

Clinical Findings with Real-Time Color B-Scan Ultrasonography*..................................471
   N.R. Bronson II and N.C. Pickering

Studies with a Real-Time Acoustical Holography System*...473
   W.W. Taylor

Transskull Ultrasonic Impediography*.........................475
   J.P. Jones and F.J. Fry

Acoustic Impedance Profiling -- An Experimental Model and Analytical Study with Implications for Medical Diagnosis*...477
   A.C. Kak, F.J. Fry and N.T. Sanghvi

Computerization of Manual Echocardiograms*...................479
   L.R. Smith and S.E. Wixson

Ultrasonic Visualization and Therapeutic
    Computer Controlled System*..........................481
  F.J. Fry, N.T. Sanghvi, R.C. Eggleton
  and W. Erdmann

How to Select Transducers to Achieve Best
    Clinical Results by Use of Transducer
    Beam Sensitivity Profile Data*.......................483
  R.E. Hileman

A Chopped Ultrasonic Radiometer Operating
    in the Milliwatt Acoustical Power
    Levels with Digital Readout*.........................485
  T. Matzuk and W.A. Lindgren

TISSUE INTERACTIONS

The Therapeutic Efficacy of Ultrasound in
    Treatment of Autoimmune Diseases.....................487
  J.A. Roseboro, A. Norman, H. Machleder,
  H. Paulus and R. Stern

Intercellular Gas: Its Role in Sonated
    Plant Tissue...501
  A. Gershoy, D.L. Miller and W.L. Nyborg

Clinical Results Obtained with an Ultrasonic
    Spectral Analysis System*............................513
  F.L. Lizzi, M.A. Laviola and D.J. Coleman

Interaction of Ultrasound with Tissues*....................517
  E.L. Carstensen

Ultrasonic Heating at Tissue Interfaces*...................518
  L.A. Frizzell and E.L. Carstensen

Ultrasonic Determination of Tissue Macro-
    structure by Frequency Sweeping*.....................519
  R.C. Waag, R. Gramiak and R. Lerner

Through Transmission Patterns in Solid
    Tumors*..521
  N. Hassani, R. Bard and L. von Micsky

Studies of Acoustical Attenuation,
    Absorption and Scattering for
    Diagnosis of Tissue Pathology*.......................523
  P.P. Lele, N. Senapati and A.I. Murphy

The Effects of Acoustic Streaming on
    Nerve Conduction*...524
  P.P. Lele and R. Mecca

Animal Studies of Cataracts Produced by
    High-Intensity Ultrasonic Energy*.................................525
  F.L. Lizzi, A.J. Packer and D.J. Coleman

The Effect of Continuous Wave Ultrasonic
    Therapy on Myocardial Infarction
    in the Dog*...527
  T.D. Franklin Jr., J.T. Fallon, R.C. Eggleton
  and F.J. Fry

Effects of Exposure of the Nine-Day Rat
    Embryo to Ultrasound*...529
  M.R. Sikov, B.P. Hildebrand and J.D. Stearns

Ultrasonically Induced Fetal Weight
    Reduction in Mice*..531
  W.D. O'Brien Jr.

Ultrasonic Toxicity Study of the Mouse
    Reproductive System and the Pregnant
    Uterus*...533
  F.J. Fry, F. Dunn, J. Brady, W.D. Erdmann,
  P. Strang, R. Kohn, I. Baird and J. Cobb

Early Postpartum Mortality Following Ultra-
    sound Radiation*..535
  K.A. Curto

Physical Basis and Necessity for Grey-
    Level Phantom Development*..537
  T. Matzuk and M.L. Skolnick

Author Index..539

Subject Index...543

Cardiology

ECHOCARDIOGRAPHY OF THE INTER-ATRIAL SEPTUM

Navin C. Nanda; Raymond Gramiak; Peter Viles;
James Manning; Charles M. Gross
Departments of Medicine (Cardiology), Radiology and
Pediatrics, School of Medicine
Rochester, New York 14642

Atrial septal identification has been carried out from a right parasternal position but this technique has been limited in its utility since only a few patients are suitable for echocardiographic examination from the right side of the sternum.[1] Echocardiographic recordings of the tricuspid valve often contain a thin linear echo complex deep to the valve which has, in the past, caused some confusion and resulted in the identification of this line as the ventricular septum. The purpose of this report is to identify this line as the atrial septum, based on correlations with known anatomy and by the use of intra-cardiac contrast injections, as well as to demonstrate its usefulness and application in various clinical settings. It confirms, in part, previous work done in this field in Japan.[2]

Material and Methods

The first part of the study included 10 patients with no known anatomic abnormalities of the inter-atrial septum. Routine echocardiographic examinations were performed and included beam angulation studies from the mitral valve to the tricuspid valve. In all, a moving structural echo could be demonstrated directly behind the tricuspid valve recording. A commercially available ultrasonoscope (Picker) and standard transducers were used in all studies. Recording was on 35 mm film run continuously in an oscilloscope record camera (Fairchild).

In four patients, ultrasonic contrast studies were obtained using indocyanine green injections. In 2 of them separate catheters were placed in the right and left atria at the time of open heart surgery, while in the remaining 2 patients the right heart

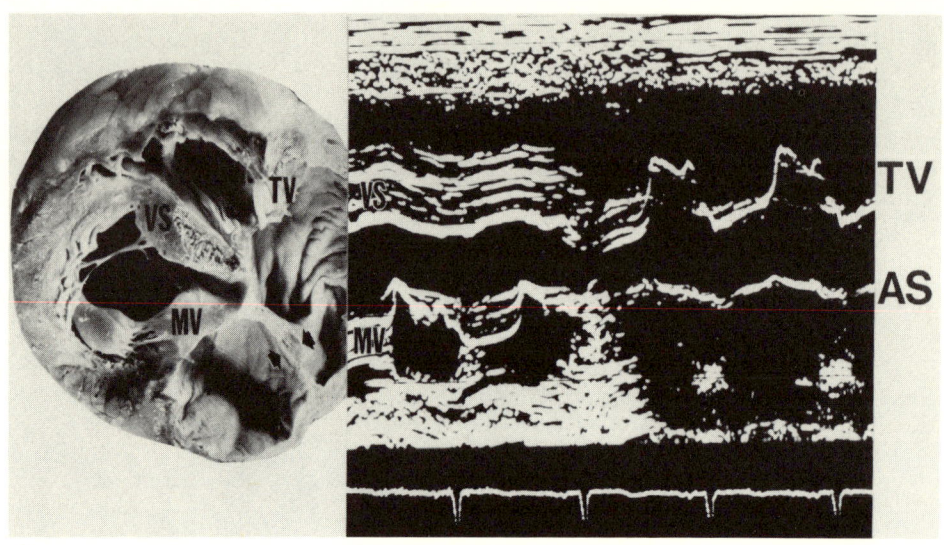

Figure 1

Identification of the atrial septum. The atrial septum (AS) is recorded during ultrasonic beam scanning from the mitral to the tricuspid valve (TV) and is continuous with the mitral valve (MV). The specimen of the heart, on the left, demonstrates the anatomic continuity between the atrial septum (black arrows) and the mitral valve. VS = ventricular septum   ECG = electrocardiogram.

catheter was passed into the left atrium through a patent foramen ovale during cardiac catheterization.

The second part of the study included 11 patients with atrial septal defects (4 with proven ostium secundum defects, 5 with proven ostium primum defects and 2 with complete atrio-ventricular canal defects), 5 patients with coronary sinus pacing catheters, 8 patients with right ventricular pacing catheters and 3 patients with large pericardial effusions.

Anatomic specimens of the heart were also studied and correlated with the echocardiographic findings.

Results

The structural echo present behind the tricuspid valve was found to be regularly thin, measuring approximately 5 mm in width. It moved anteriorly in systole and posteriorly in diastole with a maximal amplitude of 8-14 mm (average 10 mm). A small circumscribed posterior deflection occurred in diastole, in some patients, follow-

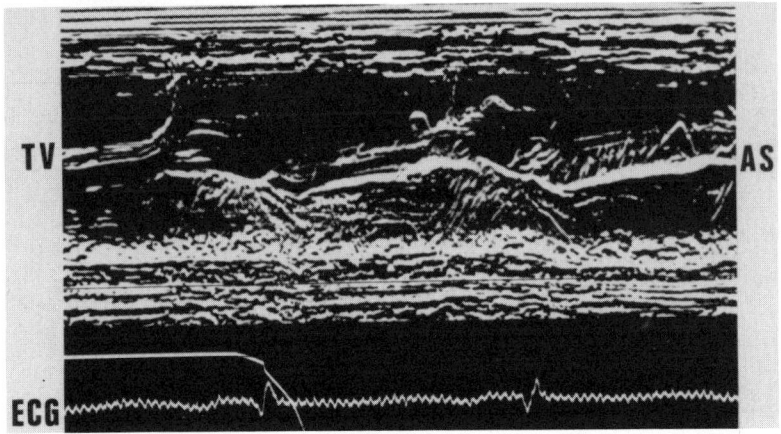

Figure 2

<u>Ultrasonic validation of the atrial septum</u>. Injection of indocyanine green into the left atrium via a catheter passed through a patent foramen ovale produced contrast echoes behind the atrial septum (AS) recorded posterior to the tricuspid valve (TV). Some leakage of the contrast agent anteriorly into the tricuspid valve region was noted during atrial systole. ECG = electrocardiogram.

ing the inscription of the P wave of the electrocardiogram. Beam angulation studies showed continuity of this structure with the mitral valve. Correlation with anatomic specimens, cut to reveal the plane of beam angulation, showed that the atrial septum is continuous with the mitral valve (Fig. 1). In 2 patients with atrial flutter, this linear echo exhibited a flutter pattern similar to that shown by the right and left atrial walls.

Ultrasonic contrast studies using indocyanine green injections into the right atrium through a catheter surgically placed in that chamber, showed contrast filling behind the tricuspid valve and limited posteriorly by the linear echo complex. When contrast injections were made into the left atrium through a separate catheter placed in that cavity during surgery, the space behind the linear structure filled with contrast echoes, delineating the atrial septum lying between the two atria. Contrast injections into the left atrium via a catheter passed through a patent foramen ovale produced echoes in the space behind the structural echo with some contrast leaking into the right atrium anteriorly, mainly during atrial systole (Fig. 2).

In the group of patients with secundum atrial septal defects,

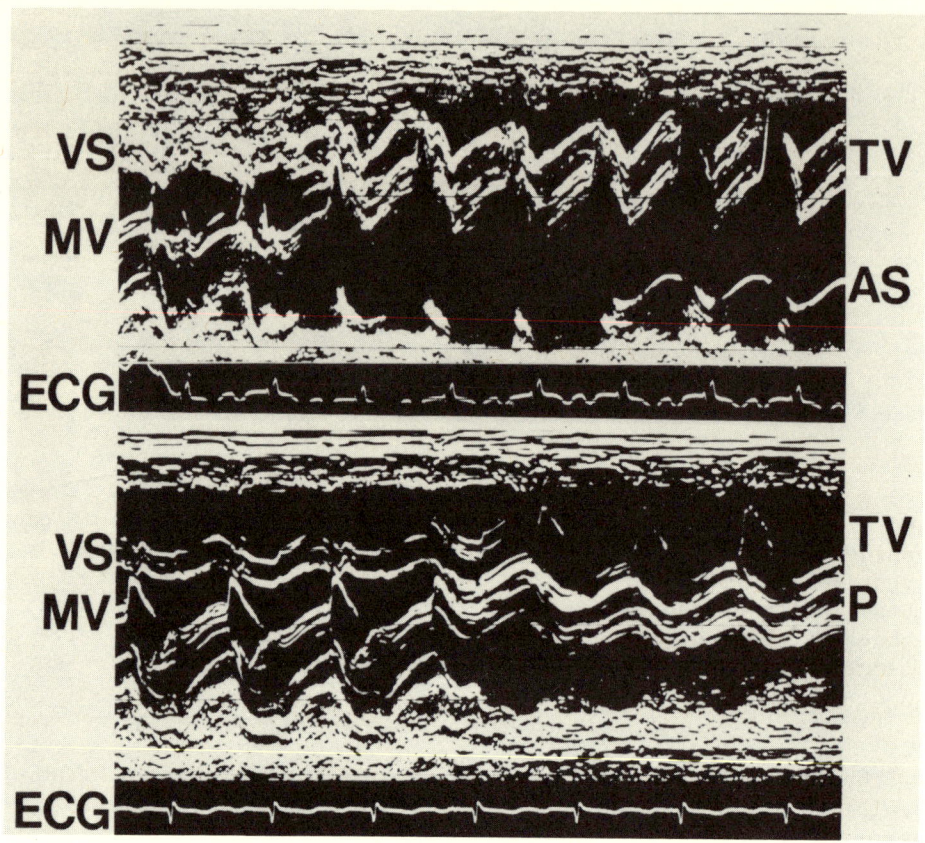

Figure 3

Pre- and postoperative studies of the atrial septal region in atrio-ventricular canal defect. Upper panel. Preoperative recording showing interruption of continuity between the mitral valve (MV) and the atrial septum (AS). Lower panel. Postoperative echogram showing continuity between the mitral valve and the synthetic patch (P) used for surgical closure of the defect. TV = tricuspid valve VS = ventricular septum ECG = electrocardiogram.

continuity could be shown between the mitral valve and the atrial septum as the beam was directed from the mitral valve to the tricuspid. In patients with atrio-ventricular canal defects, the normal continuity between the mitral valve and the atrial septum was interrupted and the atrial septum could be imaged in a deeper position relative to the mitral valve as the scan progressed more medially. In some instances, the atrial septum could not be recorded. Follow-

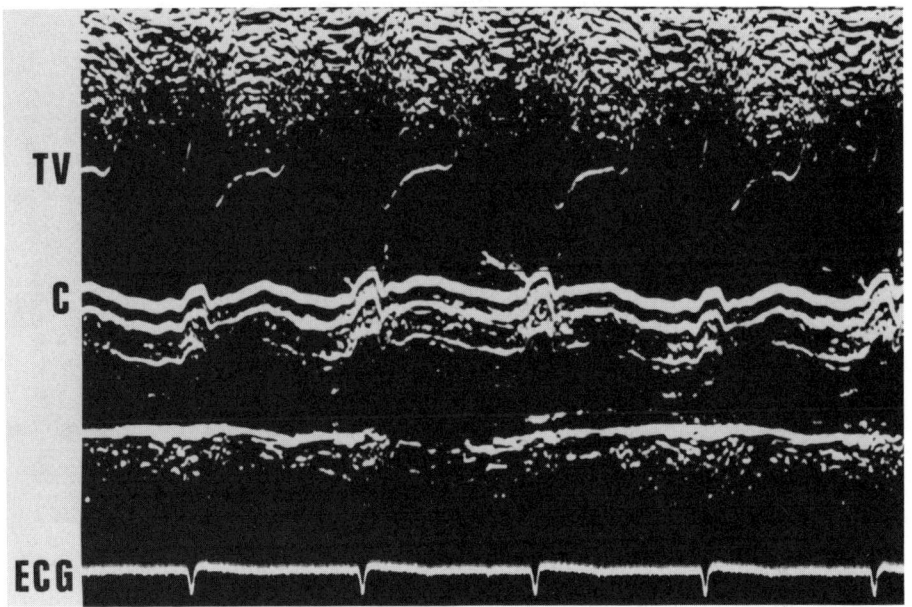

Figure 4

Demonstration of a coronary sinus pacing catheter (C) behind the tricuspid valve (TV). ECG = electrocardiogram.

ing repair of the atrio-ventricular canal defect the mitral valve could be seen to be continuous with a thick echo complex behind the tricuspid valve, probably representing the synthetic patch used for surgical closure of the defect (Fig. 3).

Pacing catheters in the coronary sinus were identified as multilayered echo complexes in the region of the atrial septum and demonstrating its motion pattern. In addition, a prominent circumscribed anterior movement of the catheter was observed with atrial systole (Fig. 4). In some instances, the catheter echoes masked the atrial septal image. Beam scanning revealed the catheter echoes to be at the same depth or slightly deeper to the echoes obtained from the mitral valve or the posterior aortic wall (Fig. 5) Right ventricular pacing catheters, on the other hand, presented as prominent complexes superimposed on the tricuspid valve recording (Fig. 6) or in front of it and could be shown in the right ventricle during mitral valve recording (Fig. 7). They were not observed in the region of the atrial septum.

In three instances, pericardial effusion could be identified be-

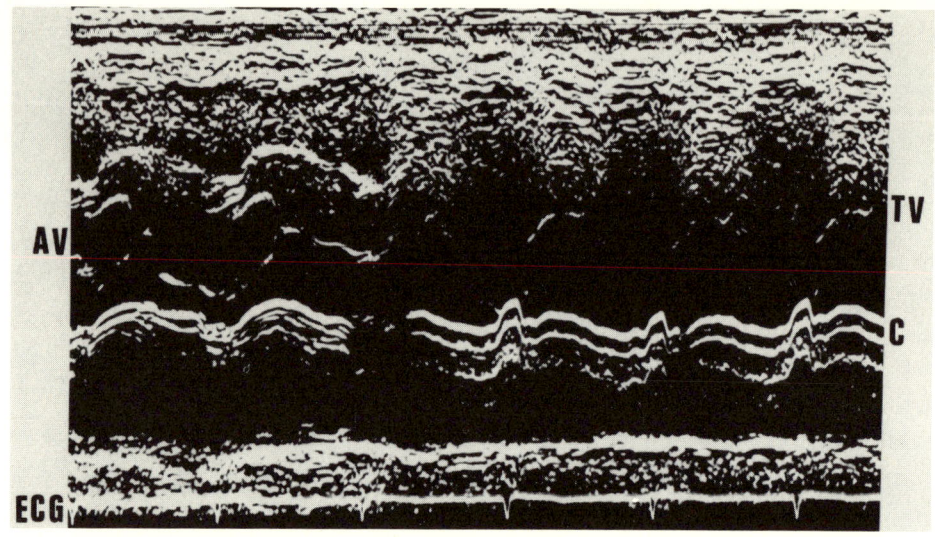

Figure 5

Relationship of the coronary sinus pacing catheter (C) to the posterior aortic wall.   AV = aortic valve   TV = tricuspid valve   ECG = electrocardiogram

hind the left atrial wall during recordings of the atrial septum (Fig. 8-9). The extension of the effusion behind the left atrium was indicated by continuity with the fluid space behind the left ventricle. None of the patients had evidence of left pleural effusion.

Delineation of the atrial septum was also found useful in the identification of the septal leaflet of the tricuspid valve. Simultaneous echocardiographic recording of two leaflets of the tricuspid valve together with the ventricular or the atrial septum identifies the posteriorly moving leaflet as the septal cusp of the tricuspid valve, since the posterior or the inferior leaflet of the tricuspid valve lies deeper to the ultrasonic plane required for simultaneous imaging of these structures (Fig. 10).

Discussion

In the present study, the atrial septum has been identified as a thin echo complex lying behind the tricuspid valve and routinely detected from a left parasternal position. The identification has

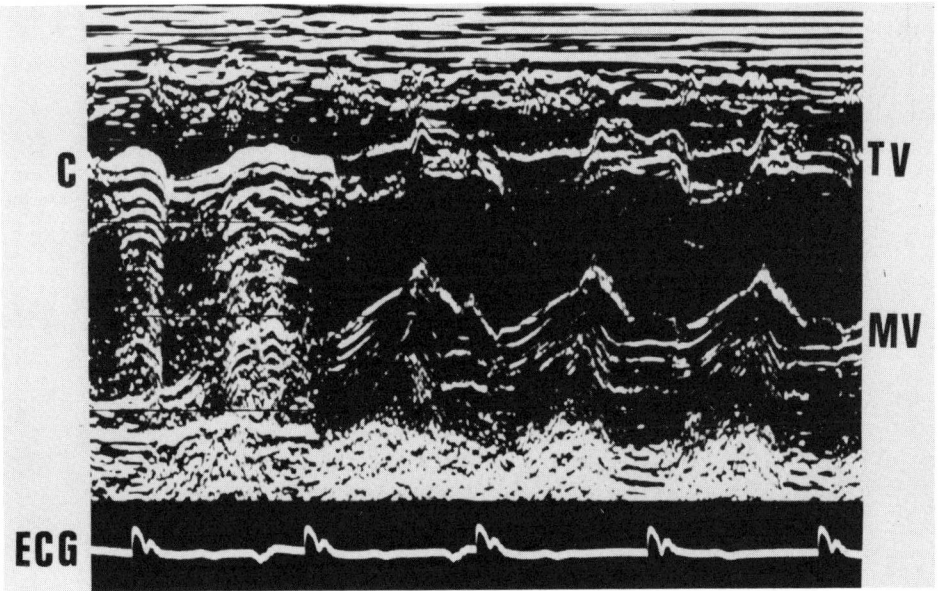

Figure 6
Relationship of right ventricular pacing catheter (C) to the tricuspid valve (TV). MV = mitral valve   ECG = electrocardiogram.

been validated using ultrasonic contrast studies. The movement pattern of the atrial septum is probably extrinsic in origin and related to the dynamics of adjacent, dominant structures as they move through the cardiac cycle. Scanning maneuvers from the mitral to the tricuspid valve show continuity between the atrial septum and the mitral valve. The atrial septum is also shown to be in close proximity to the posterior aortic wall during beam scanning from the aortic valve to the tricuspid (Fig. 11). Confusion of the atrial septum with the ventricular septum, especially in patients with congenital heart disease, can be avoided by performing mitral to tricuspid scans during every examination. The ventricular septum is regularly thicker than the atrial septum, terminates as the tricuspid valve echoes make their appearance and, in some instances, can be seen to arch posteriorly to come close to the atrial septum.

Identification of the atrial septum from the left parasternal position adds to the diagnostic armamentarium of the echocardiographer. The portion of the atrial septum examined by this technique includes the base of the septum which is deficient in partial and complete atrioventricular canal defects. This is reflected in the interruption of the normal continuity between the atrial septum and the mitral valve during beam scanning from the mitral to the tricuspid valve. Beam angulation studies should, therefore, be utilized in all

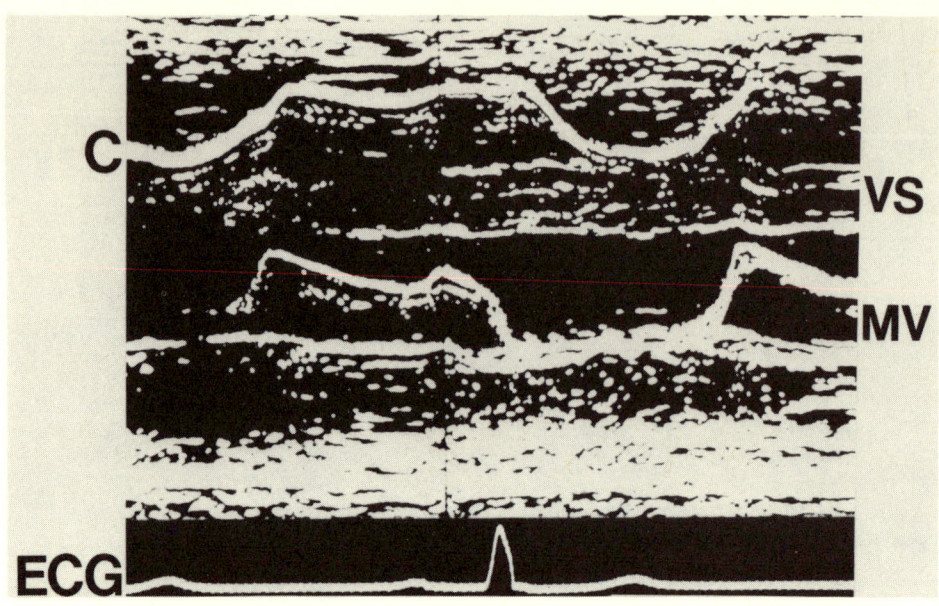

Figure 7

Demonstration of right ventricular pacing catheter (C) in the right ventricular cavity during mitral valve (MV) recording. VS = ventricular septum ECG = electrocardiogram.

patients suspected to have these conditions, since the region of the atrial septum involved in endocardial cushion defects is demonstrated by this technique.

Pacing catheters placed in the coronary sinus and right ventricle may be difficult to separate radiologically as well as electrocardiographically in some instances. The technique has already proved useful in our hands in confirming the correct position of the coronary sinus catheter despite the fact that entry into the coronary sinus is not visualized by this method. Since the coronary sinus is located at the base of the atrial septum, it is reasonable to assume that the motion pattern of the atrial septum will be imparted to a catheter which is directed into it. Right ventricular pacing catheters are imaged in front of the tricuspid valve or superimposed on it and generally move anteriorly in diastole. Furthermore, they can be shown to be located in the right ventricular cavity during echocardiographic recording of the mitral valve.

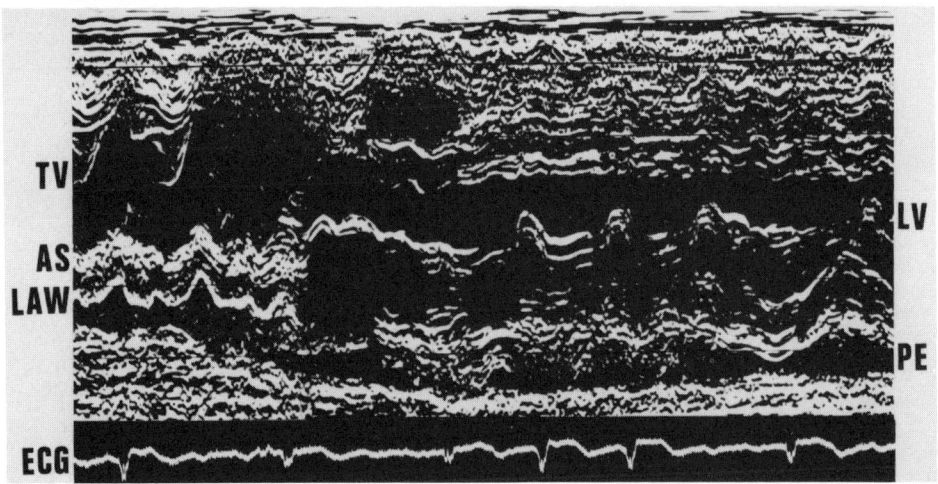

Figure 8

Pericardial effusion (PE) behind the left atrium. Extension of effusion behind the left atrial wall (LAW) is indicated by continuity with fluid space behind the left ventricle (LV). AS = atrial septum   TV = tricuspid valve   ECG = electrocardiogram.

Beam scanning from the mitral to the tricuspid valve is useful in identifying the extension of pericardial effusion behind the left atrium, as indicated by continuity with the fluid space behind the left ventricle. Detection of pericardial effusion behind the left atrial wall during aortic or mitral valve recording is generally less rewarding, probably because of the proximity of the insertion of the pulmonary veins into the left atrium in that region, resulting in a relatively small or non-existent potential pericardial effusion space. This technique can be used to differentiate pericardial from pleural fluid since the latter cannot extend behind the left atrium because of the mediastinal pleural reflections.

Although two cusps of the tricuspid valve are often recorded during echocardiographic examinations, the identity of the posteriorly moving cusp has remained unclear and has been the source of considerable confusion.[3] Correlation with anatomic specimens indicates that the ultrasonic beam traversing the anterior tricuspid leaflet and the ventricular septum or the base of the atrial septum would traverse the septal leaflet of the tricuspid valve rather than the posterior or the inferior leaflet which is located deeper and hence outside the confines of the projected ultrasonic beam pathway. Thus echocardiographic recordings of two leaflets of the tricuspid valve together with simultaneous imaging of the ventricular

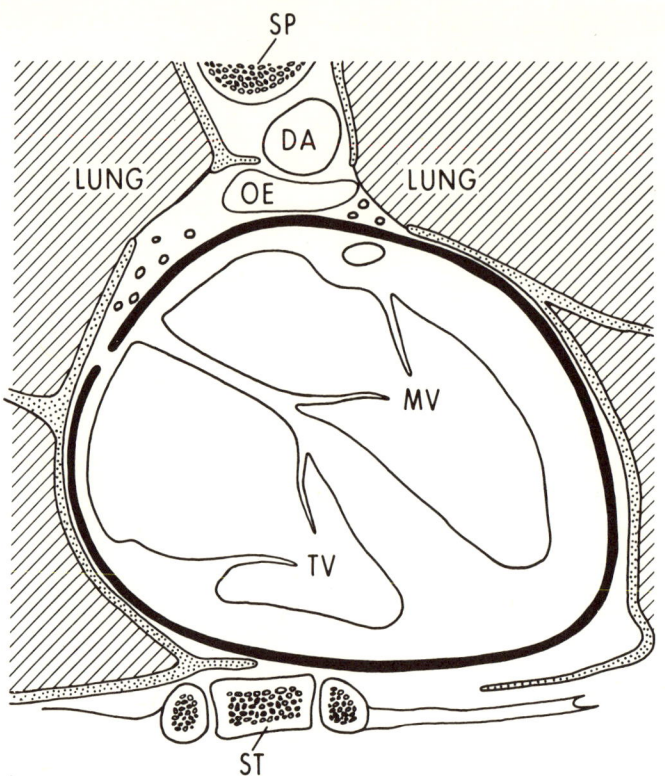

Figure 9

Schematic representation of an anatomic section demonstrating the presence of pericardial space (shown in black) behind the left atrium. The stippled area represents the pleural space which is a closed system and offers no communication to the mediastinum behind the left atrium.   MV = mitral valve   TV = tricuspid valve   SP = spine   ST = sternum   DA = descending aorta   OE = oesophagus.

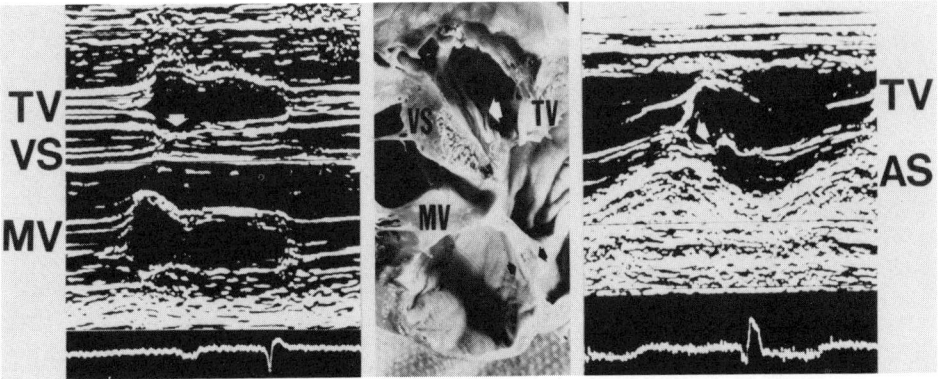

Figure 10

Identification of the septal leaflet of the tricuspid valve.
Correlation with the anatomic specimen identifies the posteriorly
moving cusp of the tricuspid valve (TV) as the septal leaflet (shown
by white arrows) when it is recorded simultaneously with the ventricular septum (left) or the atrial septum (right). The posterior or
the inferior cusp of the tricuspid valve is not recorded since it is
located deeper to the ultrasonic plane required for simultaneous
imaging of these structures. MV = mitral valve   VS = ventricular
septum   AS = atrial septum. The black arrows on the anatomic
specimen denote the atrial septum.

or the atrial septum identifies the posteriorly moving leaflet as
the septal cusp of the tricuspid valve.

   Our study indicates that echocardiographic examination of the
atrial septal region has application in the diagnosis of atrio-ventricular canal defects, detection of pacing catheters in the coronary
sinus and their differentiation from transvenous endocardial right
ventricular pacing catheters, demonstration of pericardial effusion
behind the left atrium and identification of the septal leaflet of
the tricuspid valve.

   Estimation of right atrial size may be improved by recognition
of the atrial septum. Its motion pattern could be an indicator of
the volume and direction of the atrial shunts.

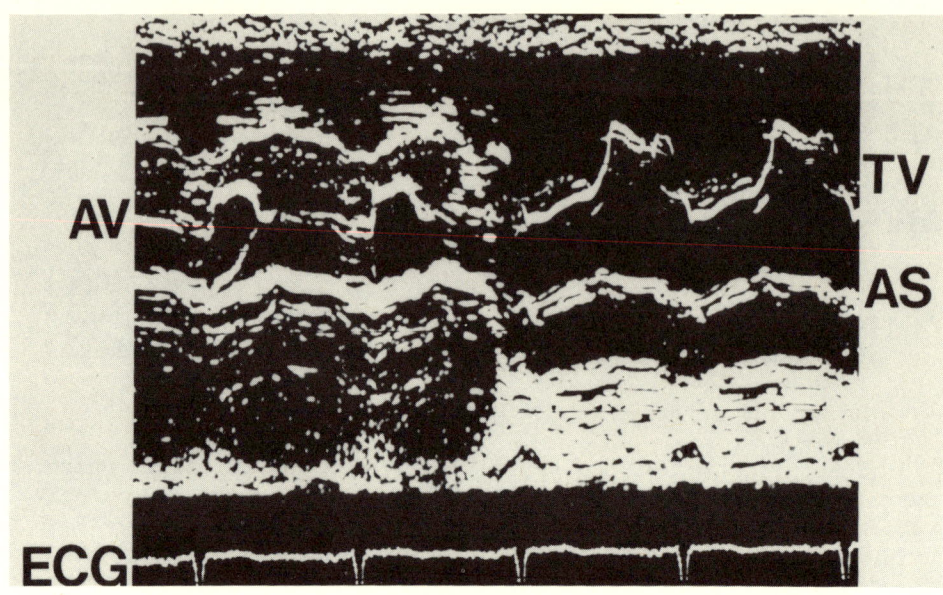

Figure 11

Beam scanning from the aortic valve (AV) to the tricuspid valve (TV) shows the close proximity of the atrial septum (AS) to the posterior aortic wall. ECG = electrocardiogram.

References

1. Gramiak R, Shah PM, Kramer DH: Ultrasound cardiography: Contrast studies in anatomy and function. Radiology 92:939, 1969

2. Matsumoto M, Nimura Y, Matsuo H, Nagata S, Mochizuki S, Sakakibara H, Abe H: Interatrial septum in B-mode and conventional echocardiograms - A clue for the diagnosis of congenital heart diseases. J Clin Ultrasound 3:29, 1975

3. Feigenbaum H: Echocardiography. Philadelphia, Lea and Febiger, 1972

ECHOCARDIOGRAPHIC RECOGNITION OF INTRA-ATRIAL BAFFLE DYSFUNCTION

Navin C. Nanda; Raymond Gramiak; Scott Stewart;
James Manning
Departments of Medicine (Cardiology Unit), Radiology,
Surgery and Pediatrics
University of Rochester School of Medicine
Rochester, New York

The outlook for children with dextro-transposition of the great vessels has improved considerably since the introduction of the Mustard procedure[1]. This technique involves the placement of a patch or baffle, constructed from the pericardium or a synthetic material, in the atria to achieve physiologic correction. A previous report from our laboratory described the echocardiographic patterns presented by the intra-atrial baffle as well as validation of its identification using ultrasonic contrast studies[2]. Complications do occur as a consequence of the use of the intra-atrial baffle. These include systemic venous and pulmonary venous obstruction as well as leakage resulting from shrinkage and detachment. It would, therefore, be useful if echocardiography could identify malfunction of the intra-atrial baffle.

Material and methods

Echocardiographic studies were performed in three patients following the Mustard procedure for dextrotransposition of the great vessels who showed hemodynamic/angiographic evidence of significant leaks (shunt ratios of 2 or more) across the pericardial baffle. All patients were male and their ages were 5, 6 and 10 years. The echocardiographic examinations were performed using a commercially available echograph (Picker) and a 2 MHz collimated transducer. Continuous records were made on 35 mm film by means of a Fairchild oscilloscope record camera and a dual beam oscilloscope operating as a slave. Routine echocardiographic recordings of the cardiac valves and chambers were obtained. Particular attention was given to the delineation of echoes from the intra-atrial baffle in the atrial chambers behind the great vessels and in the vicinity of the atrioventricular valves.

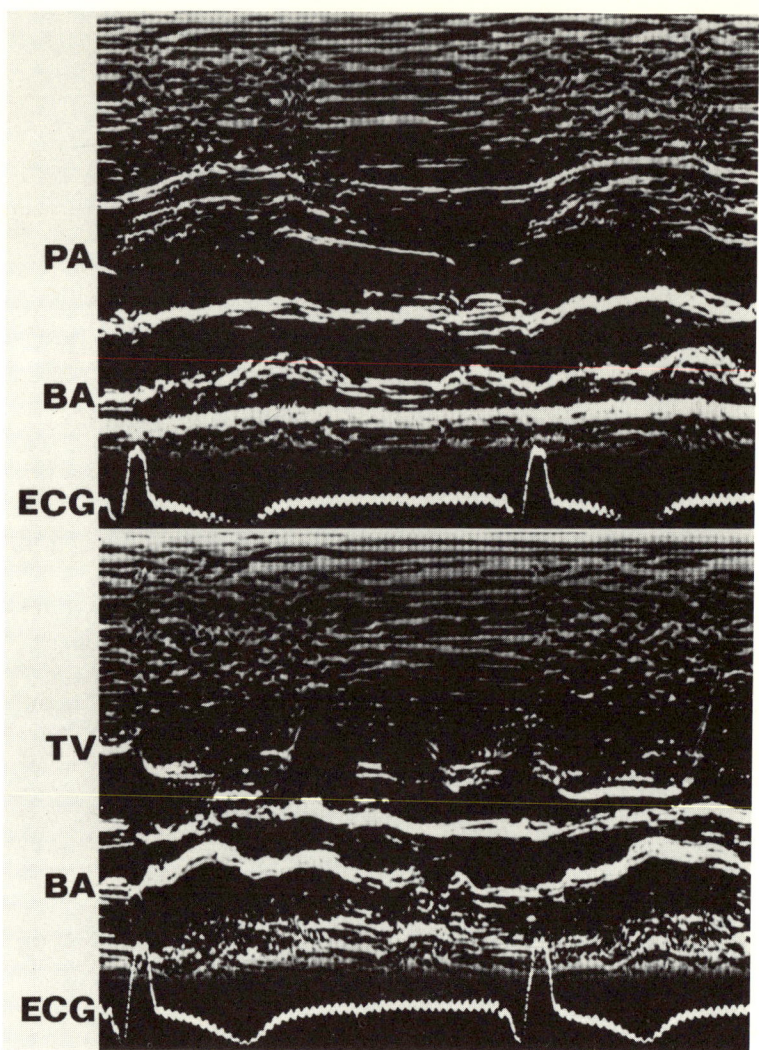

Figure 1

Echocardiographic findings in baffle incompetence. Upper panel. A prominent deflection of the baffle recording (BA) behind the pulmonary artery (PA) is observed during atrial systole ('a' wave). The pulmonary artery as well as the systemic venous atrial chamber (represented by the space between the posterior pulmonary artery wall and the baffle echo) are both large in size. Lower panel. A prominent systolic anterior motion is seen in the baffle echo (BA) behind the tricuspid valve (TV). ECG = electrocardiogram.

Results

The chief echocardiographic feature indicative of baffle dysfunction, noted in all the three patients, was a prominent anterior deflection produced by atrial systole ('a' wave) in the baffle recorded behind the pulmonary artery. One patient also demonstrated a large pulmonary artery with a large systemic venous atrial chamber imaged behind the vessel as well as a sharp prominent systolic anterior motion of the baffle echo recorded behind the tricuspid valve (Fig. 1). In this particular patient, baffle incompetence was suspected by echo contrast studies using indocyanine green within 24 hours of the Mustard procedure. Injections through a catheter placed at surgery at the lower end of the superior vena cava produced a cloud of echoes in the right ventricular outflow area consistent with a significant leak across the pericardial baffle (Fig. 2). Postoperatively he remained cyanotic with a fair amount of pulmonary venous congestion. Cardiac catheterization revealed a significant leak at the baffle site with the pulmonic to systemic blood flow ratio of 2.9:1. At re-operation, the baffle was found to have torn away from the superior aspects of the right and left atria and from the margin along the tricuspid valve. A new pericardial baffle, cut in the Brom technique, was inserted. Echo contrast studies performed within 24 hours of the second operation showed the pericardial baffle to be competent with absence of contrast echoes in the right ventricular outflow tract following systemic venous injection (Fig. 2). The baffle echo pattern was restored to normal following re-operation. Only small 'a' waves could be discerned in the baffle recording behind the pulmonary artery and the previously observed prominent systolic anterior motion of the baffle behind the tricuspid valve disappeared. Furthermore, the size of the pulmonary artery as well as the width of the systemic venous atrial chamber located behind it appeared to be significantly smaller as compared to the dimensions obtained in the presence of a malfunctioning baffle (Fig. 3).

Another finding, seen in two patients with baffle dysfunction, was the presence of coarse or fine undulations in systole (Fig. 4).

These abnormalities of the baffle motion pattern were absent in a comparison group of eight operated patients with dextrotransposition of the great vessels who showed no evidence of significant shunting across the baffle. In three of them competence of the pericardial baffle was also demonstrated using echo contrast studies in the immediate post-surgical period.

Discussion

Echoes from the pericardial intra-atrial baffle are most frequently obtained behind the pulmonary artery. Less commonly they are observed behind the aortic root and posterior to the mitral

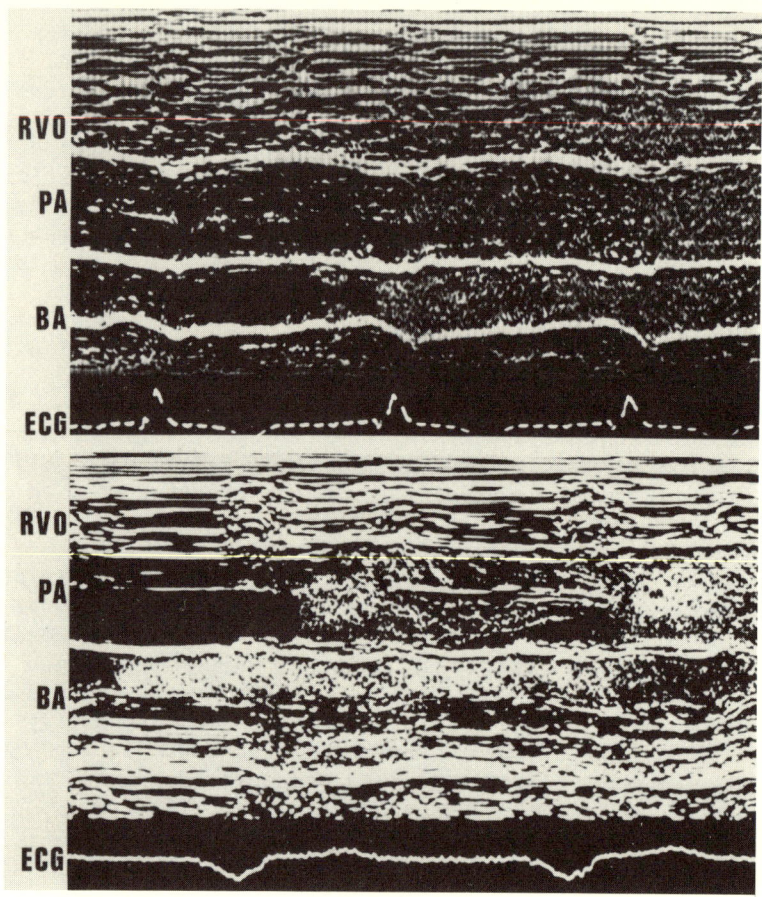

Figure 2

Echo contrast studies. Baffle incompetence is supported by the presence of contrast echoes in the right ventricular outflow (RVO) following injection into the systemic venous atrial chamber (upper panel) while their absence following placement of a new pericardial baffle denotes a competent baffle (lower panel). BA = baffle echoes PA = pulmonary artery ECG = electrocardiogram.

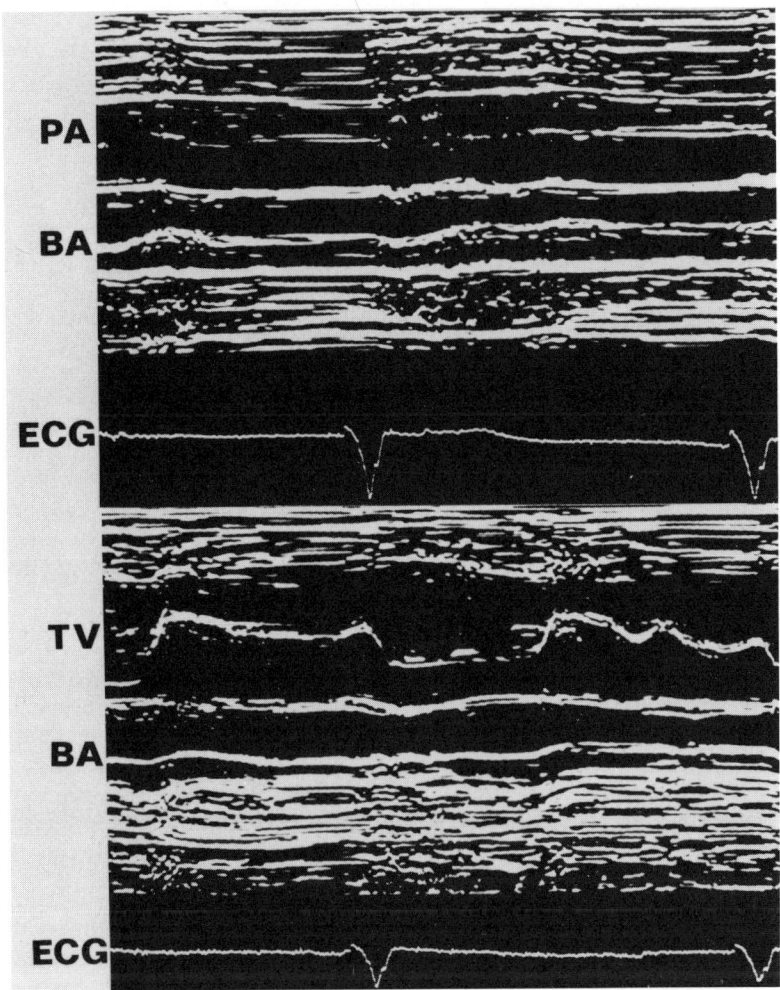

Figure 3

Echocardiographic findings following placement of a new pericardial baffle. The echo patterns have been restored to normal with virtually absent 'a' waves, decreased width of the pulmonary artery (PA) and of the systemic venous atrial chamber, and absence of abnormal systolic motion of the baffle echo (BA) imaged behind the tricuspid valve (TV). ECG = electrocardiogram.

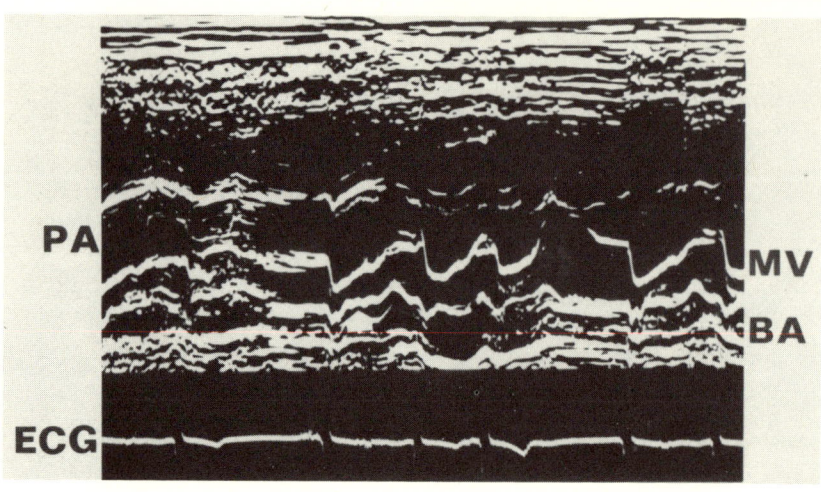

Figure 4

Systolic undulations (arrow) of the baffle echoes (BA) recorded behind the mitral valve (MV) in a patient with significant baffle incompetence. PA = pulmonary artery   ECG = electrocardiogram.

and tricuspid valves. The normal movement pattern generally resembles that produced by a stenotic atrioventricular valve. A sharp anterior movement occurs at the onset of diastole and this is followed by flattening in mid and late diastole. With the beginning of ventricular systole a rapid posterior motion is observed and during the remainder of systole the baffle echoes show no motion or very gradual anterior motion (Fig. 5). Atrial systole produces no motion or a slight anterior movement in the baffle echo recorded behind the pulmonary root. Coarse systolic undulations or low amplitude fine systolic flutter are not observed normally.

In the present study, all patients with significant baffle incompetence showed a prominent anterior deflection during atrial systole in the baffle recording obtained behind the pulmonary artery. The prominent 'a' wave probably reflects the increased mobility of the incompetent baffle resulting from significant shunting of blood across it. Increased width of the pulmonary artery as well as the relatively large dimension of the systemic venous atrium (represented by the space between the posterior wall of the pulmonary artery and the pericardial baffle echo) also appears to be related to the increased blood flow across the pericardial baffle into the systemic venous-pulmonary artery circuit. This may also explain the presence of systolic flutter observed in the baffle recording in two patients.

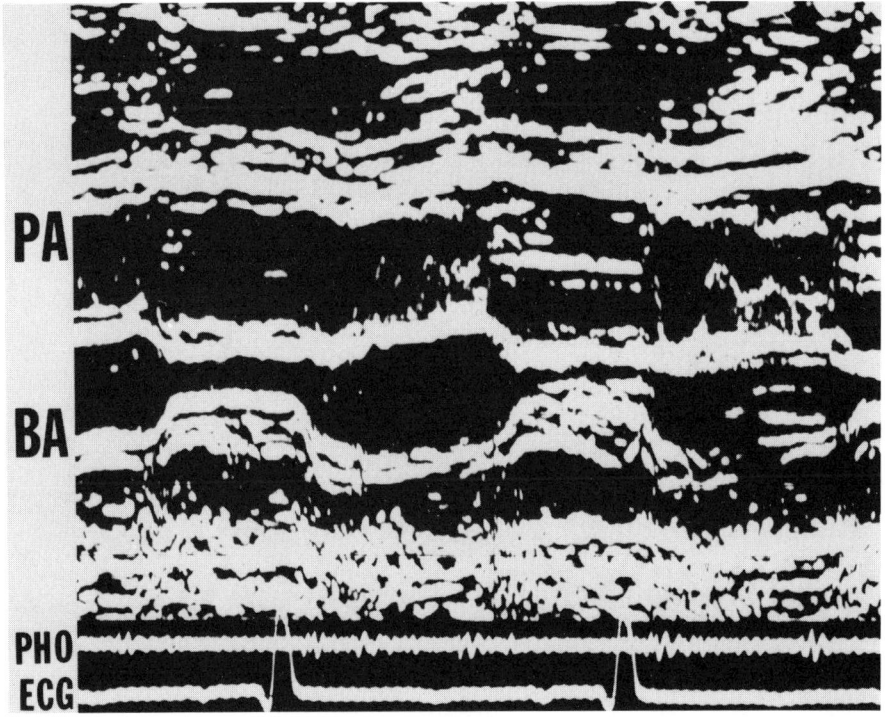

Figure 5

Normal motion pattern of the intra-atrial baffle (BA) recorded behind the pulmonary artery (PA). Note the sharp anterior movement at the onset of diastole, absence of 'a' waves and gradual anterior motion in systole. PHO = phonocardiogram ECG = electrocardiogram.

A prominent systolic anterior movement of the baffle echo seen behind the tricuspid valve in one patient was probably related to the unsupported baffle which had detached in the region of the tricuspid valve. Following placement of a new competent pericardial baffle, the echo patterns were restored to normal with only small 'a' waves, decreased width of the pulmonary artery and of the systemic venous atrial chamber and absence of abnormal systolic motion of the baffle echo imaged behind the tricuspid valve.

Ultrasonic contrast injections into the atrial cavities in the immediate postoperative period, serial studies of the size of the great vessels and of the newly constructed atrial chambers as well as observation of the motion patterns of the baffle echoes may provide indications of baffle incompetence.

References

1. Mustard WT: Successful two-stage correction of transposition of the great vessels. Surgery 55:469, 1964

2. Nanda NC, Stewart S, Gramiak R, Manning J: Echocardiography of the intra-atrial baffle in dextro-transposition of the great vessels. Circulation 51:1130, 1975

USEFULNESS OF ECHOCARDIOGRAPHIC PEAK VELOCITY OF CIRCUMFERENTIAL FIBRE SHORTENING

Derek R. Boughner, M.D., John Nolan, M.D., P. Rechnitzer, M.D., Department of Medicine, and Department of Biophysics, University of Western Ontario, London, Ontario, Canada

Echocardiography has been recommended as a valuable non-invasive technique for the assessment of left ventricular function. The motion of the endocardial surfaces of the septum and posterior wall can be recorded by directing the ultrasound beam just inferior to the mitral valve plane. From this the left ventricular minor axis diameter can be accurately measured throughout systole and the stroke volume, ejection fraction, posterior wall velocity and mean velocity of circumferential fibre shortening (mean V_{CF}) can be estimated.

The stroke volume and ejection fraction are valuable in the assessment of ventricular function but are sensitive to acute changes in both preload and afterload. In addition, these echocardiographic estimates are less reliable in dilated or small left ventricles although correction factors are available (1,2). The ejection fraction reflects only the extent of myocardial shortening not the duration of ejection and although it can, in general, separate normal from abnormal ventricles it is not sufficiently sensitive to detect mild dysfunction.

The use of left ventricular posterior wall velocity was initially recommended as a valuable method of assessing changes in left ventricular function (3,4) but subsequent studies have suggested that its value is limited in assessing total left ventricular performance, especially in coronary artery disease (5). Comparison of values between patients has proven unreliable.

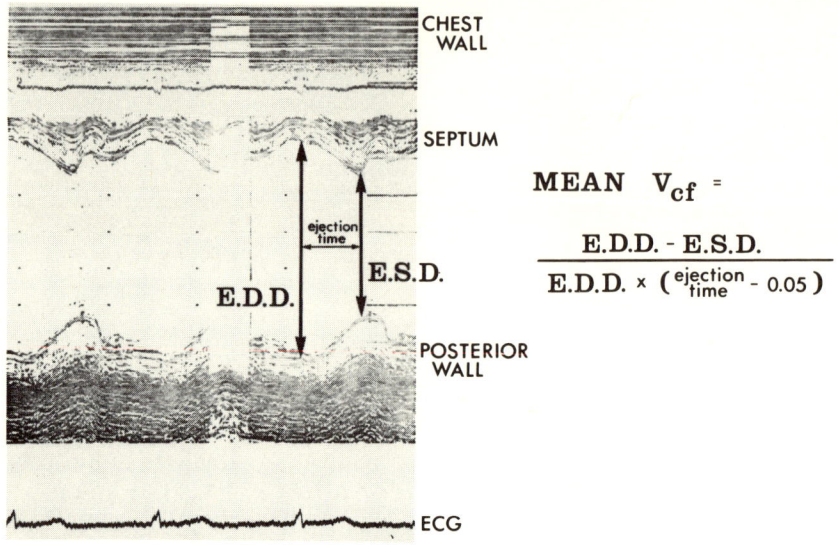

Figure 1
Echocardiogram illustrating the method used for calculating mean velocity of circumferential fibre shortening (mean V_{CF}). E.D.D. = end diastolic diameter E.S.D. = end systolic diameter

Calculation of mean V_{CF} has proven more useful and is more widely used. Mean V_{CF} calculated from the echocardiograms has correlated well with that calculated from left ventricular angiograms (6,7). Although those initial studies showed that, on the average, abnormal ventricles had a lower mean V_{CF} than normal ventricles there was significant overlap present between the two groups. Of most importance has been the tendency for some normal ventricles to give values of mean V_{CF} that fall well within the abnormal range. Thus mean V_{CF} may not be acceptable if it is used, for example, to study improvement in abnormal ventricles, after medical treatment, coronary artery by-pass procedures, or physical training. Here a clear separation between normals and abnormals would be required. For this reason we felt that a more accurate yet easily measured estimate of the velocity of circumferential fibre shortening was desirable.

In the rapid echocardiographic estimation of mean V_{CF} two difficulties arise. These primarily relate to the calculation of the ejection time, a major feature of the formula (Figure 1). The determination of the point at which minimum left ventricular diameter is achieved can be difficult as this minimum diameter is often maintained for 40-80 msec. In addition, the ejection time is measured from the peak of the "R" wave on the ECG to the point of minimum ventricular diameter, minus 50 msec. This 50 msec correction factor is to account for the pre-ejection period when no appreciable fibre shortening takes place and is arbitrarily applied to a wide variety of real values both greater or less than that approximation. Thus although the mean V_{CF} can usually separate normal from abnormal ventricles, overlap is inevitable with normal ventricles that have long pre-ejection periods being reduced to the abnormal range in particular.

Angiographic studies continue to recommend the velocity of circumferential fibre shortening as an excellent measure of left ventricular function (8,9). We therefore considered the possibility of measuring left ventricular minor axis diameters at various specific points during systole and more directly obtaining the rate of change

METHOD

Echocardiograms were obtained using a Unirad model 100 ultrasonoscope and 2.25 MHz transducer. The echocardiograms were recorded on Polaroid film and on a Honeywell #1856 strip chart recorder. Patients were receiving no medications when studied and lay in a supine position with the transducer applied to the fourth, left intercostal space. The left ventricular minor axis diameter was recorded by aiming the ultrasound beam just below the mitral valve.

Three groups of patients were studied: 14 sedentary normals, 15 athletes who exercised regularly and extensively, and 17 patients with proven myocardial infarctions within the previous three months. The group of athletes were selected since we had noted that the mean V_{CF} was most often inaccurate in young or especially active patients who had slow heart rates and prolonged pre-ejection periods. The cardiac patients were included as they represented a group with a single underlying disease process that could be expected to produce a range of left ventricular dysfunction.

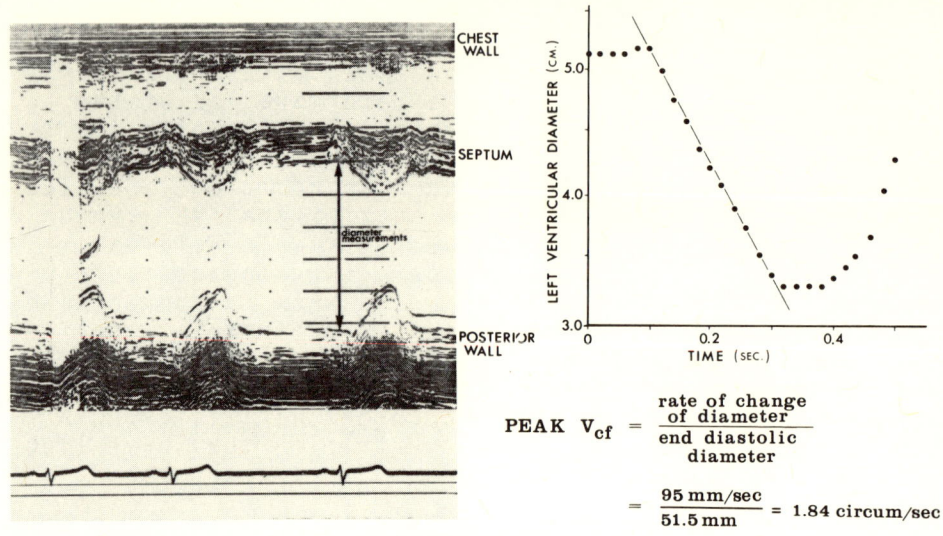

Figure 2
Echocardiogram illustrating method used for calculating peak velocity of circumferential fibre shortening (peak V_{CF}). Diameter measurements are made every 20 msec after the peak of the "R" wave on the ECG and plotted on the graph as shown. The slope of the line joining the points in midsystole represents the peak rate of change of diameter and when divided by the end diastolic diameter gives peak V_{CF} in circumferences/sec.

For each patient the mean V_{CF} was calculated from left ventricular end diastolic and end systolic diameter measurements using the formula indicated in Figure 1.

Next, using a transparent grid, the left ventricular diameter was measured every 20 msec beginning at the peak of the "R" wave in the electrocardiogram and ending at a point up to 180 msec beyond the point of minimum left ventricular diameter. These diameter measurements were then plotted versus time as illustrated in Figure 2. During mid systole they uniformly fell along a straight line and thus no difficulty was encountered in estimating the rate of change of diameter. When

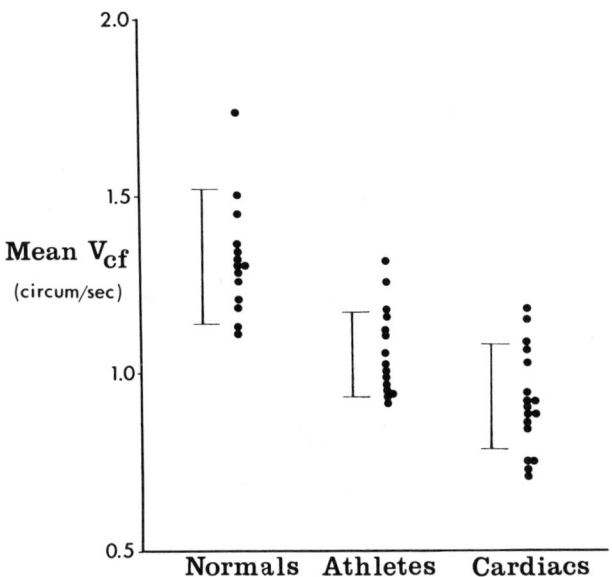

Figure 3
Mean velocity of circumferential fibre shortening (mean V_{CF}) for the 3 groups studied. There is considerable overlap between all groups and there is no significant difference between the values for the athletes and for the cardiac patients. Error bars represent standard deviation.

divided by the end diastolic diameter a normalized value representing the velocity of circumferential fibre shortening was obtained and termed the "peak V_{CF}".

RESULTS

The values for mean V_{CF} obtained for sedentary normals and athletes were significantly different ($p<0.05$) although there was considerable overlap. For normals a mean value of 1.33 ± 0.19 circum/sec was obtained (Figure 3) while athletes had a mean value of 1.05 ± 0.12 circum/sec. The cardiac patients were significantly different from normals but with some overlap and a mean value of mean V_{CF} 0.95 ± 0.15 circum/sec, and not significantly different from the athletes ($p > 0.05$).

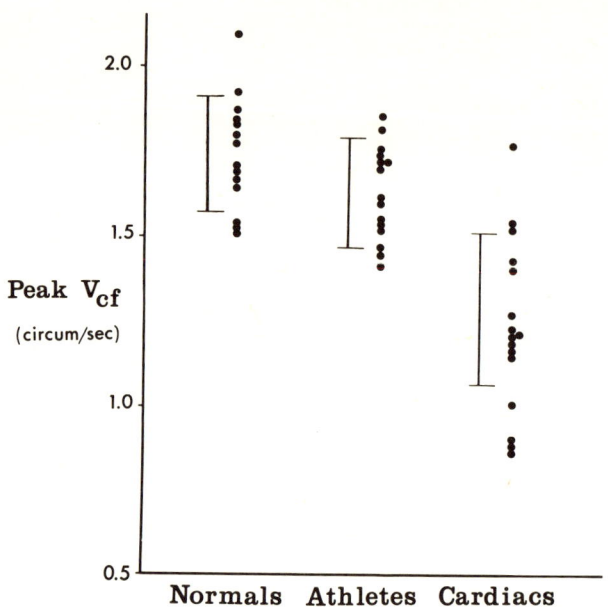

Figure 4
Peak velocity of circumferential fibre shortening (peak V_{CF}) for the 3 groups studied. There is no significant difference between the normal sedentary group and athletes. The cardiac patients show a wide distribution of values with some patients having no detectable ventricular dysfunction at rest. Error bars represent standard deviation.

The calculation of peak V_{CF} produced similar values for normals and athletes, although athletes tended to have slightly lower velocities. The mean value of peak V_{CF} for sedentary normals was 1.75 ± 0.15 circum/sec and for athletes was 1.62 ± 0.16 circum/sec (Figure 4).

The values of peak V_{CF} for the cardiac patients extended over a wide range, from 0.88 to 1.77 circum/sec, with a mean value of 1.29 ± 0.23 circum/sec. This was significantly different from both the sedentary normals and the athletes ($p<0.05$).

DISCUSSION

The velocity of circumferential fibre shortening presently appears to be a most important measure of the myocardial inotropic state. Normalized values of mean V_{CF}, determined cineangiographically, have permitted the distinction of normal from abnormal patients with complete separation among individual subjects (9) and the angiographic mean V_{CF} remains clinically useful despite chronic left ventricular dilatation. This fact is of considerable importance to the non-invasive echocardiographic technique where the estimation of ejection fraction becomes less useful under these circumstances (2). Also mean V_{CF} is not significantly affected by an acute change in preload (8,10). but is affected by changes in afterload and contractility (11). Since we can often maintain the afterload constant, changes in contractility can be assessed in response to various interventions using this measurement. Alternatively we can acutely change afterload and determine, from the new V_{CF} measurement, whether the myocardium is able to react normally.

Since echocardiography can give an estimate of the velocity of circumferential fibre shortening using the internal left ventricular minor axis diameter measurement it is a potentially valuable tool in the study of myocardial disease. However, the overlap between normal and abnormal values of mean V_{CF} reduces the application of this technique. We have illustrated the extent to which these values can, for normal ventricles, overlap with abnormal and have shown that for a selected group of athletes there may be no significant differences at all. It would appear, however, that the fault lies not with the basic echocardiographic technique but with the approximation used in the calculation. To avoid this difficulty we have illustrated that a slightly different measurement peak V_{CF}, can be a more acceptable measure of the velocity of circumferential fibre shortening. Peak V_{CF} was shown to have similar values for all normal ventricles including the athletes. This latter group did have a slightly lower mean value of peak V_{CF} indicating that their ventricles are operating more efficiently and thus at a lower point on the left ventricular force-velocity curve.

In addition, the peak V_{CF} measurement provided a wider range of abnormal values. In the cardiac patients various degrees of left ventricular impairment were suggested by a peak V_{CF} that ranged from quite low values to values that were in the normal range. These measurements could therefore have indicated the amount of myocardial damage suffered by the patient at the time of the infarction, i.e. could indicate the extent of the disease process. None of these patients had any clinical symptoms to indicate residual cardiac dysfunction.

An alternative explanation for the range of values noted in the cardiac patients must be considered. The area of myocardial injury could have influenced the value of peak V_{CF} if it was not specifically located in the path of the ultrasound beam. Thus a falsely normal left ventricular function estimate could be possible. However, no correlation was shown between the area of myocardial damage indicated by the electrocardiogram (either inferior or anterior wall) and the peak V_{CF}.

Our range of normal values obtained for peak V_{CF} was comparable to the values of peak V_{CF} calculated by Quinones et al using a somewhat different method (13). Their normal range was 2.0 ± 0.30 circum/sec. In addition, our values of peak V_{CF} were shown to change little with time. In 5 of the 17 cardiac patients both mean and peak V_{CF} were calculated seven months after the initial study and no significant differences in either value was present. The mean V_{CF} for those 5 patients in the first study was 0.95 ± 0.08 circum/sec and 7 months later was 0.96 ± 0.03 circum/sec. For peak V_{CF} the initial values were 1.25 ± 0.10 and final values 1.26 ± 0.18 circum/sec.

Since peak V_{CF} appears to have a wide range of abnormal values it is possible that this parameter could be more sensitive than mean V_{CF} to changes induced by specific interventions such as coronary artery by-pass procedures, physical training or drug administration.

For peak V_{CF} to be of practial usefulness it must be easily and quickly measured. We have found that the rate of change in diameter throughout the ejection portion of systole regularly approximates a straight line and that it is really unnecessary to measure the diameter at 20 msec intervals. Two points separated by 80 msec, measured during ejection, and joined by a straight line appeared to be adequate for establishing the rate of change of ventricular diameter and thence peak V_{CF}. With a transparent grid this can be done quickly.

From this study it appears that peak V_{CF} can distinguish more clearly than mean V_{CF} normal from abnormal ventricles on the echocardiogram. Whether it is clearly possible, as was indicated by the study, to distinguish between normal and abnormal left ventricles in coronary artery disease awaits a comparison of angiographic and echocardiographic peak V_{CF} measurements in individual patients.

REFERENCES

(1) Fortuin, N.J., Hood W.P. Jr., Sherman, M.E. Craige, E.: Determination of left ventricular volumes by ultrasound. Circulation 44: 575, 1971.
(2) Ludbrook, P., Karliner, J.S, Peterson, K., Leopold, G., O'Rourke, R.A.: Comparison of ultrasound cineangiographic measurements of left ventricular performance in patients with and without wall motion abnormalities. Brit. Heart J. 35: 1026, 1973.
(3) Kraunz, R.F., Kennedy, J.W.: Ultrasonic determination of left ventricular wall motion in normal man. Am Heart J 79: 36, 1970
(4) Fogelman, A.M., Abbassi, A.S., Pearce, M.L., Kattus, A.A.: Echocardiographic study of the abnormal motion of the posterior left ventricular wall during angina pectoris. Circulation 46: 905, 1972
(5) Ludbrook, P., Karliner, J.S., London, A., Peterson, K.L., Leopold, G.R., O'Rourke, R.A.: Posterior wall velocity: an unreliable index of total left ventricular performance in patients with coronary artery disease. Am J Cardiol 33: 475, 1974.
(6) Fortuin, N.J., Hood W.P., Craige, E.: Evaluation of left ventricular function by echocardiography. Circulation 46: 26, 1972
(7) Cooper, R.H., O'Rourke, R.A., Karliner, J.S., Peterson, K.L., Leopold, G.R.: Comparison of ultrasound and cineangiographic measurements of the mean rate of circumferential fibre shortening in man. Circulation 46: 914, 1972.
(8) Ross, J.Jr., Peterson, K.L.: On the assessment of cardiac inotropic state. Circulation 47: 435, 1973.
(9) Peterson, K.L., Skolven, D., Ludbrook, P., Uther, J.B., Ross, J. Jr.: Comparison of isovolumic and ejection phase indices of myocardial performance in man. Circulation 49: 1088, 1974.
(10) Rafflenbeul, W., Butterich, D., Muller, M., Krayenbuhl, H.P.: Einflub von akuten anderungen der vorbelastung auf die mittlere zirkumferentielle faserverkurzungsgeschwindigkeit des linken ventrikels. Z. Kardiol 64: 211, 1975.
(11) Quinones, M.A., Gaasch, W.H., Cole, J.S., Alexander, J.K.: Echocardiographic determination of

left ventricular stress-velocity relations in man with reference to the effects of loading and contractility. Circulation 51: 689, 1975.

This study was supported by grants from the Ontario Department of Health and the Ontario Heart Foundation. Dr. Boughner is an Ontario Heart Foundation Senior Research Fellow.

MYOCARDIAL CONTRACTILITY IN NORMAL AND POST INFARCTION SUBJECTS AT REST AND DURING ISOMETRIC EXERCISE

J.P. Nolan, M.D., D.A. Cunningham, Ph.D., D.R. Boughner, M.D. The University of Western Ontario, London, Ontario, Canada

Interest has developed in non-invasive techniques for analyzing left ventricular function. Echocardiography is a tool currently being used in this regard. A deficiency of the technique is its inability to study myocardial function during dynamic exercise. Isometric exercise is a useful alternative to dynamic exercise and allows ultrasound examination of the left ventricle under stress. It has been studied extensively and used in several instances to study abnormal and normal left ventricular function. Isometric exercise results in the production of two cardiovascular phenomenon; an increase in heart rate and an elevation in blood pressure both of which increase myocardial oxygen demand and the work of the heart. Its simplicity of application has allowed several recent studies of isometric exercise and its effects on myocardial force velocity relations. One recent paper has been published by Stefadouros using echocardiography to determine the normal ventricular response.

Analysis of left ventricular myocardial contractility both at rest and in response to isometric stress was studied using reflected ultrasound in two groups of subjects. Sixteen subjects considered to have normal left ventricular function were compared to sixteen post myocardial infarction patients who had made an uncomplicated recovery from an acute myocardial infarction at least twelve weeks previous to the study. The patients were evenly divided in terms of having sustained anterior or inferior wall damage.

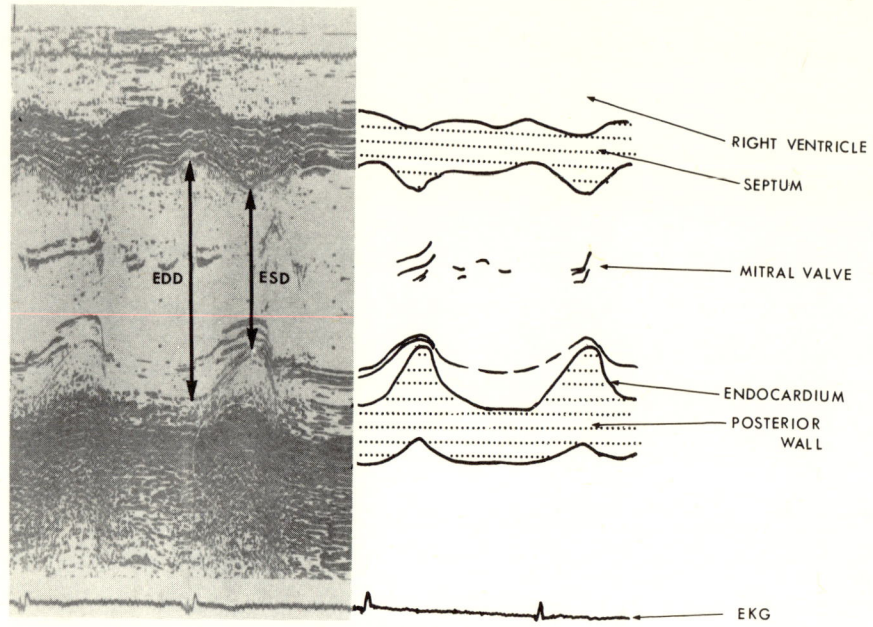

Figure 1
Echocardiogram of a normal left ventricle at rest

Echocardiographic tracings were recorded both at rest and after two minutes of isometric hand grip exercise performed at 33% of maximum voluntary contraction (Figures 1 and 2). All recordings were taken with a paper speed of 50 mm/second. A Unirad ultrasonoscope model 100 using a 3.5 MHz transducer was employed. The hand grip exercise was performed using a C.H. Stoelting Co., hand grip dynamometer.

Both mean velocity of circumferential fibre shortening (mean V_{CF}) and peak velocity of circumferential fibre shortening (peak V_{CF}) were measured. Mean V_{CF} was calculated, using for the duration of systole the peak of the R wave on the simultaneously recorded electrocardiogram to the point of maximal excursion of the endocardial surface of the posterior wall. From this interval, 50 msecs was subtracted for pre-ejection period to give the left ventricular ejection time. The end diastolic and end systolic diameters were measured at the above points. Peak V_{CF} was measured as the slope of the easily drawn line through a series of points representing minor axis diameters measured throughout

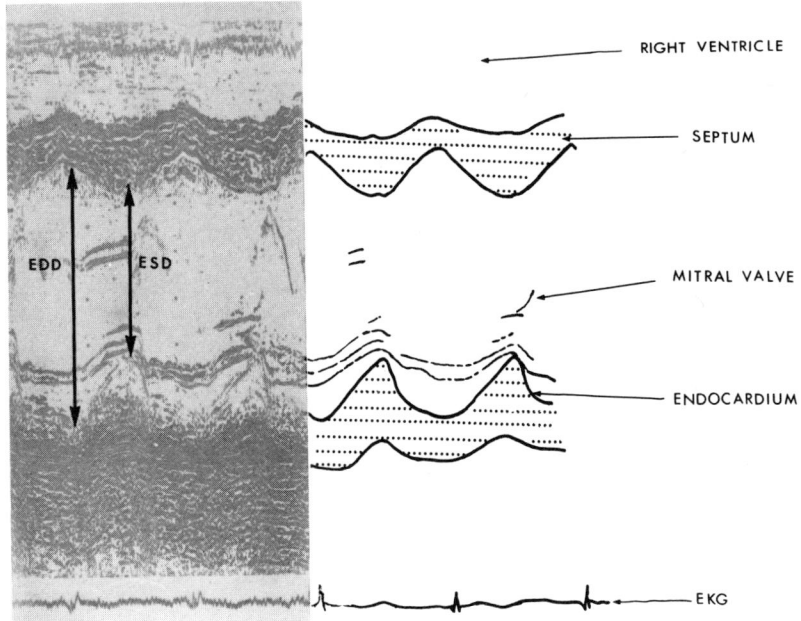

Figure 2
Echocardiogram of the left ventricle pictured in Figure 1 under isometric stress illustrating the increase in cardiac frequency.

systole at 20 msecond intervals and plotted at that interval. To allow for magnification and comparison among subjects, this velocity was normalized by dividing by the end diastolic diameter.

The normal subjects showed no significant change from resting to exercise mean V_{CF} (1.29 $\pm$ 0.05 to 1.34 $\pm$ 0.07) or peak V_{CF} (1.74 $\pm$ 0.04 to 1.77 $\pm$ 0.12). The cardiac subjects showed lower mean values for all four measurements: mean V_{CF} from resting to exercise (0.95 $\pm$ 0.04 to 0.87 $\pm$ 0.04) and peak V_{CF} from resting to exercise (1.29 $\pm$ 0.06 to 1.07 $\pm$ 0.06) $P < 0.001$. However, only the peak V_{CF} measured in the cardiac patients was consistently lower in response to the exercise (Figure 3).

The new concept of peak V_{CF} appears to be a more sensitive indicator than mean V_{CF} of the myocardial infarction patient's decreased ability to enhance myocardial contractility via inotropic mechanisms in

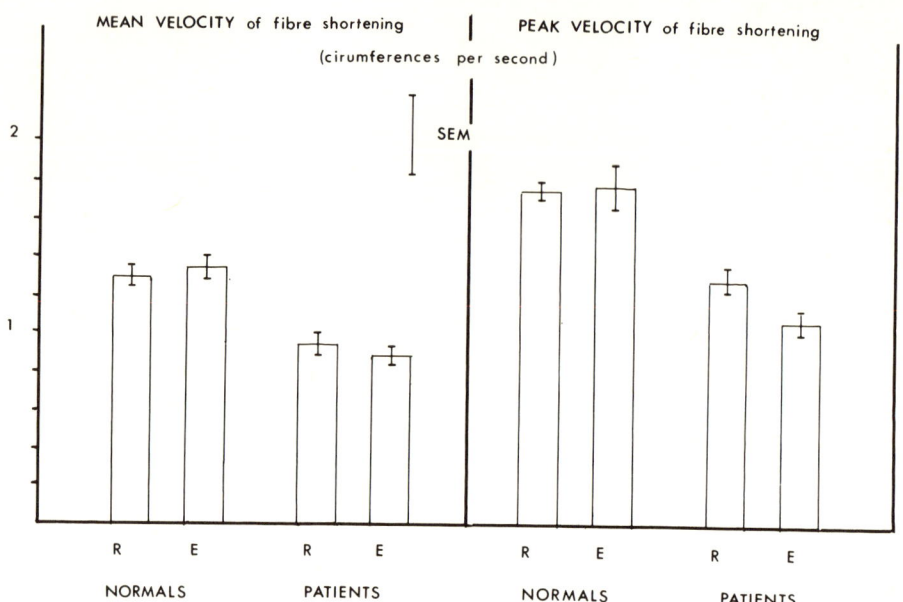

Figure 3

Left ventricular velocities in normal subjects and post infarction patients at rest and during isometric exercise.

response to the acute after-load produced by isometric stress. The mean V_{CF} concept was originally devised as a shortcut for the derivation of contractility through measurement of the velocity of circumferential fibre shortening at the point of maximum tension generated by the left ventricle. As a shortcut it produces overlap and lacks the sensitivity of the former measurement to separate patients with varying degrees of disability. The peak V_{CF} concept utilized in this paper is likely a more accurate reflection of the true mean V_{CF} concept and its general use in the assessment of left ventricular function is recommended. These results support the hypothesis that the cardiac patient functions lower on the force velocity function curve not only at rest, but has less reserve than normal subjects to the effects of isometric stress (Figure 4).

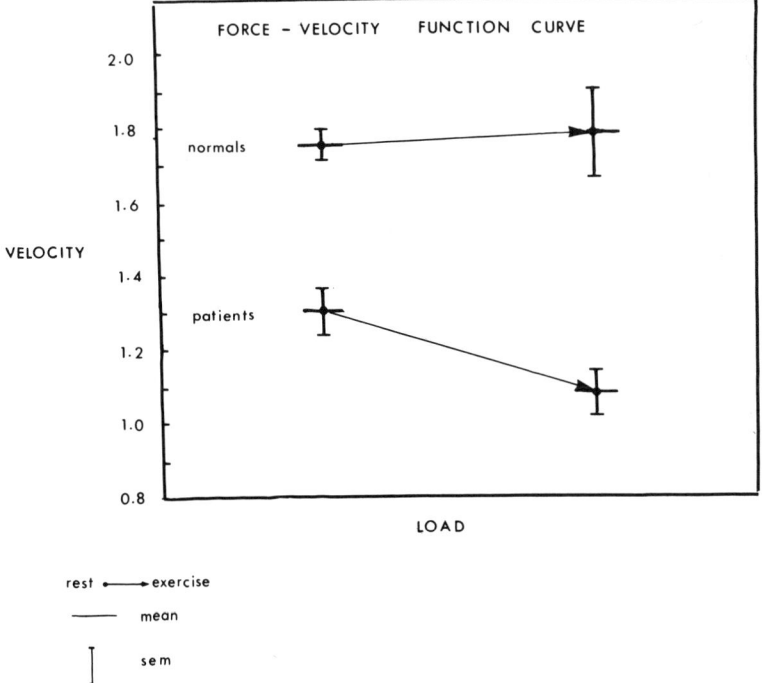

Figure 4
Comparison of the force velocity function response in normal subjects and post infarction patients in response to isometric stress.

The reason for these findings is not entirely clear. There are four possible mechanisms to account for the phenomenon. None of these patients had post infarction angina or positive stress tests and, therefore, ischemic myocardiums. Alterations in autonomic tone and circulating catecholamines are two mechanisms that are difficult to invoke as there is no evidence to suggest that the infarction patient is any different from the normal individual in this regard. The likely mechanism is a change in ventricular compliance. The scar tissue in the infarcted myocardium results in a stiff ventricle and hence not as responsive to inotropic stimuli or changes in acute afterload as the normal ventricle.

REFERENCES

(1) Glick, G., Sonnenblick, E.H., Braunwald, E.: Myocardial force velocity relations studied in intact unanaesthetized man. Journal of Clinical Investigation 44: 6: 978-988, 1965.

(2) Helfant, R.H., DeVilla, M.A., Meister, S.G.: Effect of sustained isometric handgrip exercise on left ventricular performance. Circulation 44: 982-992, 1971.

(3) Lind, A.R., McNichol, G.W.: Circulatory responses to sustained handgrip contractions performed during other exercise, both rhythmic and static. Journal Physiology 192: 595-607, 1967.

(4) Linquist, V.A.Y., Spangler, R.D., Blount, S.G. Jr.: A comparison between the effects of dynamic and isometric exercise as evaluated by the systolic time intervals in normal man. American Heart Journal 85: 2, 227-236, 1973.

(5) Mitchell, J.H., Wildenthal, K.: Static (isometric) exercise and the heart. Annual Review of Medicine 25: 369-381, 1974.

(6) Quinones, M.A., Gaasch, W.A., Cole, J.S., Alexander, J.K.: Echocardiographic determination of left ventricular stress-velocity relations in man. Circulation 51: 689-700, 1975.

(7) Sonnenblick, E.H., Braunwald, E., Williams, J.F. Jr., Glick, G.: Effects of exercise of myocardial force velocity relations in intact unanaesthetized man: Relative roles of changes in heart rate, sympathetic activity and ventricular dimensions. Journal of Clinical Investigation 44: 12: 2051-2062, 1965.

(8) Stefadouros, M.A., Grossman, W., Shahawy, M.E., Stefadouros, F., Witham, A.C.: Noninvasive study of the effects of isometric exercise on left ventricular performance in normal man. British Heart Journal 36: 988-995, 1974.

This paper is supported by the Ontario Department of Health and the Ontario Heart Foundation.

ECHOCARDIOGRAPHIC OBSERVATIONS ON SYSTOLIC CLOSURE OF THE AORTIC VALVE IN MITRAL INCOMPETENCE

P.A.N. Chandraratna, M.D., M.R.C.P.; A. Rashid, M.D.;
with the technical assistance of D. Gindlesperger
Division of Cardiology, Department of Medicine
Mount Sinai Medical Center, Miami Beach, Florida
and the University of Miami, Coral Gables

Abstract
 Systolic closure of the aortic valve has been described in patients with IHSS, discrete membranous subaortic stenosis and right coronary sinus of Valsalva fistula. We observed abnormal aortic valve motion on the echocardiogram in four patients with mitral incompetence. Two types of abnormality were noted. The first pattern consisted of partial closure of the right coronary cusp in mid systole followed by reopening later in systole. The second pattern observed was partial closure of the right coronary cusp shortly after its opening with little or no reopening in late systole. The possible mechanism of production of this abnormality is discussed. Mitral regurgitation should be included in the differential diagnosis of conditions producing systolic closure of the aortic valve on the echocardiogram.

Introduction
 The role of echocardiography in the evaluation of patients with rheumatic heart disease and coronary artery disease has been firmly established.[1-5] More recently, the value of ultrasound in the assessment of left ventricular function has been demonstrated.[6,7]

 Gramiak and Shah established the origin of aortic valve echoes by injecting indocyanine green into the aortic root.[8] They also described the abnormalities that may be observed on the echocardiogram in patients with calcified aortic stenosis.[9] Characteristic abnormalities of aortic valve motion on the ultrasound recording have been described in idiopathic hypertrophic subaortic stenosis (IHSS), discrete membranous subaortic stenosis, and right coronary sinus of Valsalva fistula.[10-11] In this manuscript, we report abnormal aortic cusp movement in four patients with mitral incompetence. The possible mechanism of production of this abnormality is discussed.

Materials and Methods

Echocardiography was performed on 18 patients with angiographic evidence of mitral incompetence. The only basis for selection was a technically adequate aortic valve echocardiogram and the absence of aortic valve disease. The patients were examined in the supine position. A 2.25 MHz, 7.5 cm focus transducer, an Ekoline 20 ultrasonoscope and an Electronics for Medicine DR8 recorder were used. The transducer was placed in the third or fourth interspace at the left sternal border and angulated superiorly and medially until the walls of the aortic root and the aortic valve cusps were seen.

Results

Seven patients had mild mitral regurgitation (MR) on the left ventricular angiogram. All of them had normal motion of the aortic valve leaflets. Eleven patients had moderate or severe MR on angiography. Abnormal aortic valve motion was noted in four, all of whom had severe mitral reflux. A brief description of the clinical findings on each case is given below.

Patient 1, H.C., a 29 year old white male was referred because of intractable cardiac failure. One month prior to admission he fell from a height of 20 feet and sustained non penetrating chest trauma. He was hospitalized elsewhere and a new murmur of mitral regurgitation was discovered. He was referred to Mount Sinai Hospital for treatment of refractory cardiac failure. Physical examination revealed signs of severe mitral insufficiency. The presence of gross mitral regurgitation was confirmed by cardiac catheterization. There was mild left atrial enlargement. At surgery, complete rupture of the anterior papillary muscle at its base was observed. He had mitral valve replacement with good results.

Patient 2, J.W., a 59 year old negro male presented with dyspnea on exertion and paroxysmal nocturnal dyspnea of six months duration. Physical examination revealed signs of severe mitral incompetence. At cardiac catheterization he was noted to have severe mitral regurgitation, marked left ventricular and left atrial enlargement. There was mild reduction of left ventricular contractility.

Patient 3, R.D. a 15 year old white female was referred for cardiac evaluation because of increasing shortness of breath on exertion. There was no past history of rheumatic fever. Physical examination revealed a blood pressure of 200/120 and signs of left ventricular enlargement and severe mitral incompetence. The presence of mitral regurgitation was substantiated at cardiac catheterization. There were no other valvular lesions.

Patient 4, W.W., a 56 year old white male was admitted to the hospital with a complaint of shortness of breath of seven months duration. He had physical signs suggestive of severe mitral regurgitation. Cardiac catheterization and left ventricular angiography revealed severe mitral incompetence, moderate enlargement of the left atrium and moderate reduction of left ventricular contractility. Coronary arteriography showed 90% stenoses of the proximal right coronary artery and the first marginal branch of the circumflex artery.

All four patients demonstrated partial systolic closure of the aortic valve. Two patterns of aortic valve motion were observed. The first type of abnormality consisted of opening of the aortic valve in systole, mid systolic partial closure of the valve, followed by reopening in late systole. This pattern was observed in two patients (H.C. and R.D.). The second pattern noted (patients J.W. and W.W.) was opening of the aortic valve in systole followed by partial closure of the valve with little or no reopening in late systole.

Figures 1 and 2 illustrate the first pattern of abnormal aortic valve motion. Partial and mid systolic closure of the right coronary cusp followed by reopening in late systole is seen in each case. The echocardiogram taken after mitral valve replacement on the patient referred to in Figure 1 is shown in Figure 3. The right coronary cusp of the aortic valve does not demonstrate the mid systolic closure that was observed preoperatively. The second pattern of abnormal aortic valve motion is depicted in Figure 4. Partial closure of the right coronary cusp is seen shortly after opening of the valve and there is little or no reopening of the cusp in late systole.

Discussion

Abnormal systolic closure of the aortic valve on the echocardiogram may be seen in patients with idiopathic hypertrophic subaortic stenosis (IHSS), discrete membranous subaortic stenosis, and right coronary sinus of Valsalva fistula.[10,11] The characteristic abnormality in IHSS is mid systolic partial aortic valve closure followed by reopening of the valve.[11] The closure of the aortic valve is due to left ventricular outflow tract obstruction with a consequent fall in the aortic flow. In discrete membranous subaortic stenosis, there is rapid partial closure of the aortic valve shortly after its opening. This is followed by rapid fluttering of the valve[10] but reopening of the valve is not seen in contrast to the pattern observed in IHSS. Johnson and his associates recently described abnormal aortic cusp motion in ruptured right coronary sinus of Valsalva

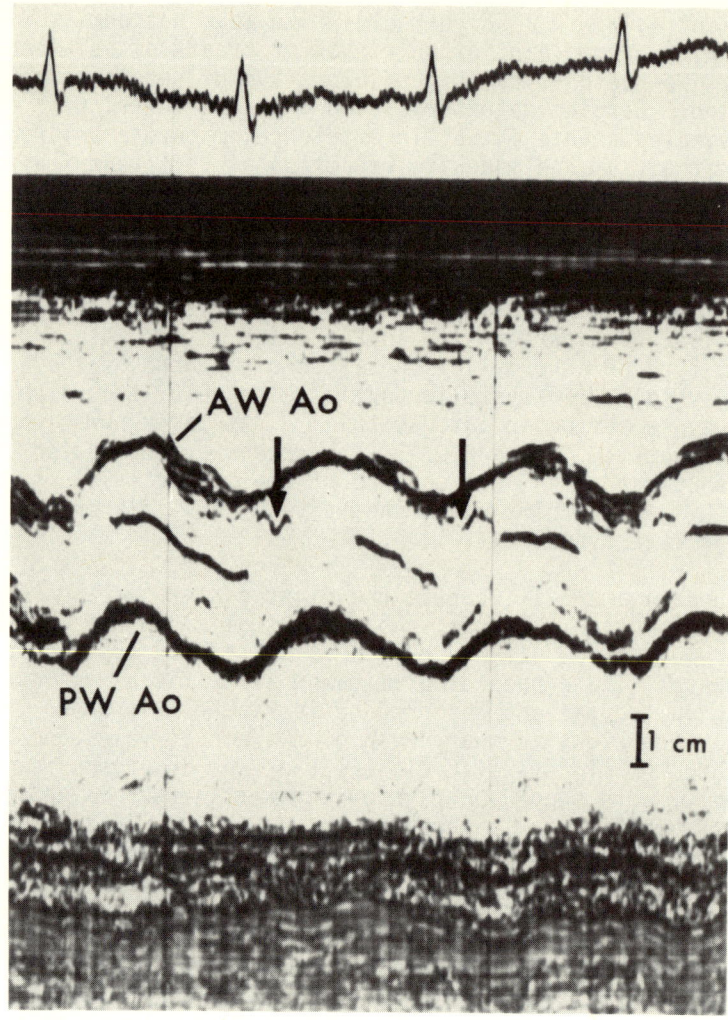

Figure 1
This illustrates the echocardiogram of the aortic valve of patient H.C. Partial closure of the right coronary cusp (indicated by vertical arrow) in mid systole is seen.
AW AO = anterior wall of aortic root
PW AO = posterior wall of aortic root

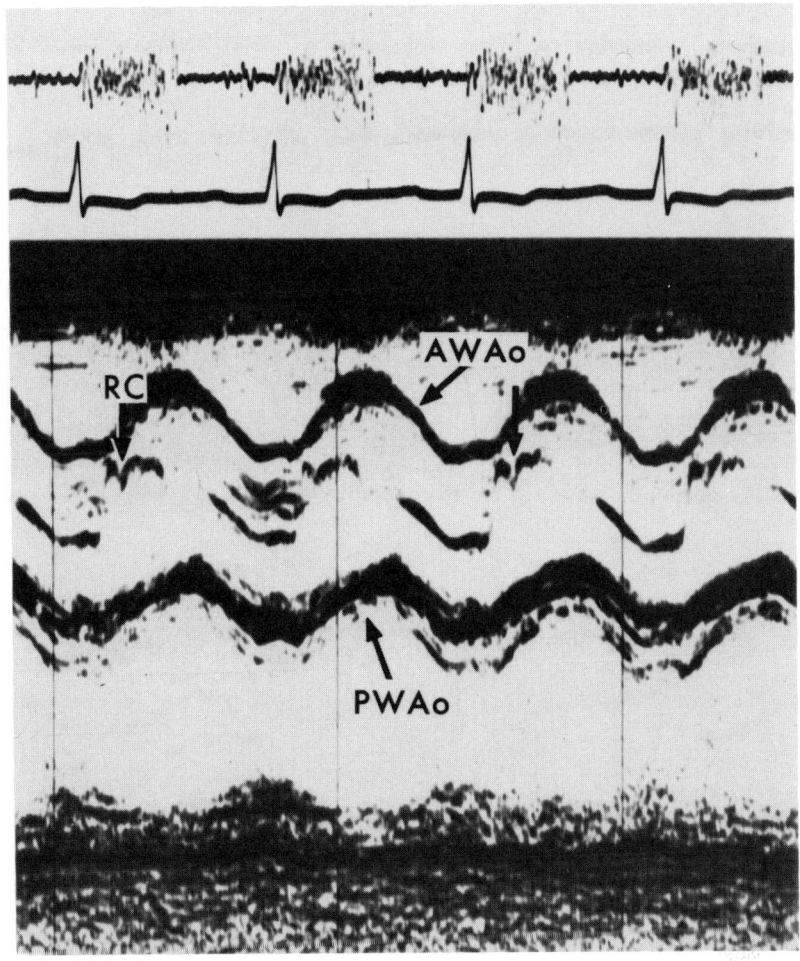

Figure 2
Ultrasound recording of the aortic valve of patient R.D. is shown. Aortic valve opening is followed by partial closure of the right coronary cusp (RC). There is reopening of the valve later in systole.
AW AO = anterior wall of aortic root
PW AO = posterior wall of aortic root

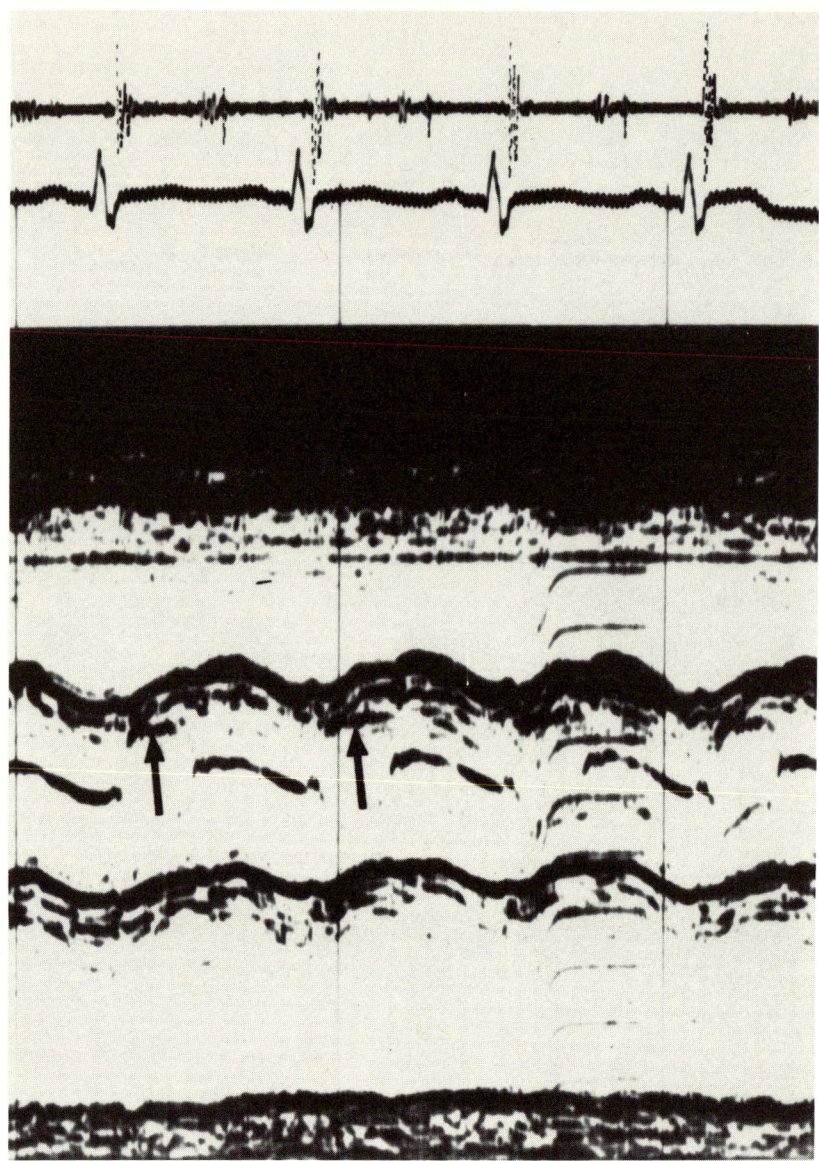

Figure 3
This depicts the aortic valve echocardiogram of patient H.C., recorded after he underwent mitral valve replacement. Motion of the right coronary cusp (vertical arrow) of the aortic valve is normal.

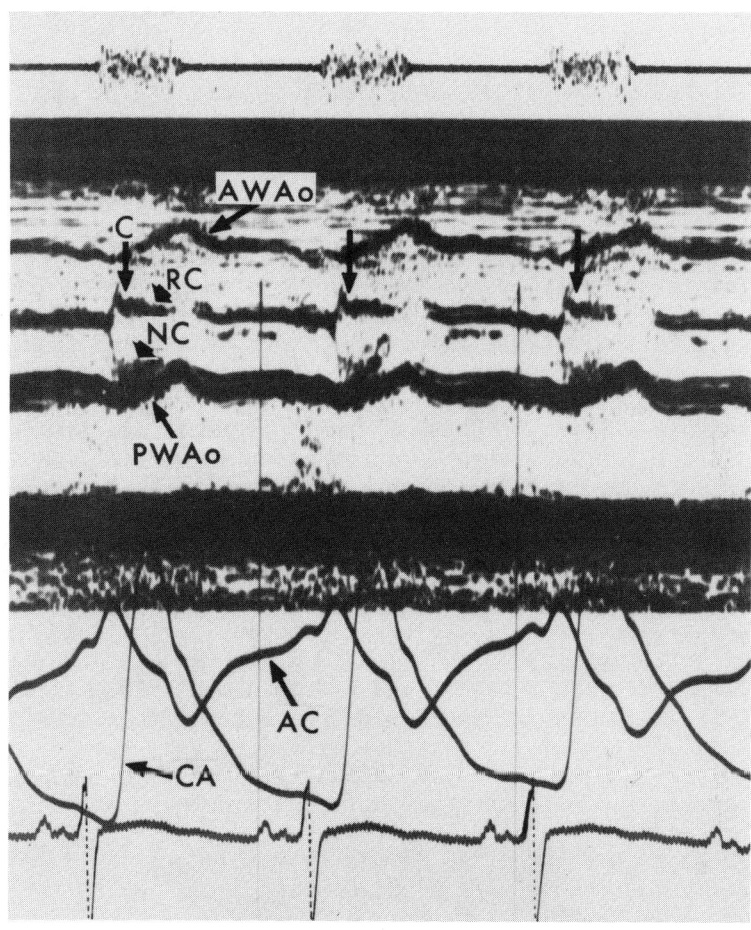

Figure 4
Echocardiogram of the aortic root of patient J.W. There is partial closure (C) of the right coronary cusp (RC) shortly after valve opening. There is little or no reopening of the cusp later in systole.
AW AO = anterior wall of aortic root
PW AO = posterior wall of aortic root
NC = non coronary cusp
AC = apexcardiogram   CA = external carotid pulse

aneurysm.[11] They observed partial closure of the right coronary cusp of the aortic valve in early systole, followed by reopening in late systole. The movement of the non coronary cusp was normal.

We observed two abnormal patterns of aortic valve movement in association with mitral regurgitation. The first type of abnormality consisted of a mid systolic closure of the aortic valve with reopening later in systole. This pattern resembled that sometimes seen in patients with IHSS. Cobbs[12] has observed a miniature pulsus bisferiens in patients with ruptured chordae tendineae. He suggests that the relatively small left atrium fills maximally in mid systole, so that there is a secondary spurt in forward aortic flow towards the end of ejection. It is of interest that the central aortic pressure pulse in the patient with ruptured papillary muscle closely resembled that seen in patients with IHSS (Figure 5). A possible mechanism for the production of mid systolic aortic valve closure and abnormal aortic pulse contour is outlined below. In the early ejection phase of systole (Fig. 6, Phase 1) there is rapid ejection of blood into the aorta. There is a reduction in aortic flow in mid systole due to severe mitral regurgitation (Fig. 6, Phase 3). This triphasic pattern of aortic flow could explain rapid opening of the aortic leaflets, partial closure in mid systole and reopening in the latter part of systole. The second pattern of abnormal aortic valve motion consisted of partial closure of the right coronary cusp shortly after its opening, with little or no reopening later in systole (J.W. and W.W.). Patient J.W. had marked left atrial enlargement and W.W. had moderate enlargement of his left atrium on the angiogram. Because of the large capacity of the left atrium, significant mitral reflux probably continued till late systole. Thus, a secondary late systolic spurt of forward aortic flow probably did not occur in these patients and hence, reopening of the aortic valve was not present. An alternative explanation for partial aortic valve closure would be a Venturi effect produced by a high velocity jet of mitral regurgitation.

In summary, partial systolic closure of the aortic valve was observed on the echocardiogram in four patients. A possible mechanism of production of this abnormality is outlined. Mitral incompetence should be included in the differential diagnosis of conditions that produce partial systolic closure of the aortic valve on the echocardiogram.

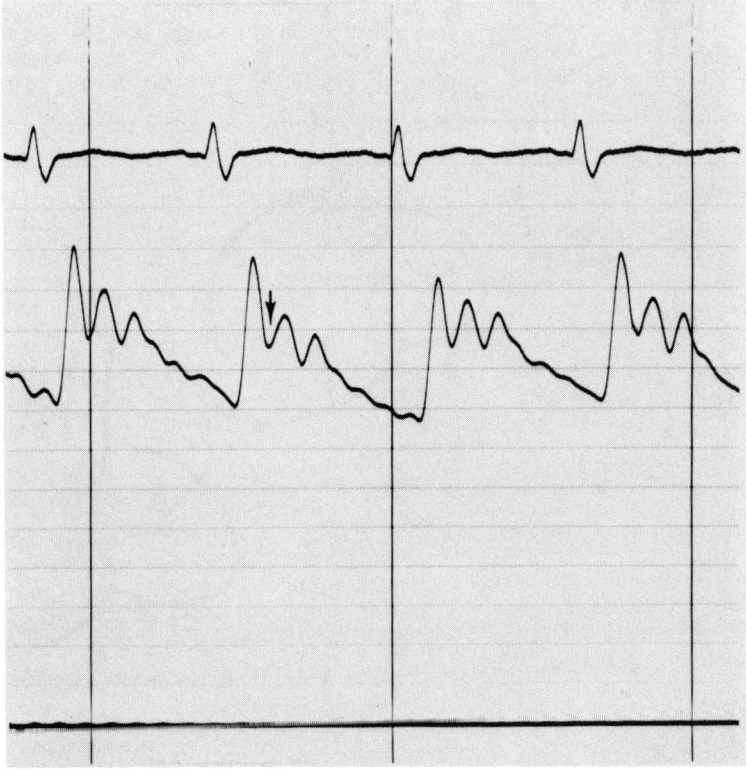

Figure 5
This shows the central aortic pressure pulse of patient H.C. Note the prominent mid systolic dip (indicated by vertical arrow) which resembles the pulse contour seen in IHSS.

SYSTOLIC EJECTION

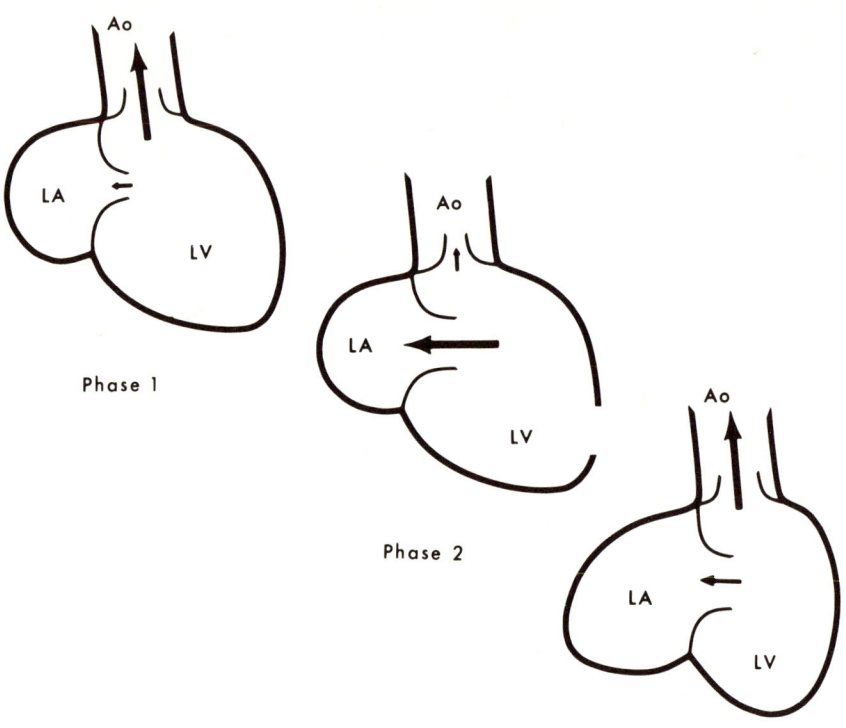

Figure 6
This is a diagram to illustrate the ejection dynamics in a patient with mitral incompetence and a relatively small, poorly compliant left atrium. In early systole (Phase 1), ejection takes place into the aorta (Ao) and into the left atrium (LA). In Phase 2 (mid-systole) the aortic flow decreases because of torrential flow into the LA. In Phase 3 (late systole) because the relatively small LA is almost completely filled, the degree of mitral incompetence decreases resulting in an increase of aortic flow.

LV = left ventricle

References
1. Joyner, C.R., Reid, J.M., Bond, J.P.: Reflected ultrasound in the assessment of mitral valve disease. Circulation 27: 503, 1963.
2. Feigenbaum, H.: Echocardiography. Philadelphia, Lea and Febiger, 1972.
3. Diamond, M.A., Dillon, J.C., Haine, C.L., Chang, S., Feigenbaum, H.: Echocardiographic features of atrial septal defect. Circulation 43: 129, 1971.
4. Lundstrom, N.R.: Echocardiography in the diagnosis of Ebstein's anomaly of the tricuspid valve. Circulation 47: 597, 1973.
5. Jacobs, J.J., Feigenbaum, H., Corya, B.C., Phillips, J.F.: Detection of left ventricular asynergy by echocardiography. Circulation 48:263, 1973.
6. Fortuin, N.J., Hood, W.P., Craige, E.: Evaluation of left ventricular function by echocardiography. Circulation 46: 26, 1972.
7. McDonald, I.G., Hobson, E.R.: A comparison of the relative value of non-invasive techniques - echocardiography, systolic time intervals and apexcardiography in the diagnosis of primary myocardial disease. Am. Heart J. 88: 454, 1974.
8. Gramiak, R., Shah, P.M.: Echocardiography of the aortic root. Invest. Radiol. 3: 356, 1968.
9. Gramiak, R., Shah, P.M.: Echocardiography of the normal and diseased aortic valve. Radiology 96: 1, 1970.
10. Davis, R.J., Konecke, L.L., Dillon, J.C., Chang, S., Feigenbaum, H.: Echocardiographic findings in discrete subaortic stenosis (Abstr).Am. J. Cardiol. 31: 127, 1973.
11. Johnson, M.L., Warren, S.G., Waugh, R.A., Kisslo, J.A., Sabiston, D.C., Lester, R.G.: Echocardiography of the aortic valve in non-rheumatic left ventricular outflow tract lesions. Radiology 112: 677, 1974.
12. Hurst, J.W.: The Heart. McGraw-Hill, 1974, p. 866.

HYPERTENSION IN ADOLESCENTS - AN ULTRASOUND STUDY

W. P. Laird and D. E. Fixler

Southwestern Medical School

Dallas, Texas   75235

Recent information suggests that ultrasound is a reliable technique to evaluate left ventricular function by non-invasively estimating left ventricular stroke volume, ejection fraction (EF), mean rate of circumferential fiber shortening (mean V_{CF}), and relative change in minor axis with systole.[1-4] In addition, ultrasound measurement of septal and left ventricular free wall thickness may provide a sensitive method for detecting early changes of left ventricular hypertrophy.[5]

The purpose of this study was to use echocardiography to study groups of hypertensive adolescents in an effort to detect subtle cardiovascular abnormalities not readily appreciated by other non-invasive tests.

METHODS AND MATERIALS

Echocardiograms were performed on 8 adolescents with mild hypertension (MHT). All are followed regularly in the Hypertension Clinic of the Children's Medical Center. Each patient has had a documented elevation in blood pressure (BP) on at least 3 separate clinic visits. For this study, an elevated BP was defined as systolic and/or diastolic pressure over the 95th percentile for age and sex.[6] Each of these hypertensive patients had been previously evaluated in an effort to define the cause of their hypertension. In none of them could an etiology be established.

The second study group consisted of 5 pediatric patients with renal hypertension (RHT) due to chronic renal disease. The control group consisted of 8 normotensive adolescents.

The techniques utilized in obtaining the echocardiograms were similar to those described by others.[7] An Ekoline 20 Ultrasonoscope was used in all cases. The transducers included both 5.0 MHz and 2.25 MHz non-focused units. With the transducer in the patient's 3rd or 4th left intercostal space at the sternal border, the characteristic echo of the anterior mitral valve leaflet was sought. From this position the transducer was rotated in order to record distinct left ventricular (LV) free wall and septal echoes. The left ventricle was then scanned inferiorly and superiorly along its major axis in order to accurately define the location of the LV minor dimension. This site was identified at a position which included portions of the anterior and posterior mitral valve leaflets. Echoes were then recorded on polaroid film.

Left ventricular dimensions were measured, the mean rate of circumferential fiber shortening calculated, and percent change in minor axis with systole determined from the echocardiograms using established methods.[3,4,7] Data were analyzed by unpaired t-tests.

RESULTS

Table 1 describes the clinical characteristics of the 3 groups. The mean age and mean body surface area (BSA) of the patients with MHT were similar to that of the normal group. However the group with RHT were slightly younger and had a smaller body surface area. The mean resting blood pressure in the MHT patients was 144 ± 5 (SEM) / 91 ± 4, compared to 104 ± 5 / 69 ± 4 in the normal group, and in the RHT group 144 ± 7 / 90 ± 6.

TABLE 1 - PATIENT CHARACTERISTICS

	NORMAL	MILD H.T.	RENAL H.T.
Number	8	8	5
Age (Yrs)	13.9 ± 1.8	12.7 ± 0.7	11.5 ± 0.7
BSA	1.56 ± 0.05	1.64 ± 0.11	1.26 ± 0.16
Systolic BP	104 ± 5	144 ± 5	144 ± 7
Diastolic BP	69 ± 4	91 ± 4	90 ± 6

Mean ± S.E.M.

Echocardiographic findings are shown in Table 2. The patients with RHT had the greatest left ventricular free wall thickness (mean = 0.84 cm ± 0.05) compared to the MHT group (0.75 ± 0.02), and the normals (0.56 cm ± 0.02). Mean LV diastolic dimensions and

TABLE 2 - ECHOCARDIOGRAPHIC FINDINGS

	NORMALS	MILD H.T.	RENAL H.T.
LV Free Wall Thickness (cms)	0.56 ± 0.02	0.75 ± 0.02	0.84 ± 0.05
LV_D (cms)	4.5 ± 0.1	4.6 ± 0.1	4.6 ± 0.3
LV_S (cms)	2.8 ± 0.1	2.5 ± 0.2	2.9 ± 0.2
% Change with systole	37% ± 2	46% ± 2	37% ± 2
LV Ejection Time (seconds)	0.32 ± 0.02	0.31 ± 0.01	0.33 ± .02
Ejection Fraction	.63 ± .03	.73 ± .03	.63 ± .02
Mean VCF	1.18 ± 0.11	1.49 ± 0.08	1.15 ± 0.10

Mean ± S.E.M.

LV ejection times were similar in all 3 groups. However the mean LV systolic diameter was smaller in the patients with MHT (2.5 cm ± 0.2) than that of the normals (2.8 cm ± 0.1), or the RHT group (2.9 cm ± 0.2).

The derived indices used in evaluating left ventricular function (Table 2) indicate that the patients with MHT had a significantly greater mean ejection fraction, mean percent change in minor axis with systole and mean velocity of circumferential fiber shortening.

DISCUSSION

Considerable attention has recently been directed to the problem of hypertension in adolescents. There has been substantial interest in the possible use of non-invasive diagnostic techniques to detect subtle changes in ventricular performance and myocardial hypertrophy in such patients. Thus far, however, studies suggest that the standard electrocardiogram and chest roentgenogram may be rather insensitive tests for detecting hypertensive cardiovascular abnormalities in adolescents. For example, one study found that only about 7% of children with sustained hypertension had electrocardiographic or X-ray evidence of left ventricular hypertrophy.[8] In another investigation 3 of 17 young patients with persistent hypertension had abnormal ECG findings.[9]

Of the electrocardiograms performed on all patients only one patient in each of the two hypertensive groups had ECG evidence of left ventricular hypertrophy. In contrast echocardiography demonstrated an increase in mean LV free wall thickness in our patients with MHT when compared with our normals. However, the mean value in the MHT group did fall within the range of published normal values according to body surface area.[10] The RHT patients showed a definitely abnormal increase in left ventricular wall thickness, which may have resulted from their having persistent hypertension for a longer period of time. These findings suggest that the echocardiogram may provide a more sensitive method for detecting early left ventricular hypertrophy.

Analysis of the internal LV diastolic (LV_D) dimensions as measured by echo showed that there was no significant difference among the 3 groups. Since the patients with RHT represented a slightly younger group of subjects with a correspondingly smaller mean BSA, the mean LV_D for this particular group may actually represent moderate LV enlargement.

An interesting difference in ventricular dimensions was found among the LV systolic (LV_S) values. Here the patients with MHT tended to have a smaller mean systolic dimension. When the percent systolic change in diameters was calculated, a significant difference was evident. This finding also accounted for the increase in ejection fraction of the MHT group since the echo derivation of EF is primarily related to the ratio of LV_S to LV_D. Furthermore, inasmuch as the LV ejection times of the 3 groups were similar, the mean V_{CF} of the MHT subjects were predictably increased.

The hemodynamics of the earliest phase of essential hypertension remain controversial and theoretical. The studies of some investigators have led them to suggest that the development of sustained arterial hypertension may possibly be preceded by a stage of labile hypertension characterized by a hyperkinetic circulation.[11,12] Their work indicates that typically the hemodynamics of such patients is characterized by an increased cardiac output and normal peripheral resistance. Later, in the phase of fixed, essential hypertension the resistance is elevated and the cardiac output normal.

It is not known whether any of our patients with MHT will ultimately develop essential hypertension; however the present study does suggest that these subjects have echocardiographic evidence of hyperkinetic LV function.

REFERENCES

1. Pombo JF, Troy BL, Russell RO Jr: Left ventricular volumes and ejection fraction by echocardiography. Circulation 43:480-490, 1971

2. Fortuin NJ, Hood WP Jr, Sherman ME, Craige E: Determination of left ventricular volumes by ultrasound. Circulation 44:575-584, 1971

3. Meyer RA, Stockert J, Kaplan S: Echographic determination of left ventricular volumes in pediatric patients. Circulation 51: 297-303, 1975.

4. Cooper RH, O'Rourke RA, Karliner JS, Peterson KL, Leopold GR: Comparison of ultrasound and cineangiographic measurements of the mean rate of circumferential fiber shortening in man. Circulation 46:914-923, 1972

5. Morganroth J, Maron BJ, Krovetz, LJ, Henry WL, Epstein SE: Electrocardiographic evidence of left ventricular hypertrophy in otherwise normal children. Clarification by echocardiography. Am J Cardiol 35:278-281, 1975

6. Lauer RM, Connor WE, Leaverton PE, Reiter MA, Clarke WR: Coronary heart disease risk factors in school children: The Muscatine study. J Pediatr 86:697-706, 1975

7. Feigenbaum H: Clinical application of echocardiography. Progr Cardiovasc Dis 14:531-558, 1972

8. Londe S, Bourgoignie JJ, Robson AM, Goldring D: Hypertension in apparently normal children. J Pediatr 78:569-577, 1971

9. Kilcoyne MM: Adolescent hypertension II. Characteristics and response to treatment. Circulation 50:1014-1019, 1974

10. Feigenbaum H: Echocardiography. Philadelphia, Lea & Febiger, 1972, p218

11. Eich RH, Peters RJ, Cuddy RP, Smulyan H, Lyons RH: The hemodynamics in labile hypertension. Am Heart J 63:188-195, 1962

12. Frohlich ED, Tarazi RC, Dustan HP: Re-examination of the hemodynamics of hypertension. Am J Med Sci 257:9-23, 1969

TWO-DIMENSIONAL ECHOCARDIOGRAPHIC ASSESSMENT OF NORMAL MITRAL LEAFLET MOTION

> Joseph Kisslo; Gregg Friedman; Michael Johnson; Olaf T. von Ramm
> Departments of Medicine and Biomedical Engineering
>
> Duke University, Durham, N.C. 27710

Measurement of quantitative data from the time-motion echocardiogram of the mitral valve is often difficult. One-dimensional echo beams usually intercept the anterior mitral leaflet in a variety of places during the cardiac cycle and, most likely, do not accurately reflect the total motion of the entirety of the leaflet. Changes in the geometric configuration of the anterior mitral leaflet and its cyclic spatial relationships to the mitral ring were studied in twenty normal volunteers using a real time, two-dimensional, phased array imaging system. All patients were in normal sinus rhythm and were studied at rest. Breath was held at end expiration. Scans were obtained through both the long and short axes of the mitral valve.

The changing spatial locations of the anterior mitral leaflet, mitral ring and aortic root were traced, frame by frame, from video tape recordings in order to construct geometric reference models for the study of mitral apparatus motion on the models. Lines perpendicular to the chest wall were drawn to the aortic root, mitral ring and anterior mitral leaflet. By measuring distances from the chest wall to the targets along these lines, time-motion echocardiograms were reconstructed. Additional lines at various angles were drawn to the anterior mitral leaflet from the chest wall in an effort to determine the effect of transducer position and angle on the resultant time-motion echo contours.

In systole, the mitral ring and anterior mitral leaflet descended caudally and anteriorly in synchrony with the contracting ventricle. Such data would indicate that the C-D portion of the time-motion echo bears little relation to primary leaflet motion and that mitral amplitude should be measured from the D to E points. With reference to the chest wall, the anterior mitral leaflet underwent a series of alternating wave-like concave and convex configurations during the cardiac cycle. In diastole, the maximum excursion and radius of curvature of the anterior mitral leaflet was most marked near its tip. This degree of curvature was also widely variant between patients. When opened at the E point the anterior mitral leaflet assumed a concave configuration. The E-F slope was determined first by the rapid cephalad and posterior ascent of the mitral ring to its starting position and second by the progressive straightening of the anterior mitral leaflet.

The various reconstructed time-motion echocardiograms of the anterior mitral leaflet were quite different in contour depending on the degree of angulation of the line of measurement and the degree of alternating curvature of the leaflet during diastole. It was additionally possible to calculate a theoretical E-F slope of the mitral leaflet by measuring the sequential positions of a fixed point on the leaflet (usually 2.5 cm. from the valve ring). Such a plot revealed a sigmoid curve, rather than straight line, for E-F slope. The degree of curvature of the theoretical E-F slope varied directly with the degree of cyclic curvature of the valve leaflet.

It must be concluded that anterior mitral leaflet motion seen on time-motion echocardiography is a composite of both mitral ring movement and alternating wavelike motions of the leaflet itself. Depending upon the degree of these alternating diastolic curvatures and the angle the echo beam makes with the mitral leaflet, a variety of one-dimensional patterns may be recorded.

QUANTITATIVE ECHOCARDIOGRAPHY: A STUDY OF CHAMPION CHILDHOOD ATHLETES

H. D. Allen; N. Schy; J. Wood; S. J. Goldberg;
D. J. Sahn; R. Wojcik
Department of Pediatrics, Arizona Medical Center,
Tucson, Arizona

Although most pediatric echocardiographic criteria have been concerned with qualitative aspects of cardiac anatomy, dimensional quantitation has demonstrated utility in children with lesions causing cardiac pressure or volume overloads. Examples of this include following left atrial dimension in children with patent ductus, or ventricular septal defect and right ventricular anterior wall thickness in cor pulmonale. In order to utilize quantitative echographic techniques, normal chamber and great vessel dimensions established during a collaborative study from the Universities of Arizona and Indiana were derived and presented last year at this meeting by Epstein. The study established percentile nomograms which compared direct echocardiographic measurements of walls, chambers and great vessels in unselected normal healthy children to the best correlate, body surface area. These nomograms have been utilized as a basis for reading echocardiograms of children evaluated for various reasons in our cardiac clinics. A number of athletic youngsters with normal hearts were found to have excessive echocardiographic dimensions. Accordingly, it became clear that more definition of the upper 5th percentile was required. In order to define this range, we selected the best available group of highly trained childhood athletes, competitive swimmers. Competitive swimming is a major sport in Arizona. Tucson has 60 competitive teams, each composed of approximately 100 youngsters.

We selected as subjects for our investigation the city championship team. These athletes, ages 5 through 17, train for approximately two hours a day, six days a week and some time considerably more. Training, much of which is against the clock, consists of swimming several miles each day. Mean training duration was two years although many children had participated much longer. Each child had a standard echocardiogram performed. Echocardiographic measurement accuracy was increased by utilizing calipers combined with a variable scale ruler, as in the previous normal study. Echocardiograms were measured by an unbiased observer without reference to normal nomograms.

Seventy children were studied. Adequate results were obtained in all children except two in whom the right ventricular anterior wall could not be adequately visualized. In comparison to the normal nomograms, 100% of the swimmers had right ventricular anterior walls thicker than the 95th percentile of normal ("percentile" refers to normal distribution). Eighty-nine percent had septal thickness > 50th percentile and 84% had septal thickness > 95th percentile. Seventy-nine percent had left ventricular posterior wall thickness > 50th percentile and 76% had thickness > 95th percentile. Eighty-six percent of the children had aortic root dimensions > 50th percentile and 74% exceeded the 95th percentile. Similar increases were found for aortic leaflet separation. In contrast, 64% of the children had left atrial dimensions which were less than the 50th percentile. Left ventricular end diastolic and end systolic dimension showed a wider scatter, although the median for these measurements was approximately equal to the 50th percentile for the normal distribution. Right ventricular cavity was considerably larger than normal as 97% of the children exceeded the 50th percentile and 91% exceeded the 95th percentile. Comparison of cardiac dimensions did not correlate to fastest swimming times for various events.

We conclude from these data that cardiac mass and certain cardiac chamber and great vessel dimensions are significantly different in trained childhood athletes as compared to unselected normal youngsters. Knowledge of the effect of training on cardiac dimensions is essential for quantitative pediatric echocardiography.

THE ECHOCARDIOGRAPHIC SPECTRUM OF MITRAL VALVE (MV) MOTION IN

CHILDREN WITH AND WITHOUT MITRAL VALVE PROLAPSE (MVP)

D. J. Sahn; J. Wood; H. D. Allen; W. Peoples;
S. J. Goldberg
Department of Pediatrics, University of Arizona Medical
Center, Tucson, Arizona

Recent concern has been expressed over the sensitivity and specificity of echocardiography for the diagnosis of MVP. Accordingly, the purpose of the present study was to define the single crystal and multiple crystal cross-sectional echo spectrum of mitral valve motion in 68 asymptomatic children (age 3-15 years) without abnormal physical findings who constituted the normal group, and 26 children (age 2-10 years) with physical findings of systolic click murmur (CM). From M-mode echoes, mitral valve systolic posterior motion was defined as minor if it was $>10\%$ of the E-F excursion and significant if it was more than 20%. Mitral valve echoes were evaluated only where anterior and posterior leaflet were simultaneously visualized. Of 45 normal children studied by single crystal echo 9 had minor mid to late systolic dips (MSD) of both leaflets, 3 had minor holosystolic "hammocking" (HH) while 3 patients had significant MSD. These findings represent the normal spectrum of mitral valve motion for M-mode and do not represent MVP. There were no dimensional abnormalities in the normal group. Real time cross-sectional studies on 23 normal patients demonstrated a spectrum of mitral valve motion in which the bodies of the anterior and posterior leaflets (defined as that portion of the leaflets occupying a distance halfway between the free edge and the annular insertions) become horizontal with systolic ejection as the aortic root moves anteriorly and the posterior atrio-ventricular junction moves inferiorly. The coaptation line at the free edges of the leaflets gradually moves anteriorly during systole. There was little superior motion of the mitral apparatus which assumed a curvilinear funnel shape with slight arching of both leaflets. Studies of single crystal M-mode outputs selected from within the array showed that 7 of 23 normal patients had various combinations of HH and MSD of significant degree on tracings obtained from the body of the mitral valve leaflets while only one patient showed minor MSD when outputs were selected from the free edge where the leaflets coapted. Multicrystal studies in the 26 patients with CM and MVP demonstrated significant arching of the bodies of the leaflets superiorly and posteriorly towards the left atrium. The findings of MVP could be confirmed easily in these patients by single crystal element M-mode outputs selected from the array at the free edge as well as at the body of the leaflets. M-mode findings were most striking when outputs were selected from the area of maximal mitral arching. Twenty-one of these 26 patients had aortic root dimensions which exceeded 95th percentile by more than 2 mm. Five patients had Marfan's Syndrome and an additional six had minor musculo-skeletal deformaties. The results of this study indicate that the demonstration of the echo findings of MVP in normal patients as well as patients with physical findings of CM are highly dependent on transducer angulation and the portion of the valve examined. Cross-sectional echocardiography was of significant utility in demonstrating the superior and posterior arching of leaflets present in patients with MVP. The presence of aortic root dilatation or physical findings of musculo-skeletal abnormalities were suggestive that the echocardiographic findings demonstrated were associated with abnormal cardiac connective tissue. A spectrum of normal mitral valve motion was defined for both single and cross-sectional echocardiographic studies and it was documented that abnormal M-mode studies could often be derived from single crystal outputs receiving echoes from the body of the mitral valve leaflet even in normal patients. It is therefore suggested that the critical differentiation of the spectrum of normal mitral valve motion from MVP requires careful evaluation of echoes derived from the free edge of the leaflet where the anterior or posterior leaflet echoes coapt in early systole. Echoes obtained with a superior angulation such that the left atrium is visualized behind the mitral valve are much less satisfactory in achieving this differentiation in children than those obtained with the transducer perpendicular to the chest wall and the beam passing through the two mitral leaflets and the posterior left ventricular wall. The study should allow a standardized approach to echocardiography in these patients and reduce overdiagnosis.

CROSS-SECTIONAL ECHOCARDIOGRAPHIC ASSESSMENT OF SEVERITY OF

AORTIC STENOSIS IN CHILDREN

A. E. Weyman; H. Feigenbaum; R. A. Hurwitz;
D. A. Girod; J. C. Dillon; J. Stewart
Department of Medicine
Indiana University, Indianapolis, Indiana 46202

In a recent report we described the relationship of the maximum aortic cusp separation determined during long axis cross-sectional scanning of the aortic valve to the severity of aortic stenosis in adults. In order to utilize this measurement in children some correction for body size is obviously necessary. Because aortic size increases relative to body surface area as patient size decreases, routine correction of aortic valve orifice diameter for body surface area is misleading. We therefore elected to relate maximum aortic cusp separation (MACS) as an expression of aortic orifice size to the diameter of the aortic root (AO) at the valvular level. Thus the estimated aortic valve orifice diameter is expressed as a percentage of the aortic diameter. In this study MACS was determined in 14 children, ages 4 to 14 years, with valvular aortic stenosis and in 22 normal subjects. In normal subjects the aortic leaflets open freely with ventricular contraction and assume a position parallel and in close apposition to the walls of the aorta. In normals the maximum aortic cusp separation therefore should approach the aortic diameter. In the 22 normal subjects the MACS averaged 73% of the aortic diameter (range 63 to 92%). The data for the 14 children with aortic stenosis is listed in table I.

TABLE I

	No.	MACS/AO	Range
Severe	1	21%	-
Moderate	4	34%	31 - 40%
Mild	9	53%	42 - 63%

The reliability of this ratio was then evaluated in a larger combined group of 44 children and adults. The results of the combined group is listed in table II.

TABLE II

	No.	MACS/AO	Range
Severe	16	25%	13 - 31%
Moderate	9	34%	24 - 45%
Mild	16	55%	40 - 63%

Based on this preliminary data the ratio of MACS to AO appears to be helpful in correcting for body size in children and in relating MACS to the severity of aortic stenosis.

ECHOCARDIOGRAPHIC OBSERVATIONS REGARDING PULMONARY VALVE MOTION IN CHILDREN WITH PULMONARY VASCULAR OBSTRUCTIVE DISEASE

S. J. Goldberg; H. D. Allen; D. J. Sahn

Department of Pediatrics, University of Arizona Medical Center, Tucson, Arizona

Pulmonary valvular motion has recently been characterized for adults with pulmonary vascular obstructive disease (PVOD). Echocardiographic features of PVOD include loss of the presystolic posterior motion (the pulmonary valve "a wave") flattening of the diastolic segment and premature systolic anterior motion (PSAM) of the pulmonary valve, which is almost always followed by a secondary systolic posterior motion. The systolic pulmonary valve motion thus inscribed resembles the letter "w". We postulated that PSAM would occur earlier in children with a site for right to left shunting. Our study population consisted of 8 children with ventricular septal defect plus PVOD of severe degree, 18 patients with cor pulmonale and pulmonary hypertension due to cystic fibrosis and 500 children with various other forms of congenital cardiac disease studied by consecutive examination, approximately 20% of whom had pulmonary vascular obstruction of some degree. All children with ventricular septal defect and severe PVOD had PSAM of the pulmonary valve. Those with combined cor pulmonale and PVOD had variable pulmonary valve motion, but most were not separable from normals. Two of those children had PSAM. Of the 500 consecutive examinations of children, we found only 8 with PSAM of the pulmonary valve. With respect to PSAM, two groups of children emerged with differences, those with severe PVOD plus VSD (group 1) and those with PVOD without VSD (group 2). Group 2 could further be broken down into children with high pulmonary pressure on the basis of flow, and high pulmonary pressure on the basis of pulmonary vascular obstruction. We have thus far found no examples of children with PSAM on the basis of high pulmonary blood flow causing high pulmonary pressures without PVOD. Only those children with some degree of pulmonary vascular obstruction demonstrated PSAM. On the basis of echo derived right ventricular systolic time, PSAM occurred in the first 35% of systole in group 1 children and later in systole in group 2 children. This finding is consistent with hemodynamics in group 1 children, in whom right ventricular blood can be diverted into the left ventricle via the VSD after initial pulmonary blood flow fills the available pulmonary circulatory space and lung circulatory resistance to further filling exceeds systemic resistance. In group 2 children, no diversion path is available and the right ventricle must continue to extrude blood despite the reflected waves and the high flow resistance. The echocardiographic features permit the separation of group 1 and group 2 children and verifies the utility of echocardiography of the pulmonary valve in the study of ventricular ejection dynamics.

ECHOCARDIOGRAPHIC FEATURES OF COMMON VENTRICLE

J. B. Seward; A. J. Tajik; D. J. Hagler; D. G. Ritter

Division of Cardiovascular Diseases and Internal Medicine
Mayo Clinic and Mayo Foundation, Rochester, MN 55901

Single or common ventricle is a rare and complex form of congenital heart disease in which the ventricular chamber receives blood from both atrioventricular valves, either separately or as a common atrioventricular valve. Cardiac catheterization and selective angiocardiography are required to establish the diagnosis.

We wish to report on a series of 25 patients (ages 1.5 through 28 years) who had common ventricle, with reference to distinctive features, contrast studies with indocyanine green, and differential diagnosis. Diagnosis was established in all cases by cardiac catheterization. Surgical or autopsy (or both) confirmation was available in 7 of the 25 cases. With these diagnostic methods, 16 patients had type A common ventricle (outflow chamber present), and 9 had type C common ventricle (no outflow chamber); 20 of the 25 patients had two atrioventricular valves.

M-mode echocardiograms were obtained with a Smith-Kline instrument (Ekoline 20 Ultrasonoscope) interface to a Honeywell or Cambridge multichannel strip chart recorder. A 2.25-MHz transducer was used. Five of the initial echograms were recorded on Polaroid film.

The echocardiographic features of common ventricle with two atrioventricular valves (20 patients) included (1) absence of a bona fide septal echo on a base-to-apex sector scan; (2) ability to simultaneously record echoes (in the same sound beam) of an anterior and a posterior atrioventricular valve without an intervening septal echo (this feature was recorded in 16 of the 20 patients who had angiocardiographic documentation of two atrioventricular valves); and (3) normal motion of the atrioventricular valves.

The echocardiographic features of common ventricle with a common atrioventricular valve (five patients) included (1) a single atrioventricular valve located posteriorly in the ventricle and which had a large amplitude of excursion during diastole and (2) absence of a demonstrable second atrioventricular valve and definite ventricular septal echo.

Continuity of the posterior (mitral) atrioventricular valve and great artery was an unusual echocardiographic finding in our series of common ventricle. In six patients with type C common ventricle (no outflow chamber), continuity between the mitral valve and the posterior great artery (pulmonary artery) was demonstrated.

In the nine patients with type C common ventricle, scanning toward the apex of the ventricle revealed an intraventricular echo. This echo was seen intermittently and only on isolated views in seven patients but was noted consistently in two patients. These two patients subsequently underwent surgical exploration, which revealed a large papillary muscle receiving chordae from both atrioventricular valves, presumably the structure producing this intraventricular (pseudoseptal) echo.

In seven patients, contrast echocardiograms with indocyanine green were obtained at cardiac catheterization. With caval, atrial, or ventricular injections of dye, a cloud of echoes filled the entire ventricular chamber, with no evidence of a ventricular septum. In the presence of intraventricular (pseudoseptal) echoes, the cloud of echoes appeared to engulf the echo and aided in differentiating this echo from a true ventricular septal echo.

In contrast to the findings of others, we noted that the simultaneous echocardiographic appearance of two atrioventricular valves with no intervening septal echo in a base-to-apex scan was the most characteristic feature of common ventricle. Using this feature and contrast echocardiography with indocyanine green, we differentiated common ventricle from large ventricular septal defect, complete atrioventricular canal, and straddling tricuspid valve. When only one atrioventricular valve is demonstrated, common ventricle can be difficult to differentiate from hypoplastic right and left heart syndromes. In this regard, our recent experience with contrast echocardiography has been helpful in making this distinction.

DETECTION OF INTRACARDIAC RIGHT TO LEFT SHUNTING BY

ECHOCARDIOGRAPHY

L.M. Valdes-Cruz, M.D.; D.R. Pieroni, M.D.;
J.M. Roland, M.D.; P.J. Varghese, M.D.
Department of Pediatrics
The Johns Hopkins Hospital
Baltimore, Maryland 21205

The clinical diagnosis of minimal cyanosis in the pediatric patient is often difficult. A simplified technique for identifying intracardiac right to left shunting would be of great value. In previous studies, intracardiac injections have been used to produce ultrasonic reflections (UR) which outline cardiac structures and intracardiac flow patterns. In this study peripheral vein injections (PVI) were used as a modified technique to produce UR. The UR were followed echocardiographically to detect intracardiac right to left shunts.

Cardiac catheterization and echocardiographic studies were performed on 29 patients ages 5 to 15 years. Indicator dilution techniques, oximetry and angiocardiography documented a right to left shunt in 10 patients, an isolated left to right shunt in 6 children and no intracardiac communication in 13 patients.

Two and five cc of normal saline were injected by hand through a #16F intracath placed in the right antecubital vein. A strip chart echocardiogram was recorded simultaneously with each injection. In the normal circulation venous injections produce UR which traverse only the right heart chambers. Presence of UR within the left heart or aorta indicates right to left shunting.

This study revealed that PVI consistently produced detectable UR in the right heart chamber in every patient. UR were recorded within the left heart in all 10 patients with documented right to left shunts. In the 13 patients without shunts and in the 6 patients with isolated left to right shunts, UR were found only in the right heart chambers.

Thus PVI is a simple, reliable and minimally invasive technique for identifying R to L intracardiac shunting. This method is of value in the diagnostic evaluation of minimal desaturation in the post operative and ambulatory patient.

THE UTILITY AND VALIDITY OF SUPRASTERNAL NOTCH (SSN) ECHOCARDIO-

GRAPHY IN CONGENITAL HEART DISEASE (CHD)

D. J. Sahn; H. D. Allen; S. J. Goldberg; T. Ovitt;
B. Goldberg
Department of Pediatrics and Radiology, University of
Arizona, Tucson and Episcopal Hospital, Philadelphia

Echocardiographic imaging of the transverse aortic arch (TAA) and right pulmonary artery (RPA) may be obtained from the SSN. Nevertheless, the quantitative accuracy and utility of this technique has not been assessed in children. Accordingly, the present study was designed to validate echocardiographic measurement of these structures, define normal values, and abnormal variations in patients with CHD. For 10 patients undergoing cardiac catheterization suprasternal notch echo-angiographic correlation for inner-diameter measurements produced correlation coefficients of 0.96 for the TAA and 0.95 for the RPA establishing the quantitative accuracy of echo visualization. Further, ultrasonic opacification by selective saline injection validated the identification of these vessels. Twenty normal newborns (aged 24-72 hours, weight 2-3.5 kg) were shown to have RPA = 0.90 ± 0.09 cm (SE), TAA 1.07 ± 0.07 cm and TAA/RPA ratio 1.16 ± 0.04. TAA/RPA ratio was not significantly different (1.21 ± 0.04) in 50 normal children aged 2 to 10 years but the ratio was increased in patients with catheterization proved Tetralogy 2.21 ± 0.3 ($p < 0.005$)(n=10) and in aortic stenosis 1.55 ± 0.18 ($p < 0.05$) (n=7). The Tetralogy patients had increased TAA and decreased RPA while the patients with aortic stenosis had post stenotic dilatation of the ascending aorta extending to the TAA. The ratio was decreased in patients with VSD, $1.07 \pm .07$ ($p < 0.05$)(n=16), ASD 1.01 ± 0.06 ($p < 0.05$)(n=13), and pulmonic stenosis is 0.94 ± 0.08 ($p < 0.005$) (n=8). Patients with left to right shunts had increased dimension of the RPA while those with pulmonic stenosis had post stenotic dilatation of the main pulmonary artery extending into the RPA. The specific utility of the technique was demonstrated in the differential of the diagnosis of mild pulmonic stenosis versus mild aortic stenosis which may be difficult both clinically and echocardiographicly. SSN echo was also useful as an adjunct to standard M-mode echocardiography in the evaluation of patients with pseudo-truncus arteriosus for Waterston shunt and in the diagnosis of the hypoplastic left heart syndrome. Thus, these reliable noninvasive measurements of TAA and RPA are of significant utility in the diagnosis and management of CHD in children and infants.

CORRELATION OF DIAGNOSTIC ECHOGRAPHIC FEATURES OF MITRAL STENOSIS

WITH FINDINGS AT CATHETERIZATION AND SURGERY

J. H. Horgan; V. E. Kemp; W. E. Holland; R. R. Lower;
L. Bosher; R. Centor; A. Goodman
Division of Cardiology
Medical College of Virginia, Richmond, Va. 23298

The accuracy of echocardiography (E) in predicting the degree of mitral stenosis (DMS), pliability of valve leaflets (P) and the presence of calcification (C) was prospectively tested by comparison with catheterization data and measurements at open commissurotomy in 26 patients. Echographic categorization of MS as severe (E-F slope $<$ 15 mm./sec.), moderate (15-25 mm./sec.), and mild (25-35 mm./sec.) was compared with mitral valve area calculated by Gorlin's formula (G) and measured by calibrated probes at surgery (S) (Severe: area $<$ 0.5 cms. sq. Moderate: 0.5-1.0 cms. sq. Mild: 1.0-1.5 cms. sq.) In 15 patients there was agreement between the echographic and surgical estimation of DMS. 11 patients were categorized by E as more stenosed than was found by S. 21 patients had valve areas calculated by G. In 6 patients there was agreement between E and G estimation of DMS. 13 were categorized by E as more stenosed than was found by G. 2 were more stenosed by G than E. In these 2 patients DMS by E and S were in agreement. The presence of low cardiac index, atrial fibrillation and mitral regurgitation did not significantly contribute to these relationships. Surgical assessment of impaired P was related to anterior mitral leaflet excursion (ALE) of $<$ 20 mm. and $<$ 15 mm. 10 of 14 considered to have impaired P had ALE $<$ 20 mm. 1 with pliable leaflets had ALE $<$ 20 mm. $P<.01$. No patients with normal P had ALE $<$ 15 mm. 4 of 14 with impaired P had ALE $<$ 15 mm. $P<.05$. C at surgery was detected at fluoroscopy in all but one case. ALE $<$ 20 mm. detected C in 5 of 9 cases and the absence of C in 11 of 17 cases $P>.32$. ALE $<$ 15 mm. detected C in 3 of 9 cases and the absence of C in 16 of 17 cases $P>.06$. The observation of increased density (D) of mitral echoes as an index of C detected 7 of 9 surgically calcified valves and 13 of 17 noncalcified valves $P<.01$. D detected 7 of 7 valves considered calcified at catheterization and 14 of 18 noncalcified valves $P <$ .001. These data suggest: 1) That DMS is overestimated by current criteria. 2) That ALE <20 mm. is a more sensitive indicator of impaired P than ALE <15 mm. 3) That increased D is an accurate indicator of the presence of C.

THE EFFECT OF TRANSDUCER PLACEMENT ON THE ECHOCARDIOGRAPHIC
PATTERN OF MITRAL VALVE PROLAPSE

W. Markiewicz; J. Stoner; S. Hunt; E. London; R. Popp

Cardiology Division

Stanford University Medical Center, Stanford, Ca. 94305

Specific patterns of mitral valve prolapse have been identified with echocardiography. The variability of presentation of these patterns within a single patient has been noted in our laboratory. In an attempt to clarify this variability, echocardiographic studies were carried out in 100 presumably normal females aged 18 to 35. Echocardiograms of the mitral valve were performed from the second, third, fourth, and fifth intercostal spaces and orientation of the transducer in each of these interspaces was noted. Subjects with no evidence of mitral valve prolapse show a flat or posterior systolic segment from the second intercostal space with caudal transducer direction. Perpendicular placement of the transducer in the third intercostal space shows a gradual anterior migration of the mitral valve during systole. Cephalad direction of the transducer from the fourth intercostal space or below shows a markedly anterior systolic segment of the mitral valve. This pattern is apparently related to descent of the mitral annulus towards the apex during ventricular contraction and the component of this motion registered along the path of the sound beam. The posterior motion of the mitral valve seen in mitral valve prolapse can be reliably recorded only when the transducer is perpendicular to the chest wall as caudal direction of the transducer gives false positive records and cephalad direction of the transducer gives false negative records. These findings have been incorporated into our analysis of patients with a clinical syndrome of mitral valve prolapse.

CROSS-SECTIONAL ECHOCARDIOGRAPHY IN EVALUATION OF PATIENTS WITH DISCRETE SUBVALVULAR AORTIC STENOSIS

A. E. Weyman; H. Feigenbaum; J. D. Dillon;
S. Chang
Department of Medicine
Indiana University, Indianapolis, Indiana 46202

Ten patients with discrete subvalvular aortic stenosis were examined using a real-time, high resolution, cross-sectional echocardiographic sector scanner. There were two patients with a thin discrete subvalvular membrane, group I; five patients with a more extensive area of subvalvular narrowing, group II; and three patients in whom a residual area of outflow tract obstruction remained following prior surgical revision, group III. In the two patients with a thin obstructive membrane, group I, two distinct linear echoes were observed in the outflow tract. These echoes were located immediately beneath the aortic valve, were not continuous with the walls of the outflow tract and showed some dynamic motion during the cardiac cycle. In four of five patients with diffuse outflow tract narrowing, group II, a relatively extensive area of inward bowing of both anterior and posterior margins of the outflow tract was noted. In the fifth case, a prominent localized, shelf like increase in thickness of the basal portion of the muscular septum along with a corresponding echo projecting anteriorly from the mid portion of the anterior mitral leaflet was present. The septal thickness in this case at the level of the free edge of the mitral valve, along with the septal posterior wall ratio was normal. In each of the three cases examined following surgical revision of the outflow tract, group III, a different pattern of outflow tract narrowing was observed. In each case, however, the presence of outflow tract narrowing itself was clearly demonstrated. This study suggests that cross-sectional echocardiogra offers an alternative and probably improved method for the non-invasi visualization of the left ventricular outflow tract.

THE COMPARATIVE UTILITIES OF REAL TIME CROSS-SECTIONAL ECHOCARDIOGRAPHIC IMAGING SYSTEMS IN COMPLEX CONGENITAL HEART DISEASE

D. J. Sahn; W. L. Henry; H. D. Allen; J. M. Griffith; S. J. Goldberg
Department of Pediatrics, Arizona Medical Center, Tucson, Cardiology Branch of the National Heart and Lung Institute, Bethesda

Of the currently available real time cross-sectional echocardiographic techniques, the multiple crystal system and the mechanical sector-scanner differ significantly with regards to the images produced. Their comparative utility for the diagnosis of congenital heart disease has yet to be evaluated simultaneously. Accordingly, the present study was designed to compare imaging characteristics and describe diagnostic criteria in 44 children (age 6 months-18 years) with known congenital heart disease who were studied with both systems. In 8 patients with "corrected" transposition, the multiple crystal system imaged a large area of cardiac anatomy in the transverse plane to demonstrate the abnormal septal orientation and side by side atrio ventricular valves while the sector-scanner allowed a detailed analysis of insertion of the mitral and tricuspid valves. Although the abnormal great artery orientation could be assessed by both systems, different diagnostic criteria were relied upon; with the sector-scanner, diagnosis was based on the absence of the normal spiraling pattern in the transverse plane while with the multiple crystal system the course and contour of the anteriorly placed aorta was used. The presence of dextrocardia (n=2) did not preclude these observations. Similiar observations of great artery relations were made in 6 patients with d-transposition and in 6 patients with single ventricle (2 with dextrocardia). In 4 patients with Ebstein's malformation, the leftward and inferior displacement of the septal leaflet of the tricuspid valve was identified by the multiple crystal system, whereas an abnormal insertion tricuspid leaflet was visualized by the sector-scanner. With the multiple crystal system, the changes of orientation and contour of mitral valve leaflets in the sagittal plane supplemented by transverse plane observations of leaflet orientation allowed the diagnosis of endocardial cushion defect in 8 patients, while the transverse plane visualization of the alignment of tricuspid and mitral valve insertion was the major diagnostic criteria identified by the sector-scanner. Both systems were equally insensitive to the visualization of ventricular septal defect or subtle abnormalities of the aortic valve and left ventricular outflow tract (12 patients). The large area of cardiac visualization obtained with the multicrystal system allowed rapid determination of positional relations of the atrio-ventricular valve and great artery orientation. In contrast, higher resolution visualization of smaller areas of the heart, such as details of atrio-ventricular valve insertion and great artery shape in the transverse plane provided the major diagnostic criteria for the sector-scanner. The two methods of ultrasonic cardiac imaging were complimentary. The sagittal and transverse plane images obtained rapidly with the multicrystal system were valuable indicators of areas for further study by the sector-scanner. Thus, the multicrystal and mechanical sector-scanner systems are synergistic in echocardiographic evaluation of alterations of cardiac anatomy in complex congenital heart disease.

SPECTRUM OF ECHOCARDIOGRAPHIC FINDINGS IN BACTERIAL ENDOCARDITIS

P. Roy; A. J. Tajik; E. R. Giuliani; T. T. Schattenberg;
G. T. Gau; R. L. Frye
Division of Cardiovascular Diseases and Internal
Medicine
Mayo Clinic and Mayo Foundation, Rochester, MN 55901

Forty-six echocardiograms were obtained from 32 patients with bacterial endocarditis (BE), using a commercially available, single probe instrument (Ekoline Model 20) interfaced on a strip chart recorder (Honeywell Model 1856 or Cambridge Multichannel Physiological Recorder). A 2.25-MHz, ½-inch-diameter, 5.0- or 7.5-cm focused transducer was used. The group included 23 males (72%) and 9 females (28%) with an average age of 53 years. Twenty-nine patients (91%) had active BE, whereas 3 were referred for valve replacement after successful medical treatment. All had endocarditis on natural valves. No patient was included whose clinical findings could be explained entirely by sustained bacteremia without cardiac involvement. Twenty-nine patients (91%) had consistently positive blood cultures and 29 (91%) had congestive heart failure. Fourteen patients (44%) had systemic embolic episodes. Nineteen patients (59%) had surgical interventions related to their BE: 5 had embolectomy and 14 had valve replacement. In two cases, autopsy was performed. The echocardiograms were interpreted without knowledge of surgical or autopsy findings. Correlation was good between echocardiographic and anatomic observations.

The spectrum of echocardiographic findings included three categories: (1) Preexistent abnormalities were seen in 13 patients (41%). Five of the 13 patients were initially thought to have BE on normal valves; in them echo showed mitral stenosis (1 patient), bicuspid aortic valve (AV) (2 patients), and prolapse of the mitral valve (MV) (2 patients). Echo confirmed clinically suspected preexistent abnormalities in eight other patients. Six of the 13 patients had MV prolapse but any or all of them could have been secondary to MV involvement by the BE process and not constitute a preexisting disorder. (2) Characteristic valvular vegetations (VG) (irregular shaggy thickening of leaflets or mass of fuzzy echoes) were seen in 28 patients (88%), on AV in 6, on MV in 9, and on both valves in 13. In 14 patients, echo findings were confirmed by surgery or autopsy. Fourteen patients had embolic episodes and all had VG on echo. (3) Abnormalities (other than VG) secondary to BE were commonly seen. Twenty-three patients (72%) showed increased septal and posterior wall excursion consistent with volume overload of the left ventricle (LVVO). Eight patients (25%) had a flail posterior mitral leaflet and two of these were confirmed surgically. Five patients (16%) had a coarse fluttering echo in the outflow tract of the left ventricle consistent with a prolapsing aortic cusp or aortic vegetation and two had surgical confirmation. Five patients (16%) had signs of severe aortic regurgitation (AR) of recent onset (premature MV closure) and all had surgical confirmation of severe AR. Echocardiographic abnormalities persisted after successful medical treatment.

We conclude that echocardiography is helpful in patients with BE: (1) it shows the characteristic vegetations; (2) it permits recognition of unsuspected preexistent lesions; and (3) it demonstrates the extent and nature of valvular damage secondary to BE and some of the pathophysiologic consequences (e.g., LVVO). However, it does not differentiate active diseases from healed vegetations. Our study does not permit precise definition of the sensitivity and specificity of the echo findings in BE.

ECHOCARDIOGRAPHIC FEATURES OF STRADDLING TRICUSPID VALVE

J. B. Seward; A. J. Tajik

Division of Cardiovascular Diseases and Internal Medicine
Mayo Clinic and Mayo Foundation, Rochester, MN 55901

The straddling or overriding tricuspid valve is an extremely rare cardiac anomaly in which the tricuspid valve straddles a large ventricular septal defect that opens partly into the morphologic right ventricle and partly into the morphologic left ventricle. The mitral valve opens directly into the morphologic left ventricle. Both the inflow (sinus) and outflow portions of the right ventricle can be recognized, and this feature allows the straddling tricuspid valve to be differentiated from type A common ventricle in which the sinus portion of the right ventricle is not formed. Angiographic differentiation of the straddling tricuspid valve from type A common ventricle (with outflow chamber) is difficult. The echocardiographic features of straddling tricuspid valve have not been previously described. We wish to present the salient echocardiographic features of four patients (ages 4 through 23 years) with proved straddling tricuspid valve.

M-mode echocardiograms were obtained with a Smith-Kline instrument (Ekoline 20 Ultrasonoscope) interfaced with a Honeywell or Cambridge multichannel strip chart recorder.

The echocardiographic features of straddling tricuspid valve included the following. When the sound beam was directed toward the basal aspect of the left ventricle, echoes of two atrioventricular valves could be simultaneously recorded without an intervening septal echo. As the transducer was tilted inferiorly and the sound beam was directed through the body of the left ventricle, a distinct ventricular septal echo could be recorded. The most distinctive feature of straddling tricuspid valve, however, was apparent on the continuous scan from base-to-apex of the left ventricle. The septal echo appeared at a level that corresponded to the midportion of the tricuspid valve echo, with the posterior tricuspid valve leaflet located posterior to the septal echo. This feature was noted in the echocardiogram of all four patients and is consistent with the straddling anatomic position of the tricuspid valve relative to the ventricular septum.

Using these echocardiographic features, we correctly predicted the presence of a straddling tricuspid valve in the last two patients of our series before confirmation by cardiac catheterization. Because common ventricle and tricuspid atresia are the two most frequent conditions with which straddling tricuspid valve is angiographically confused, the echocardiogram is of paramount importance in differentiating these entities. Moreover, since common ventricle at our institution has become amenable to complete anatomic repair, the distinction between common ventricle and straddling tricuspid valve has assumed greater importance because complete repair thus far has not been feasible in the latter condition.

DETECTION OF CONGENITAL VENTRICULAR DIVERTICULUM BY CROSS SECTIONAL ECHOCARDIOGRAPHY

E. S. Williams; A. E. Weyman; C. M. Estevez;
H. Feigenbaum
Department of Medicine
Indiana University School of Medicine
Indianapolis, Indiana   46202

This report describes a 47 year old white female with recurrent cerebral embolization in association with a 2 cm. diameter submitral valvular intramural ventricular diverticulum. There was no history of coronary artery disease, myocarditis, or chest trauma. The cardiovascular examination, electrocardiogram, and standard M-mode echocardiogram were normal. Tests for the presence of collagen-vascular and inflammatory disease were negative. Although the diverticulum was not visible on chest x-ray or fluoroscopy, it was readily demonstrable with real-time, cross-sectional echocardiography. Through the use of ultrasound we were able to define the location and extent of the diverticulum and record the effect of ventricular contraction on its configuration. Angiography, and subsequently surgery, confirmed the nature of the diverticulum and normalcy of adjacent myocardium and coronary arteries. At surgery, the diverticulum was found to have a wide ostium and its inner surface was continuous with the endocardium - as predicted by the echocardiogram. The walls and floors were smooth and white, and appeared to be composed of fibrous tissue.

While M-mode echocardiography satisfactorily evaluates ventricular motion and dimension, it does not allow adequate analysis of ventricular shape. This patient demonstrates a type of problem in which shape or contour is the critical problem and for which the mechanical sector scanner is better suited. In addition, the high line density (120 lines/frame) permitted precise localization of the diverticulum and suggested that its walls and floor were smooth.

This is an unusual case but further demonstrates the value

of cross-sectional echocardiography in the study of ventricular anatomy. In this instance, it provided the only non-invasive evidence suggestive of aneurysm or diverticulum.

EVALUATION OF LEFT VENTRICULAR APICAL ANEURYSMS BY CROSS SECTIONAL ECHOCARDIOGRAPHY

A.E. Weyman; H. Feigenbaum; J. C. Dillon;
S. Chang
Department of Medicine
Indiana University, Indianapolis, Indiana 46202

Shape and contraction pattern of the left ventricular apex were examined in 25 consecutive patients with angiographically demonstrated apical aneurysms and 15 normal subjects using a real-time high resolution mechanical sector scanner. Examinations were conducted with the probe placed directly over the left ventricular apex with the sweep of the scan parallel to the long axis of the left ventricle. In normal patients the anterior and posterior walls of the left ventricle tapered to a rounded tip. At the onset of systole the apical segment showed initial motion toward the base of the heart followed by an inward motion of the anterior and posterior wall. When endocardium and epicardium were recorded, systolic thickening of the walls of the apical segment was also observed. In patients with apical aneurysms the normal tapering of the ventricular apex was lost and the apex became rounded and dilated. In addition normal contraction toward the base of the heart was either absent or motion of the apical segment was in a direction opposite to the base of the heart. Recognition of apical aneurysms was facilitated by the observation of a hinge point seperating normal muscular contraction from the akinetic or dyskinetic segment. This hinge point was most frequently observed along the inferior surface of the heart. In addition to changes in contraction pattern, no endocardium could be recorded in the area of the ventricular aneurysm. In a number of cases the intensity of the echos from the aneurysmal segment was greater than that observed from normal endocardium or epicardium, suggesting the presence of scar tissue. This study suggests that cross - sectional echocardiography may provide a rapid and non-invasive means for determining the presence of apical aneurysms.

Echocardiography in Patients with Marfan's Syndrome and Their Asymptomatic Relatives

M.N. Payvandi; R.E. Kerber; F.M. Abboud

University of Iowa Hospitals

Iowa City, Iowa 52242

    The purpose of this study was to evaluate the frequency of cardiovascular abnormalities in patients with Marfan's syndrome and their asymptomatic relatives by use of echocardiography. We studied 6 patients with skeletal and opthalmologic evidence of Marfan's syndrome; 19 asymptomatic first degree relatives were also studied. All subjects underwent a complete history, physical exam, electrocardiogram, phonocardiogram and chest x-ray in addition to echocardiography.

    Echo evidence of mitral prolapse was present in all 6 of the Marfan's patients. Two of the 6 had palpitations, 5 of the 6 had systolic clicks and/or murmurs confirmed by phonocardiography, 3 of the 6 had EKG abnormalities and none had left atrial enlargement on chest x-ray or echo. Of the 19 asymptomatic relatives 8 had echo evidence of mitral valve prolapse, 3 of the 19 had clicks and/or murmurs, 3 of the 19 had EKG abnormalities, and none had left atrial enlargement.

    None of the Marfan's patients or their relatives had aortic insufficiency murmurs. Two of the six patients had dilated aortic roots on echo which were not apparant on chest x-ray. Five of the 19 relatives had dilated aortic roots on echo, but similarly none were apparant on chest x-ray.

    Conclusions: patients with Marfan's syndrome have a high incidence of mitral prolapse and aortic abnormalities. A large number of asymptomatic relatives of Marfan's patients have similar mitral and aortic abnormalities. Reliance on physical exam (i.e. clicks or murmurs) chest x-ray and EKG to detect these abnormalities may be misleading as many were apparant only on echo. Echocardiography should be used routinely in the assessment of patients with Marfan's syndrome and their first degree relatives.

Echocardiography in Wolff-Parkinson-White Syndrome.

M.S. Chandra; R.E. Kerber; D.D. Brown; D.C. Funk;
F.M. Abboud
University of Iowa and Veterans Administration
Hospitals
Iowa City, Iowa   52242

    Twenty-three patients with Wolff-Parkinson-White (WPW) syndrome were studied by echocardiography to assess interventricular septal motion and to detect associated cardiac abnormalities. All patients underwent physical examination, scalar electrocardiogram, Frank system vectorcardiogram, phonocardiogram and chest x-ray; 6 had cardiac catheterization.
    The patients were classified according to Boineau into the following WPW types: anterior right ventricular pre-excitation (Type I) - 6 patients, posterior right ventricular pre-excitation (Type II) - 5 patients, posterior left ventricular pre-excitation (Type III) - 12 patients. No patients with lateral left ventricular pre-excitation (Type IV) were encountered.
    Twenty patients were in WPW at the time of the echocardiographic study. Five patients had abnormal interventricular systolic septal motion: 3 type A (anterior in systole) septal motion and 2 type B (flat in systole) septal motion. All 5 of these patients had WPW Type I. All of the 15 Type II and Type III WPW patients had normal septal motion. Three patients were not in WPW during the study; 2 of them had abnormal IVS motion: 1, with Type A septal motion, had WPW Type II and the other, with Type B septal motion, had WPW Type III. This latter patient had an atrial septal defect. Two patients had intermittent WPW, Type II and III; in both septal motion remained within normal limits on WPW beats, although minor changes in motion were apparant. Associated cardiac abnormalities were evident in 6 patients: mitral valve leaflet prolapse (2 patients); hypertrophic obstructive cardiomyopathy (1 patient), congestive cardiomyopathy (1 patient), hypertrophic nonobstructive cardiomyopathy (1 patient), atrial septal defect (1 patient). The patient who had hypertrophic nonobstructive cardiomyopathy also had a calcified mitral annulus.

We conclude that abnormal interventricular septal motion is associated with the WPW abnormality and appears to be encountered primarily in Type I WPW. In addition, echo and other noninvasive diagnostic procedures reveal associated cardiac abnormalities in a high proportion of WPW patients and should be routinely performed.

ECHOCARDIOGRAPHIC INDOCYANINE GREEN (ICG) DYE FLOW PATTERNS IN
PATIENTS WITH TRUNCUS ARTERIOSUS (TA), TETRALOGY OF FALLOT (TF),
AND PULMONARY ATRESIA WITH VENTRICULAR SEPTAL DEFECT (PA)

A. J. Tajik; J. L. Assad-Morell; J. B. Seward;
D. J. Hagler; E. R. Giuliani; D. G. Ritter
Division of Cardiovascular Diseases and Internal
Medicine
Mayo Clinic and Mayo Foundation, Rochester, MN 55901

In 21 patients (pt)--8 with TA, 6 with TF, and 7 with PA--
echocardiograms were performed while injecting ICG dye during
cardiac catheterization. The concentration and amount of dye
injected and the technique of injection have been previously
detailed. In each patient, three to five injections of dye were
recorded and the flow patterns were analyzed. The usual sites of
injection of the dye were the superior and the inferior vena cava,
right ventricle, and aortic or truncal root.

After the caval injection of dye, a cloud of echoes first
appeared in the right ventricle during diastole and outlined the
right ventricular cavity. During subsequent systole, no echoes
appeared in the left ventricle; instead, the cloud of echoes was
seen in the left ventricle during the early diastolic phase of the
subsequent cardiac cycle. These echoes appeared anterior to the
mitral valve (left ventricular outflow tract) and the mitral valve
funnel remained echo-free. Further elucidation of the phase of
the cardiac cycle during which this intracardiac right-to-left
shunt occurred was obtained with use of simultaneous phonoecho-
cardiography in conjunction with ICG dye injection. This approach
clearly revealed that this right-to-left shunt at ventricular
level commenced after the aortic closure and prior to opening of
the mitral valve, representing the isovolumic relaxation phase of
the cardiac cycle.

In all three conditions, similar dye flow patterns were
recorded when dye was injected in the superior and the inferior
vena cava, except for six patients (three with TA and three with
TF) in whom the caval injection of dye produced a different type
of flow pattern. In these patients, the cloud of echoes appeared

simultaneously in both right and left ventricular chambers during diastole; however, unlike the above described pattern of diastolic right-to-left shunting at ventricular level, in these six patients the cloud of echoes appeared in the left ventricular chamber after opening of the mitral valve, posterior to the anterior mitral valve leaflet and filled the mitral valve funnel. This type of flow pattern was indicative of a right-to-left shunt at the atrial level in these entities. Despite the fact that such a defect could not be demonstrated during cardiac catheterization, an interatrial communication was found in all patients at subsequent operation.

A selective right ventricular injection of ICG dye revealed the simultaneous appearance of a cloud of echoes in the left ventricle in all three conditions. Truncal valve incompetence was assessed by supravalvular injection of dye in five patients. In four of the five, a cloud of echoes appeared in both ventricular chambers (R>L) during diastole, indicating a preferential regurgitant flow into the right ventricle and confirming previously observed angiocardiographic findings.

Our studies have proved helpful in detection of associated atrial septal defect and have provided a better insight into the physiology of intracardiac right-to-left shunt flow dynamics.

QUANTIFICATION AND PROGNOSIS OF ACUTE MYOCARDIAL INFARCTION:
COMPARISON OF ECHOCARDIOGRAPHIC AND CATHETERIZATION INDICES

A. DeMaria; J. Angel; E. Amsterdam; D. Mason

Section of Cardiovascular Medicine
University of California, Davis, Calif. 95616

Stroke work index (SWI), obtained by right heart catheterization as the product of stroke index (SI), and the difference of mean arterial blood pressure (BP) and mean pulmonary artery wedge pressure (PAW) SWI=SI(BPxPAW)1.36 has been demonstrated to accurately reflect the extent and prognosis of acute myocardial infarction. Echocardiography provides an atraumatic technique by which many parameters of cardiac function may be assessed. Therefore we attempted to utilize echocardiography to construct an index of ventricular performance of quantitative and prognostic value. Echocardiography and right heart catheterization were performed simultaneously in 38 patients within 36 hours (average 12 hours) of acute myocardial infarction. The patient population consisted of 31 males and 7 females with a mean age of 60. Echoes were performed in a standard fashion with a commercially available ultrasonoscope while right heart catheterization was performed using a Swan-Ganz catheter. 10 patients suffered pump failure and death following infarction and were classified as non-survivors (NS) while 28 patients survived (S) the infarction. Clinical data, including chest x-ray and physical examination could not distinguish NS from S. SWI, determined by catheterization was markedly reduced in NS 10.5 as compared with survivors 33.3 ($p<.001$). No separation could be found between NS and S in echographic stroke volume and cardiac output, although echo end diastolic dimension (EDD) was greater 6.4 to 5.2, ejection fraction (EF) (EdD-EsD/EdD) less 35 to 55% and VCF less 0.71 to 0.96 in NS (all $p<.01$). Subsequently a non-invasive index was formulated (NI) as NI=EF (BP/EdD) where EF and EdD were obtained by echo and BP by cuff sphymomanometer. NI correlated very well with SWI ($r=0.83$, $p<.001$) and was markedly reduced in NS (18.1) as compared with S (44.6 $p<.001$). Moreover only 1 NS had an NI of above 22 whereas only 1 S had NI below this value (p<.001). Thus, echocardiography may be employed to calculate an index of ventricular performance in patients with myocardial infarction which correlates well with that obtained by cardiac catheterization. This non-invasive index provides a sensitive method to assess the prognosis in infarction patients.

RIGHT VENTRICULAR COMPRESSION: A RELIABLE ECHOCARDIOGRAPHIC

SIGN OF CARDIAC TAMPONADE

N.B. Schiller, E. Botvinick

Department of Medicine - Division of Cardiology

University of California, San Francisco, CA

Early canine studies of the hemodynamics of cardiac tamponade predicted compression of the thin-walled right ventricle. In over 2,000 echocardiograms performed in our institution, pericardial effusion was identified in 172, collected prospectively over a 30 month period. Of these, 15 (8.7%) showed compression of the right ventricle when measured in the left ventricular minor axis. Compression was defined as contact of the right ventricle and septum during all or part of the cardiac cycle or as maximal narrowing of the right ventricle to 1.0 cm or less. All 15 patients had large effusions.

Fourteen of the 15 patients with compression had or subsequently developed frank tamponade and underwent pericardiocentesis. One with equivocal clinical findings is currently being followed. Echocardiograms were obtained in 10 patients pre and post tap. Simultaneous hemodynamic and echocardiographic data was obtained pre and post pericardiocentesis in 5 of these patients. In all 5, removal of a small amount of pericardial fluid (100 cc or less) was associated with immediate reversal of the clinical and hemodynamic abnormalities and of the echocardiographically demonstrated right ventricular compression. Identical echocardiographic changes were observed in the other 5 tamponade patients studied post pericardiocentesis and all patients improved clinically following fluid removal. One patient in this group was particularly noteworthy in that compression was present despite pulmonary hypertension. His pulmonary artery systolic pressure was 60 mm Hg pretap and rose to 95 mm Hg post tap concurrent with a dramatic expansion of the right ventricle (1.0 to 3.1 cm). We have seen no patient with tamponade in whom right ventricular compression was absent. In three of our 15 patients, tamponade, not initially obvious, became clinically evident within four weeks of the observation of right ventricular compression. In 4 patients presenting with a benign effusion, serial echocardiographic examination revealed progressive right ventricular compression and pericardial fluid accumulation as clinically apparent tamponade developed.

While compression was the most reliable sign of tamponade in our 14 patients, other echocardiographic findings were often found to accompany it. These findings were: decreased left ventricular minor axis diastolic diameter (mean 4.0 cm with a normal value of 4.3 - 5.5 cm in our laboratory; decreased right ventricular diameter at the level of the aortic root (mean 2.9 cm with our normal value 3.5 - 5.0 cm); and swinging heart (parallel motion of the anterior and posterior cardiac walls) in 6 of 14 patients. In all patients with "swinging", a form of electrical alternans was present on simultaneous ECG. However, we have seen patients with effusion with each of these findings who were not in tampoade.

We conclude that in the setting of a large and progressively increasing pericardial effusion the echocardiographic demonstration of minor axis right ventricular compression is a sensitive (94%) and specific (100%) sign of frank or impending cardiac tamponade.

PRE- AND POSTOPERATIVE ECHOGRAPHIC INVESTIGATION OF LEFT

VENTRICULAR FUNCTION IN AORTIC STENOSIS (AS)

Richard A. Meyer; Joan Korfhagen; Gregory L. Johnson;
Samuel Kaplan
Department of Cardiology

Children's Hospital, Cincinnati, Ohio   45229

The purpose of this study was to serially evaluate non-invasively the results of surgery upon left ventricular function in children with significant AS. Six groups of patients were evaluated: aortic stenosis -36 (age 7-19 years), coarctation of the aorta 17 (age 2-17 years), patent ductus arteriosus (PDA) 8 (age 6 mos-13 years), valvar pulmonic stenosis (PS) 7 (age 2-9 years), tetralogy of Fallot (TOF) -16 (1-13 years) and ventricular septal defect (VSD) 7 (1-10 years).

The following parameters of left ventricular function were evaluated with ultrasound: shortening fraction which is percent shortening of the left ventricular internal dimension during contraction (SF); velocity of circumferential fiber shortening (Vcf), stroke volume (SV), ejection fraction (EF) and systolic time intervals (STI) of the left ventricle. All examinations were performed using a Hoffrel ultrasonoscope which has a peak power output of $5W/cm^2$.

Preoperatively, all patients with significant AS (gradients greater than 50 mm Hg) demonstrated shortening fractions greater than 40% (range 41%-60%; mean 47%); whereas, patients with gradients of 50 mm Hg or less had high normal SF (36%-40%). Of the 56 patients in the other groups studied, only four had shortening fractions of greater than 40% (range 22%-43%). The rest had normal SF (mean 32%). In addition, the patients with significant AS had decreased left ventricular end diastolic volumes and stroke volumes for age and size. Prolongation of the left ventricular ejection time occurred only in patients with severe obstructions (gradients + 60 mm Hg).

Vcf, SV, and STI were not helpful in distinguishing mild AS from the other groups of patients nor did they show any consistency for the patients with AS. Therefore, only SF was evaluated following surgery.

Post-operatively, patients who were evaluated serially fell into two groups: those with residual gradients (measured on the operating table) of 20 mm Hg or less and those with gradients of 25 mm Hg or greater. Those with insignificant gradients had normal or slightly decreased SF as well as decreased SV within the first 12 months following surgery. The patients with residual gradients of 35 mm Hg or greater (35-75 mm Hg) had mean SF of 54% (47-63%) within the first month after surgery. At 9 months following surgery, the mean SF was 45% (41-49%) and one patient had a SF of 49% at 5 years post-op.

This study has demonstrated that a SF of greater than 40% is strongly suggestive of AS, since the SF in other cardiac lesions rarely exceeded 40%. In addition, it is possible to separate patients with valvular gradients of greater or less than 50 mm Hg. Further, if patients have residual gradients of 35 mm Hg or higher following surgery, their SF remain persistently high; whereas, those with gradients less than 20 mm Hg had normal SF. Thus, with the use of echocardiography, it is possible for the clinician to follow the clinical course of valvular AS and to obviate the need for serial cardiac catheterization in these patients as well as to follow the post-operative course of these patients.

LEFT VENTRICULAR VOLUME DETERMINATIONS OF CANINE MODELS

Olaf T. von Ramm; David R. Cannon; Joseph A. Kisslo

Departments of Medicine and Biomedical Engineering

Duke University, Durham, N.C.   27710

Current techniques of left ventricular performance assessment involve angiographic determinations of ventricular volumes. Echocardiography offers an alternative non-invasive means of determining these volumes. However, current one dimensional techniques, ie.time-motion (T-M) methods, are inherently limited in accuracy because of uncertainties in determining the orientation of the interrogating ultrasonic beam in relation to the spatial geometries of the ventricle. The high resolution, real time, two-dimensional ultrasound imaging system, known as Thaumascan, was utilized in determining left ventricular volumes of canine models in vitro to ascertain this system's capabilities in volumetric determinations.

Freshly excised canine hearts were prepared by clamping the aorta and occluding the mitral orifice in an effort to eliminate leakage from the filled left ventricle. A mixture of water and Renografin radio opaque dye was then injected into the left ventricular cavity and the preparation suspended in a water tank. The preparation was then scanned with the Thaumascan imaging system to produce long axis images of the ventricle in two orthogonal planes. At the completion of the echo examination, biplane cinefluoroscopic images of the preparation were taken. Finally, the ventricle was drained and the volume of the liquid measured. Echo and angiographic volumes were calculated by means of the area length method.

For the seventeen canine hearts in this study, the correlation coefficient for the drained fluid versus echo volumes was .94 whereas a value of .96 was determined for the drained fluid versus angiographic volumes. In this experiment the correlation coefficient of echo versus angiographic volumes was .91.

Although good agreement between echo and measured volumes was obtained, it is not possible, in general, to obtain two orthogonal long axis views in humans. However, a correlation coefficient of .92 with the drained fluid volume was obtained by using only one long axis view to compute the ventricular volume and, at this time, it seems reasonable that it may be possible to determine left ventricular volumes in humans utilizing this two dimensional ultrasound imaging system.

ROLE OF ECHOCARDIOGRAPHY IN THE ASSESSMENT OF LEFT VENTRICULAR

FUNCTION IN PATIENTS WITH CORONARY ARTERY DISEASE

P. Chandraratna, M.D., A. Rashid, M.D., A. Tolentino, M.D.,
F. Hildner, M.D., A. Fester, M.D., B.B. Littman, M.D.

Division of Cardiology, Mount Sinai Medical Center
Miami Beach, Florida

The usefulness of echocardiography in the detection of wall motion abnormalities in patients with coronary artery disease has been demonstrated by several workers. This investigation was designed to determine the role of echocardiography in the assessment of left ventricular function in patients with significant narrowing of their coronary arteries. A recent report stated that patients who have a low left ventricular ejection fraction have a significantly higher mortality following aorto-coronary bypass graft surgery. Hence the ability to predict a poor ejection fraction by a non-invasive technique is of great prognostic importance. Echocardiography was performed on 42 patients with coronary artery disease. The only criterion for selection was a technically satisfactory echocardiogram. Left ventricular dimensions and wall motion were measured at a point just caudal to the mitral valve. The echocardiographic left ventricular end diastolic dimension (LVED) was increased above the upper limits of normal for our laboratory (>5.4 cm) in 16 patients. Fifteen of these patients had an angiographically measured ejection fraction of 0.45 or less. Three patients had a normal left ventricular end diastolic dimension i.e. <5.4 cm but ejection fractions of <0.45. Twenty two patients had ejection fractions of >0.45 and normal LVED. Two patients had a LVED >5.4 cm with an ejection fraction of >0.45. The left ventricular end diastolic dimension index (LVEDI) was increased (>3 cm/M^2) in 14 patients all of whom had ejection fractions of <0.45. Three patients had a normal LVEDI with an ejection fraction of <0.45. Twenty five patients had a LVEDI of 3 cm/M^2 or less and an ejection fraction of >0.45. The excursion of the interventricular septum was diminished in 13 patients, all of whom had significant stenosis of the left anterior descending coronary artery. The excursion of the left ventricular posterior wall was decreased (<0.9 cm) in 11 patients. In summary, increase of the left ventricular end diastolic dimension or the LVED index is usually associated with a critical reduction of the ejection fraction. Since the ejection fraction is an important determinant of mortality related to aorto-coronary saphenous vein graft surgery, echocardiography should play a useful role in the detection of patients with a poor prognosis.

EFFECTS OF SODIUM NITROPRUSSIDE ON LEFT VENTRICULAR SIZE AND
PERFORMANCE IN MYOCARDIAL INFARCTION DETERMINED BY ULTRASOUND

J. Angel; A. DeMaria, E. Amsterdam; A. Neumann;
R. Miller, D. Mason
Section of Cardiovascular Medicine
University of California, Davis, California 95616

Sodium nitroprusside, a peripheral arteriolar and venous vasodilator, has been extensively applied in the treatment of congestive heart failure accompanying acute myocardial infarction. Although nitroprusside has been documented to reduce left ventricular volume by cineangiography in patients with chronic congestive heart failure secondary to coronary artery disease, no data is available regarding left ventricular volume changes induced by nitroprusside in acute myocardial infarction patients. Therefore we evaluated the effects of nitroprusside upon intracavitary left ventricular size and cardiac performance by echocardiography in 10 acute myocardial infarction patients, and compared these results to data obtained by simultaneous right heart catheterization. Echocardiographic scans were obtained in a standard fashion with a commercially available echograph with patients in the 10° total body tilt position, and catheterization was performed utilizing a Swan-Ganz catheter. Nitroprusside infusion (30-200 micrograms/minute) produced a fall for the group of patients in mean pulmonary wedge pressure (20-13 mm Hg $p<.01$) and a reduction in mean systemic blood pressure (90 to 80 mm Hg, $p<.01$), but did not alter heart rate (98.9) or either cardiac output (4.1) or stroke index (26.1) obtained by dye dilution techniques. Cardiac output and stroke index obtained by echocardiography were also unaltered by nitroprusside. Nitroprusside produced a fall in echocardiographically determined end diastolic dimension (5.99→5.64cm, $p<.01$), and end systolic dimension (4.97→4.44cm, $p<.01$), and a concomitant increase in ejection fraction ($\Delta D/EdD$) (41-51%, $p<.01$) and mean fiber shortening velocity (EdD-EsD/ET·EdD) (0.82 to 1.05 circumferences/second, $p<.05$). Attempts to relate reduction in pulmonary wedge pressure to decrease in end diastolic dimension yielded a correlation coefficient of only

0.61. Thus, this echocardiographic data indicates that the peripheral vasodilator effects of nitroprusside reduce left ventricular end diastolic dimension, while augmenting cardiac performance by increasing left ventricular ejection fraction and mean fiber shortening velocity in the setting of acute myocardial infarction.

ECHOCARDIOGRAPHIC AND ULTRASONO-TOMOGRAPHIC STUDY OF THE LEFT VENTRICULAR DYNAMICS IN LBBB

J. FUJII, H. WATANABE, T. WATANABE, N. TAKAHASHI, A. OHTA, K. KATO

The Cardiovascular Institute
8-1-22, Akasaka, Minato-ku, Tokyo

Echocardiogram and ultrasono-cardiotomogram(UCTG) of 21 patients with complete LBBB were compared with those of 5 with right ventricular pacing, 7 with PVC induced by catheter tip in right ventricle(RV), 40 with myocardial infarction and 20 normal subjects. Cross sections were made through the long axis of the left ventricle at end-diastole, early systole and end-systole, respectively.

There were delayed onset of posterior wall contraction and three types of abnormal septal motions(type A, B, C) in patients with LBBB. In type A and B, early and abrupt posterior-directed motion of the septum occured during pre-ejection period. This abnormal motion was remarkable at the upper part of the septum in some cases and at the middle part of the septum in the others. Following this early posterior directed motion, the septum moves anteriorly with the delayed onset of left ventricular contraction in type A. This paradoxical septal movement was not remarkable in type B. Type C exhibits almost flat septal motion. All patients with RV pacing and PVC of RV origin showed abnormal septal motion of type A or B. Abnormal septal and posterior wall echograms in type A and B can be explained by asynchronous contraction of the left ventricle, with early activation of the right side of the septum but delay in activation and contraction of the left ventricular free wall. The septal motion of type C is almost the same as that of septal infarction. Moreover, most of these cases have ECG and VCG findings indicating massive septal infarction, such as Q in I, V_{5-6}, or QS in V_{1-3}, and initial vector directing right anteriorly or left posteriorly. These findings suggest that type C shows the massive septal infarction complicated with LBBB.

Echocardiography and ultrasono-tomography are considered to be useful in evaluating abnormal contraction of the left ventricle and diagnosing myocardial infarction with LBBB.

THE EFFECT OF PHASIC RESPIRATION AND ATRIAL SYSTOLE ON THE
ECHOCARDIOGRAPHIC DETERMINATION OF LEFT VENTRICULAR FUNCTION

J. I. Brenner and R. A. Waugh

Departments of Pediatrics and Medicine
National Naval Medical Center
Bethesda, Maryland 20014

Introduction. Echocardiography is an established technique for evaluating left ventricular (LV) function with numerous studies showing an excellent correlation between echocardiographic and cineangiographic dimensions in patients without regional dyskinesia. There are several explanations for some of the minor discrepancies that exist, and it is the purpose of this investigation to systematically analyze the variable effects of respiration and the point selected as "end diastole" on echocardiographic LV dimensions.

Materials and Methods. A standard echocardiographic evaluation of 20 subjects ranging in age from 12 to 40 years with no evidence of cardiovascular disease was obtained utilizing a commercially available Ekoline 20 ultrasonoscope and Smith-Kline-French 2.25 MegaHerz transducers focused at 5 and 10 cm. All recordings of LV function were made with the transducer at an approximate right angle to the plane of the chest wall in the third, fourth or fifth left intercostal space adjacent to the sternum. The echocardiographic beam was directed inferolaterally beneath the mitral valve and optimum definition of the septal and posterior left ventricular wall endocardial surfaces was obtained. Recordings, which included an ECG and respirometer, were made using an E for M DR-8 recorder at a paper speed of 50 mm per second. Left ventricular diastolic dimensions (LVDD) were measured at both the peak of the R wave ($LVDD_R$) as well as at the maximal separation of the septal and posterior left ventricular wall endocardial echos ($LVDD_{max}$). Systolic dimensions were measured on a vertical axis at the peak anterior movement of the posterior left ventricular wall. For each subject, three respiratory cycles were measured at peak expiration and peak inspiration and the beat to beat variation in heart rate noted. Subjects with a pronounced sinus arrhythmia were excluded. Left ventricular volumes were calculated using the formula of Teicholtz, et al., wherein:

$$\text{Volume} = \frac{7}{2.4 + \text{LV Dimension}} \times (\text{LV Dimension})^3$$

Results. In 8 of 20 patients, the LVDD_{max} was greater by 2 mm or more than the LVDD_R. These variations ranged from 2 to 5 mm with a commensurate variation in the calculated volumes. In 12 of 20 patients, there was a phasic inspiratory decrease in the diastolic left ventricular dimension which averaged 6%. Depending on the absolute chamber dimension, this respiratory variation accounted for up to a 30 cc. variation in the calculated stroke volume. The ejection fraction and systolic dimension did not vary consistently with respiration. For those subjects with a larger LVDD_{max}, the ejection fraction was, of course, greater when this dimension was used to calculate volumes in comparison to the LVDD_R.

Discussion. These data show that within this group of normal subjects, variations in the point selected as end diastole and phasic respiratory changes are two potential sources of discrepancies in correlative echocardiographic left ventricular dimension studies. The variation in "end diastolic" dimension relates at least in part to the timing of the atrial contribution to ventricular filling. This late diastolic increase in the LVDD frequently preceeds the beginning of the QRS complex and is absent in atrial fibrillation. With shorter PR intervals, this increase in LVDD may follow the R wave peak and thus contribute to a difference in the LVDD_{max} as compared to the LVDD_R. The significance of the respiratory variation in LVDD's is unknown but the well documented inspiratory decrease in left ventricular filling is a possible physiologic correlate. A respiratory variation in the position of the entire heart relative to the echocardiographic beam is another possible factor. The relatively constant ejection fraction may relate to the excellent cineangiographic-echocardiographic correlations reported in the literature. Given that these variations in LVDD exist in a normal population, then an even more cogent question relates to whether or not changes of a similar or even greater magnitude might exist in various cardiovascular pathological conditions.

ECHOCARDIOGRAPHIC (ECHO) METHOD OF SCINTILLATION PROBE PLACEMENT FOR RADIOCARDIOGRAPHIC ASSESSMENT (RCG) OF LEFT VENTRICULAR EJECTION FRACTION (LVEF)

N. Kallos; A. R. Ghahramani; M. Groch, A. Miale, Jr.; S. Gottlieb
University of Miami, Miami, FL., and Searle Radiographics, Inc., Des Plaines, Ill.

Measurement of LVEF can be accomplished with a scintillation probe and an intravenous bolus of radiotracer. A newly developed scintillation probe system permits a major improvement in this technique by simultaneously recording the high frequency count variations which occur as a result of left ventricular volume changes in systole and diastole along with the non-left ventricular background activity. The accuracy of the method depends on precise positioning of the detector over the left ventricle (LV). The conventional method for probe placement utilizing portable chest radiographs usually requires 30 to 45 minutes. A rapid bedside method for probe placement over the midpoint of the LV utilizing echocardiography has been proposed and is being tested. This technique involves a modification of conventional T-scanning. The largest internal dimension of the LV is established by manipulation of the sound beam perpendicular to the long axis immediately inferior to the mitral valve leaflets. The transducer is then translocated inferiorly along the anterior chest wall in the long axis until the sound beam is approximately perpendicular to the posterior LV wall immediately inferior to the mitral leaflets. A mark is then placed on the chest wall at the point of contact with the transducer for probe placement. Comparison of echocardiographic (ECHO) with fluoroscopic localization of the LV midpoint showed a difference of no greater than 12mm in 12 patients. There was a correlation coefficient of 0.98 when LVEF was measured after probe placement by both techniques. LVEF measurements after repetitive ECHO placements were highly reproducible with a correlation coefficient of 0.98. In 25 patients with coronary artery disease, the radiotracer method was compared to LVEF obtained by cineangiocardiogram and found to correlate at the 0.92 level. The time required for probe placement by ECHO was 2 to 6 minutes, thereby facilitating clinical application of the procedure. The ECHO placement and radiotracer study can be performed at the bedside in 10 to 15 minutes.

MEDIUM FOR EXTERNAL ACOUSTIC TRANSMISSION

H. D. Allen; S. J. Goldberg; D. J. Sahn; W. L. Henry;
J. M. Griffith
Department of Pediatrics, Arizona Medical Center, Tucson
Cardiology Branch of the National Heart and Lung Institute
Bethesda

The transducer-skin interface artifact makes single crystal, sector-scanner and multicrystal echocardiographic assessment of anterior cardiac structures technically more difficult than posterior structure evaluation. Furthermore, because of transducer fulcrum effect (pie wedge), relatively less area of the anterior heart can be evaluated with standard single crystal echocardiography during a sweep or with use of sector-scanners. In smaller children, further problems exist with two dimensional instruments. These include the sector-scanner transducer vibrations which might frighten children and loss of transducer-skin contact with small degrees of transducer angulation from multicrystal instruments.

A substance inserted between the transducer and skin should be non-toxic, pliable yet not easily deformed, easily available, inexpensive, and capable of transmitting sound at the same speed as tissue.

We tested a number of substances for these qualities. Quantitation of the three types of echo - single crystal, sector-scanner and multicrystal - was evaluated with a test block with and without substance insertion. Measurements were compared and were equal with one medium.

Standard single crystal echocardiograms were performed on 6 children. Echocardiography was then repeated with a medium inserted between the transducer and skin. Coupling was accomplished with standard acoustic transmitting gel. Echocardiographic measurements with and without one substance were identical. Anterior cardiac structures were frequently better seen and more anterior area could be assessed by single crystal and sector-scanner techniques by use of the medium. Examinations were quickly and easily performed. Vibrations from the moving transducer of the sector-scanner instrument were damped. Angulation of the large multicrystal transducer was easier.

The major disadvantage of using this medium was a "reflection" - a thin non-moving band of echoes, presumably from the medium which was usually seen in the right ventricular cavity. This posed no problems with qualitative or quantitative assessment.

Thus, a practical, safe, inexpensive and useful means for improving and simplyfing echocardiography can be gained by use of this medium for external acoustic transmission.

Abdominal

DIFFERENTIAL DIAGNOSIS OF ECHO-FREE RENAL MASSES

William M. Green, M.D., Donald L. King, M.D.
William J. Casarella, M. D.

Department of Radiology
The Presbyterian Hospital & The College
of Physicians and Surgeons
Columbia University
New York, N. Y. 10032

The clinical value of the ultrasonic examination of renal masses is well established. Use of ultrasound scanning to distinguish renal cysts from solid tumors has been described by many authors [1-5] and is the most frequent use of renal sonography. Since most cystic lesions are benign and since solid masses large enough to be clinically apparent are often malignant, the usefulness of the technique has been to distinguish between these two general groups. The accuracy of differentiating between cystic and solid renal masses has been reported to range from 75-96% [3-7].

The ultrasonic diagnosis of a simple cyst rests on three basic criteria: 1) the mass must be completely devoid of internal structure (echo free); 2) it must have smooth, sharply-defined margins, and, 3) there must be strong through-transmission with build up of sound energy from the far wall as demonstrated by a dense echo pattern [8-10]. If all these criteria are not met, the lesion should not be considered a simple cyst and warrants further study.

Complex or solid renal masses while classically associated with tumors have been described for a variety of benign and malignant entities. Despite occasional previous caveats, the tacit assumption in renal ultrasound heretofore has been that sonolucent masses are simple cysts. Although this is true in the vast majority of cases, recent experience with echo free renal masses suggests that a more sophisticated approach to their diagnosis is warranted.

RESULTS

This report is based on two hundred forty seven consecutive renal sonograms performed in the past twenty months. Out of one hundred forty three echo free renal masses, fourteen were not simple renal cysts. The majority of these did, however, meet all the ultrasonic criteria for cysts. Four of these fourteen cases demonstrated various aspects of hydronephrosis. There were four inflammatory masses, four malignant neoplasms, one renal artery aneurysm and one patient with a coincident cyst and tumor.

The following examples demonstrate patients with obstructive uropathy.

Illustrative Cases: A 16 year old boy who had had multiple operative procedures for exstrophy of the bladder and had had a pyelo-ileal conduit was scanned. A round, central echo free mass meeting all the criteria for a renal cyst was identified (Figure 1). His urogram and ileal conduit exam revealed obstruction at the anastomosis. The echo free renal mass in this case was produced by the obstructed, dilated renal pelvis.

A 16 year old girl with fever, CVA tenderness and a left upper pole mass on urography was examined. The sonogram demonstrated an echo free mass fulfilling all the criteria for a renal cyst. Final diagnosis was an obstructed upper

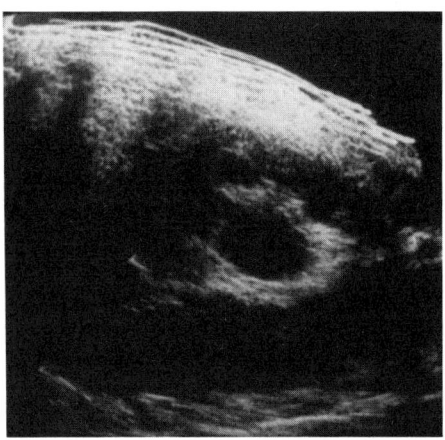 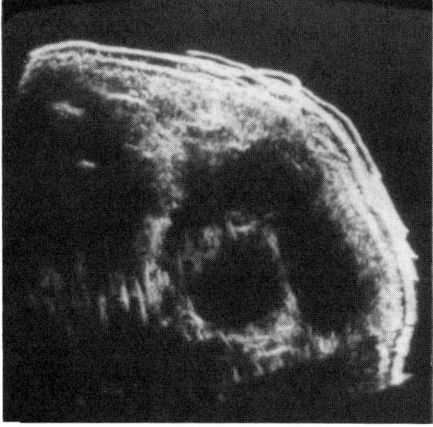

Figure 1A and B. Longitudinal and transverse scans in a 16 year old boy with an obstructed pyelo-ileal conduit. The echo free mass represents the dilated renal pelvis.

pole collecting system of a partial renal duplication.

Comment: Various stages of hydronephrosis, from a dilated renal pelvis to the functionless sac of end-stage obstruction will of course demonstrate sonolucent renal masses. The amount of remaining renal cortex and the surrounding dilated calyces should assist in suggesting the correct diagnosis on sonography. Close attention to the delayed films of intravenous urography will usually be confirmatory. However, since this is not always true, hydronephrosis should be included in the differential diagnosis of echo free renal masses.

Four patients with echo free renal masses had inflammatory lesions, three were abscesses and the fourth a xanthogranuloma. Again an abscess is not always a diagnostic problem, and we should not be surprised that it may mimic a cyst ultrasonically.

Illustrative Cases: A 20 year old man and a 3 year old girl each had fever, flank pain, and a renal mass on IVP. Both were felt clinically to have renal abscesses. The ultrasound examination demonstrated echo free masses, but in the young man it was not completely round and smooth on transverse sections (Figure 2). Angiography showed fine neovascularity in both patients and both had renal abscesses at surgery.

Comment: The two young patients were not in the appropriate age group for renal cysts. The clinical and radiographic workup suggested abscess, and although the masses were echo free they were suspicious because they did not strictly meet all the criteria for renal cysts. These discrepancies led to further evaluation and correct diagnosis.

Illustrative Case: A 44 year old man with a nine month history of fever and weight loss and a twelve centimeter renal mass was studied ultrasonically. The mass was completely echo free, round and smooth and met all the criteria for a renal cyst and was so diagnosed. However, nephrotomography yielded a thick walled mass. Because of this discrepancy and the clinical expectation of a tumor, angiography was performed. A large neovascular mass was shown which strongly suggested a malignant neoplasm. At surgery the mass was also thought to be a malignancy. However the pathology was xanthogranulomatous pyelonephritis.

Comment: Discrepancy between ultrasonic, nephrotomographic and clinical study led to angiography and subsequently to surgery. Thus, despite the incorrect ultrasonic impression of a cyst,

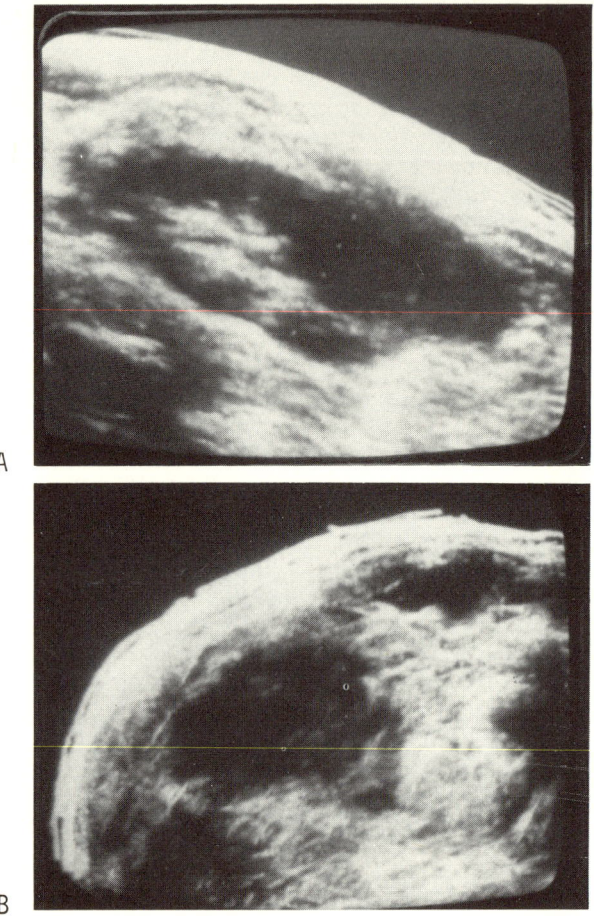

Figure 2A and B. Longitudinal and transverse scans of a 20 year old man with a renal abscess. The scans demonstrated an echo free mass in the lower pole which is somewhat irregular.

the correct diagnosis was made. The specimen was indeed a relatively cystic mass filled with mucoid debris, which apparently was too homogeneous to produce echoes on the sonogram.

Four malignant neoplasms appeared sonolucent on ultrasound examinations.

Illustrative Cases: An otherwise healthy 43 year old man with left flank pain and hematuria had a left lower pole mass on urography. The mass was echo free, but its borders were irregular (Figure 3). Therefore angiography was performed demonstrating a hypovascular mass which was poorly

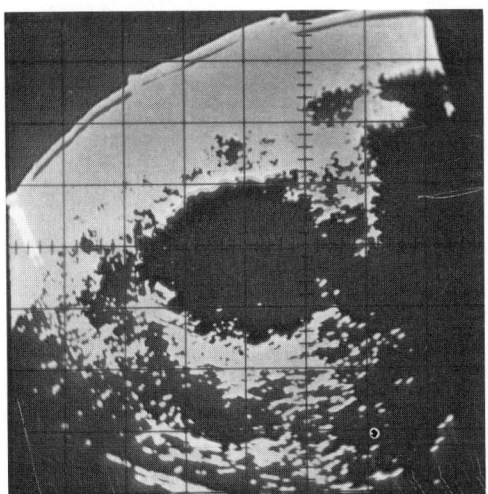

Figure 3. Transverse scan of an echo free lower pole renal mass which was a malignant melanoma.

demarcated from the surrounding cortex. Nephrectomy revealed malignant melanoma. No primary was found and the patient died shortly thereafter of diffuse disease.

A ten centimeter left upper pole renal mass with stippled calcification was discovered in a 50 year old man with flank pain and hematuria. At sonography the mass was completely round, echo free and met all the criteria for a cyst. The inconsistency between the calcifications, the hematuria and the sonogram led to angiography. A vascular tumor thought to probably be adrenal in origin was demonstrated. At surgery a large papillary cystadenocarcinoma of the kidney was found with central foci of hemorrhage and necrosis.

A 31 year old woman with the acute onset of flank pain had a flat upper pole with a lucent perirenal collection on nephrotomography. This was felt to possibly represent a subcapsular hematoma. At sonography the entire kidney was echo free and consistent with a cyst. However there also was a sonolucent envelope surrounding the echo free lower pole. Angiography demonstrated a vascular upper pole tumor with extrinsic compression of the lateral aspect of the kidney. A hypernephroma with subcapsular hematoma was removed.

Comment. Despite echo free appearances on sonography, the patients all came to angiography and surgery because of inconsistencies in their workup. The sonogram met all cystic criteria in two of these four cases, but both had hematuria, one with malignant cytology and the other with a large mass which had stippled calcification. Angiography was performed on the melanoma patient because of the irregular appearance on sonography and in the young woman because of a suspected hematoma. Of the four malignancies only the cystadenocarcinoma was a fluid filled neoplasm, explaining its ultrasound appearance. It must be recalled that ultrasound is not a histologic method and that tumors may be necrotic or homogeneous. The latter is especially true of lymphomas, melanomas, some sarcomas and some Wilm's tumors. The correct diagnosis will usually be derived if the criteria for a renal cyst are rigidly applied; and if all inconsistencies in the workup are completely resolved.

The following patient had a renal artery aneurysm.

Illustrative Case: A 23 year old woman experienced the acute onset of flank pain and had microscopic hematuria. Urography showed a three centimeter mid pelvic renal mass which on sonography appeared to be two small masses meeting the criteria for renal cysts. Because of the rarity of cysts in her age group and the hematuria, angiography was performed and demonstrated two saccular renal artery aneurysms in the hilus. Nephrectomy was performed.

Comment: Renal artery aneurysms are rare [11], but would be expected to be echo free. They therefore would have an ultrasonic appearance similar to a parapelvic cyst or a dilated renal pelvis. Hematuria or hypertension may be the only clues.

The final patient had a tumor and a cyst.

Illustrative Cases: A 68 year old man with painless hematuria and malignant urine cytology had a right upper pole renal mass which met all the ultrasonic criteria of a renal cyst (Figure 4). However, the hematuria and cytology prompted angiography which demonstrated the characteristic findings of an upper pole cyst and a small vascular tumor in the renal pelvis. The nephrectomy specimen confirmed the upper pole cyst and a transitional cell epithelioma of the renal pelvis.

Comment: The only mass identified urographically and ultrasonically was the cyst. The cytology and hematuria demanded further evaluation and the correct diagnosis was made. The simultaneous occurrence of a cyst and a tumor is often cited to serve a variety of viewpoints. The incidence has been said to range from less than one to approximately seven percent. These will continue to be a diagnostic pitfall for ultrasound,

DIFFERENTIAL DIAGNOSIS OF ECHO-FREE RENAL MASSES

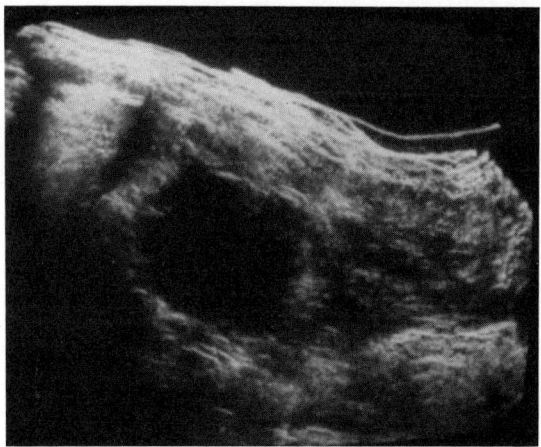

Figure 4. Longitudinal scan demonstrating an upper pole renal cyst in a patient with a synchronous tumor.

but close attention to the clinical situation and the insistence on confirmation with other studies will lead to the correct diagnosis in most patients.

DISCUSSION

Examination of renal masses with diagnostic ultrasound has become a standard part of their evaluation because of its accuracy and safety. The basic principle of the technique is that the proportion of total sound energy reflected at an interface is directly related to the magnitude of difference in the acoustic impedance of the two media. This explains the sonolucent appearance of a cyst and the internal echoes derived from the blood vessels, connective tissues and necrotic areas of tumors. However, it should not be surprising that an occasional physically homogeneous solid mass can be trans-sonic and mimic a cyst. Perhaps some of the cases illustrated which were performed on bistable equipment might have presented a different appearance on grey scale instruments.

Since most renal masses are cystic and the over whelming majority of these are benign, the tendency has been to equate these and assume that all echo free renal masses are simple cysts. However, there is a differential diagnosis, as demonstrated, and it includes most of the entities that can affect the kidney. Pitfalls can usually be avoided if all the criteria for ultrasonic diagnosis of renal cysts are scrupulously observed.

After urography has demonstrated a renal mass, ultrasound evaluation should be performed, followed by a coordinated approach utilizing nephrotomography, cyst puncture and angiography. Insistence that the diagnosis be confirmed by more than one study, should result in a diagnostic accuracy approaching 100 percent [10,12,13].

In summary:
1) Not all echo free masses are simple cysts;
2) All three criteria for renal cysts must be rigidly met before that diagnosis can be confidently made;
3) Failure to meet these criteria, or discrepencies with clinical or other diagnostic studies demands further evaluation;
4) In all cases, diagnosis should be confirmed by more than one modality.

REFERENCES

1. Asher Wm and Leopold GR: A Streamlined Diagnostic Approach to Renal Mass Lesions with Renal Echogram. J Urol. 108:205-208, August 1972.

2. Kristensen JK, Gammelgaard PA, Holm HH, and Rasmussen SN: Ultrasound in the Demonstration of Renal Masses. Br J Urol 44: 517-527, Oct. 1972.

3. Schreck WR and Holmes JH: Ultrasound as a Diagnostic Aid for Renal Neoplasms and cysts. J Urol. 103: 281-5, March 1970.

4. Goldberg BB and Pollack HM: Differentiation of Renal Masses Using A-mode Ultrasound. J Urol. 105: 765-771, June 1971.

5. Romeiser RS, Walls WJ and Valk WL: B-scan Ultrasound in the Evaluation of Renal mass Lesions. J Urol. 112:8-12, July 1974.

6. King DL: Renal Ultrasonography: An Aid in the Clinical Evaluation of Renal Masses. Radiology. 105: 633-640, Dec. 1972.

7. Hately W and Whitaker RH: How Accurate is Diagnostic Ultrasound in Renal Disease? Br J Urol. 45: 468-473, Oct 1973.

8. Doust VL, Doust BD and Redman HC: Evaluation of Ultrasonic B-mode Scanning in the Diagnosis of Renal Masses. Am J Roentgen 117: 112-118, Jan 1973.

9. Freimanis AK and Asher WM: Development of Diagnostic Criteria in Echographic Study of Abdominal Lesions. Am J Roentgen. 108: 747-755, April 1970.

10. Becker A and Schneider M: Simple Cyst of the Kidney. Seminars in Roentgen. 10: 103-111, April 1975.

11. Cerny JC, Chang CY and Fry WJ: Renal Artery Aneurysms. Arch Surg. 96: 653-663, April 1968.

12. Pollack HM, Goldberg BB and Bogash M: Changing Concepts in the Diagnosis and Management of Renal Cysts. J Urol. 111: 326-329, March 1974.

13. Smith EH and Bennett AH: The Usefulness of Ultrasound in the Evaluation of Renal Masses in Adults. J Urol. 113: 525-529, April 1975.

ULTRASOUND DIAGNOSIS IN RENAL TRANSPLANTS

Timothy G. Lee, M.D. and Janice M. Anderson, M.D.

Division of Ultrasound, Department of Diagnostic Radiology
University of Oregon Health Sciences Center
Portland, Oregon

The diagnosis of complications following renal transplantation requires the combined skills of ultrasonography, radiography and nuclear medicine. Since Leopold first described renal transplant size measured by ultrasound, [1] this modality has become increasingly important in the management of renal transplants [2,3]. A previous report by Maklad et al shows the ultrasound scan to be highly accurate in the detection of abscess following abdominal surgery [4]. This report describes 56 postoperative renal transplant patients recently examined by the division of ultrasound during the period from March 1974 to September 1975. Nineteen of the 56 patients had positive scans covering a wide variety of pathology, the most common finding being a collection of fluid. The purpose of this paper is to present the various diagnoses made ultrasonically in the post-transplant period.

MATERIALS AND METHODS

A total of 56 patients were examined over a 19 month period, the time after transplantation varying from 1 week to 2 years. In doing the scan, as many surgical dressings were removed as possible. Mineral oil was applied to the skin where feasible and viscous Aquasonic gel was applied around open wounds. Ultrasound scanning was initially done thoroughly over the pelvis and the renal allograft area, and then over the remainder of the abdomen as indicated. If the findings were uncertain or if there was a large amount of interfering gas, the patient was examined a second and sometimes a third time. Interfering bowel gas could usually be removed after a course of simethicone.

TABLE I

Patient	History	Ultrasound Findings	Final Diagnosis
1. M.S.	Hemorrhagic pancreatitis	Large pancreas, ascites, possible pseudocyst	Pancreatitis, ascites, loculated fluid with high amylase
2. W.H.	RIQ pain	Fluid-filled mass adjacent to allograft	Urinoma
3. H.P.	Fever, back pain	Sonolucent mass, posterior to allograft, probably hematoma	Autopsy - no abscess resolving hematoma
4. F.L.	Pancreatitis	Large collection fluid LIQ ant. to allograft	600 cc seroma
5. W.B.	Fever	Large fluid collection adjacent to allograft	Lymphocele
6. J.S.	Fever	Fluid pockets around allograft	Surgery - probably resolving urinomas
7. S.E.	Fever	Fluid-filled mass displacing bladder	Infected hematoma
8. D.S.	Fever, pain	Fluid-filled mass in allograft bed	Necrotic hematoma
9. A.W.	Fever	Sonolucent mass posterior to allograft - probable hematoma	Large hematoma
10. N.Y.	Pain, allograft removed	Fluid adjacent to iliac artery	Seroma
11. G.R.	Fever	Fluid around allograft	Surgery - abscess around allograft
12. L.D.	Fever	Fluid between allograft and bladder	Urinoma
13. D.L.	Painful mass	Fluid-filled mass near allograft	Needle aspiration - seroma
14. D.B.	Rejection	Small fluid collections around allograft	Seroma
15. R.E.	Pain, fever	Free pelvic fluid	Autopsy - ascites, peritonitis
16. M.C.	Asymptomatic	Fluid-filled mass anterior to bladder	Lymphocele by aspiration under ultrasound
17. M.B.	Asymptomatic	Anterior fluid collection between allograft and bladder	Lymphocele by aspiration under ultrasound
18. J.B.	Rejection	Fluid-filled mass between allograft and bladder	Seroma
19. D.G.	Rejection, oliguria	Dilated calyces of allograft	Obstruction at ureteral anastomosis

RESULTS

In 19 of the 56 patients, positive findings were obtained which were of value in the clinical management of the patient (Table I). No false positives or negatives were reported. The most common finding was a collection of fluid, and a differential diagnosis was usually given, with an impression of the most likely etiology. Follow up of the 37 negative cases has shown no subsequent abscess or other abnormality apparent clinically or by angiography, isotope scan or other diagnostic tests. The use of ultrasonography in serial scanning of the renal allograft for detection of acute rejection with increasing allograft size has been well documented[1] and will not be discussed here.

DISCUSSION

The etiology of the fluid collections seen in our patients was varied. Although the most commonly given indication for the study was suspected abscess, in only two was the fluid collection actually shown to be abscess (Fig. 1). Other causes, therefore, should be considered in the differential diagnosis, including seroma, lymphocele, urinoma, hematoma and loculated fluid due to ascites. In this series, the most frequent finding was seroma or lymphocele (Fig. 2). Since these types of fluid collections are usually sterile, needle aspiration for diagnosis and treatment after ultrasound localization is now commonly employed, rather than surgical exploration (Fig. 3).

A fluid-filled space which increases progressively in size during the examination may represent a urinoma, particularly if it is adjacent to the bladder. Patient L.D. had a 5 x 3 cm fluid-filled mass located between the bladder and the allograft, which gradually increased in size during the scan. Since urinoma was suspected, an excretory urogram was done, which proved negative. At our insistence, a retrograde cystogram was then done. Urinoma was proven surgically (Fig. 4). The retrograde cystogram is not only valuable in the diagnosis of a urinoma, but is also essential in excluding a bladder diverticulum which may present with similar findings.

A sonolucent mass which does not appear to be fluid may represent a hematoma or postsurgical edema. In patient F.P., a sonolucent mass of the same density as the renal cortex was seen posterior to the renal allograft and thought to be a hematoma. Rescan two weeks later showed a marked decrease in the size of the mass. This was felt to be a resolving hematoma and was so proved at autopsy.

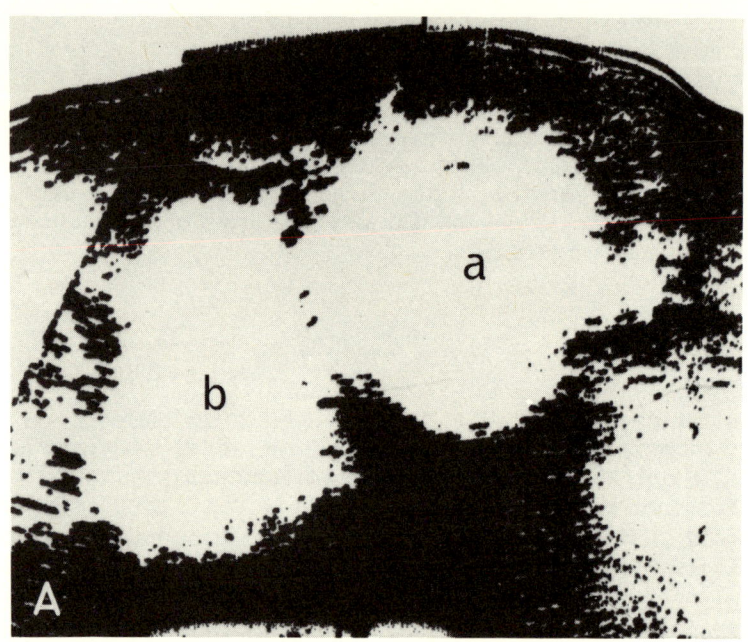
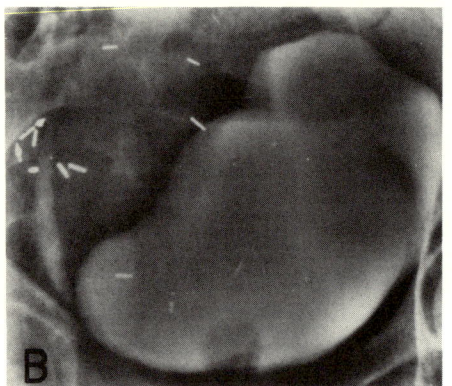
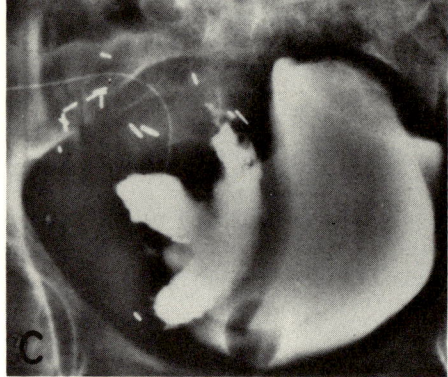

Fig. 1. Pt. S.E. (A) Transverse scan. Abscess (a) to the right of the bladder (b); the bladder was identified by a post-voiding scan. (B) Cystogram. Pressure defect on the bladder. (C) Contrast injected into abscess cavity.

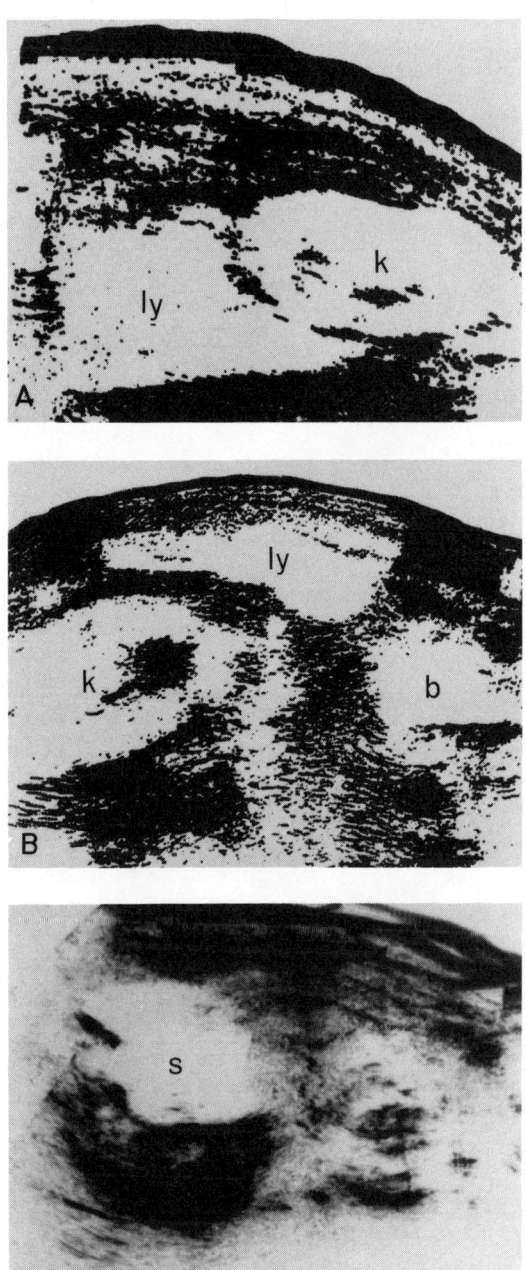

Fig. 2. (A) Pt. W.B. Lymphocele (ly) adjacent to allograft kidney (k). (B) Pt. M.B. Anterior lymphocele. Bladder (b). (C) Pt. J.B. Seroma (s).

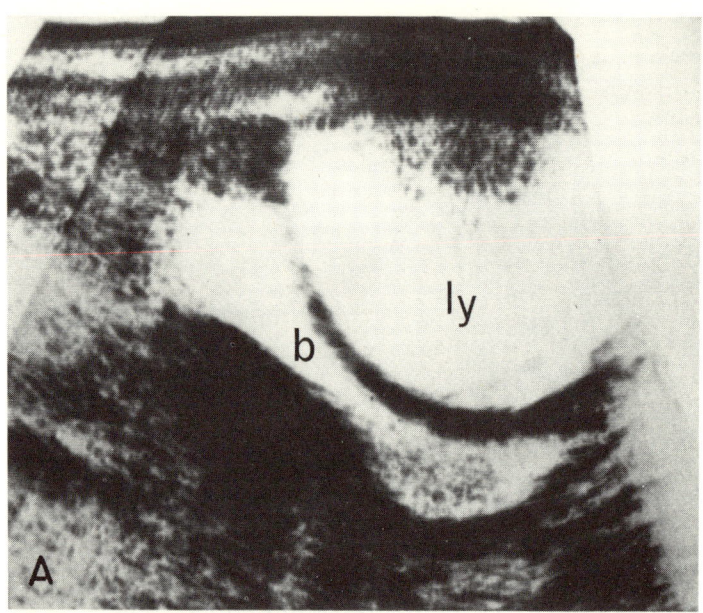

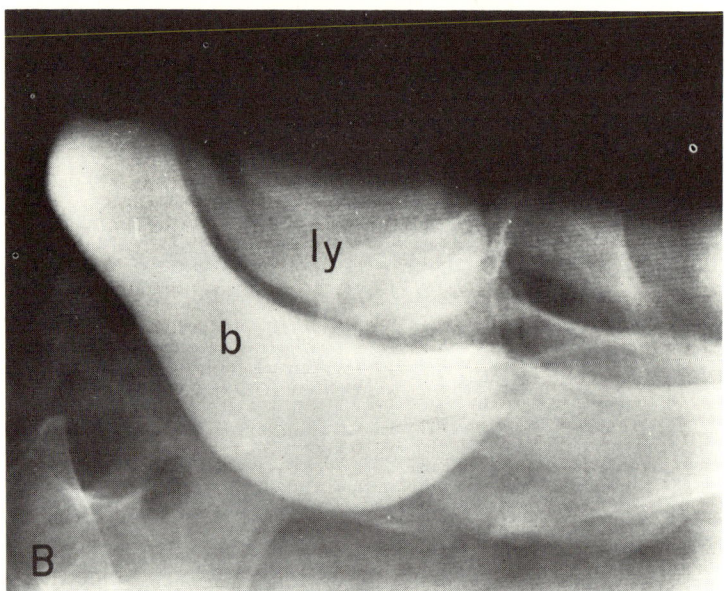

Fig. 3. Pt. M.C. (A) Saggital scan. Bladder (b). Lymphocele (ly). (B) Contrast agent injected into lymphocele after needle aspiration under ultrasound localization. Bladder visualized by cystogram.

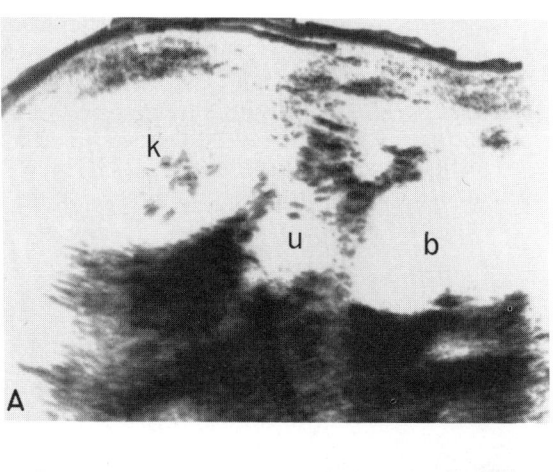

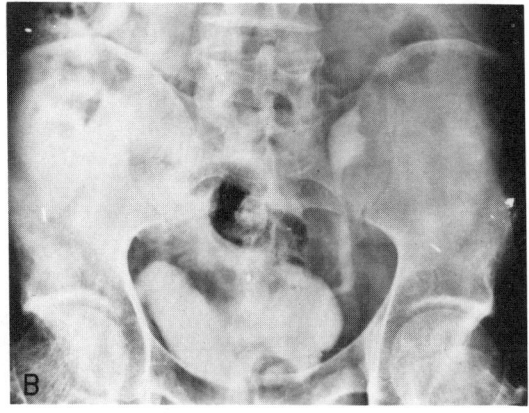

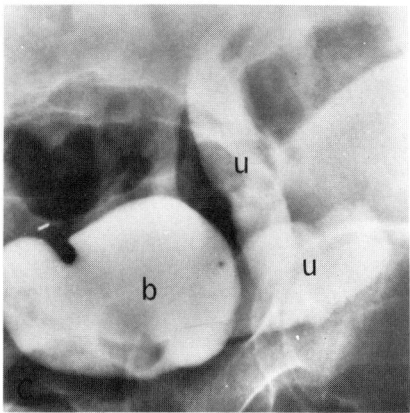

Fig. 4. Pt. L.D. (A) Urinoma (u) increased in size during scan. Allograft (k). Bladder (b). (B) Pyelogram shows no leakage of urine. (C) Cystogram demonstrated urinoma.

If ascites is suspected, a search for fluid, particularly in the pelvis, around the bladder and the liver, is useful. Patient M.S. had clinical pancreatitis; an ultrasound scan showed ascites, which changed in amount and location in serial scans. Fluid was visible around the bladder, as well as elsewhere in the abdomen. At one time the fluid collection appeared very round, and the possibility of a pseudocyst was felt likely (Fig. 5). Surgery demonstrated loculated fluid with high amylase content, which was drained, and the patient subsequently did well.

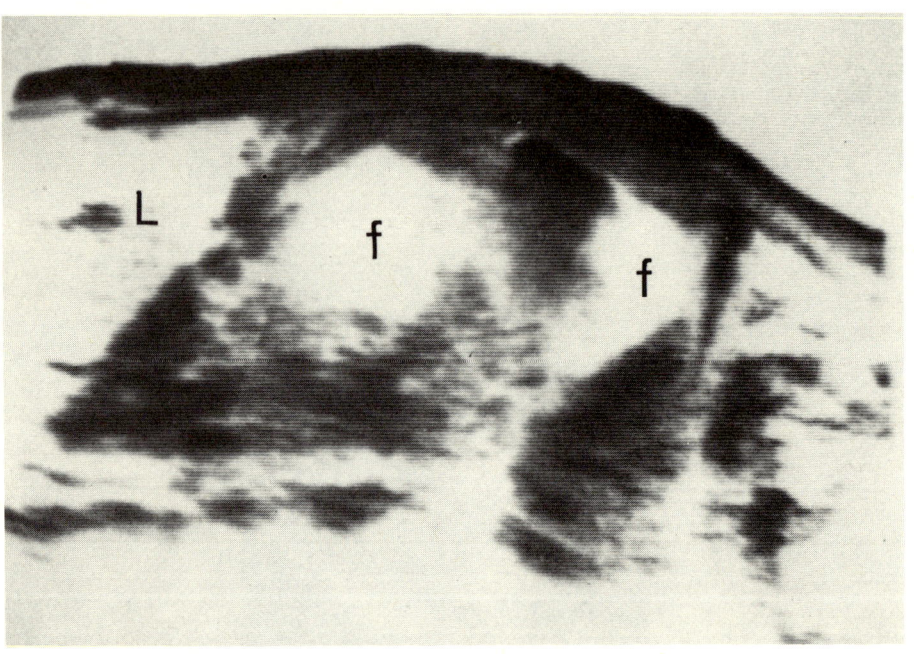

Fig. 5. Pt. M.S. Saggital scan shows rounded epigastric fluid (f), as well as fluid in the pelvis. Liver (L).

ULTRASOUND DIAGNOSIS IN RENAL TRANSPLANTS

If an allograft has been removed, a fluid collection in close proximity to the iliac artery should suggest the possibility of an aneurysm at the ligated stump. Patient N.Y. had previous bilateral allograft removals. The left side had a fluid collection adjacent to the iliac artery (Fig. 6). At the time of surgery, this proved to be seroma. Aneurysm, however, should always be included in the differential diagnosis (this patient subsequently developed one on the right side).

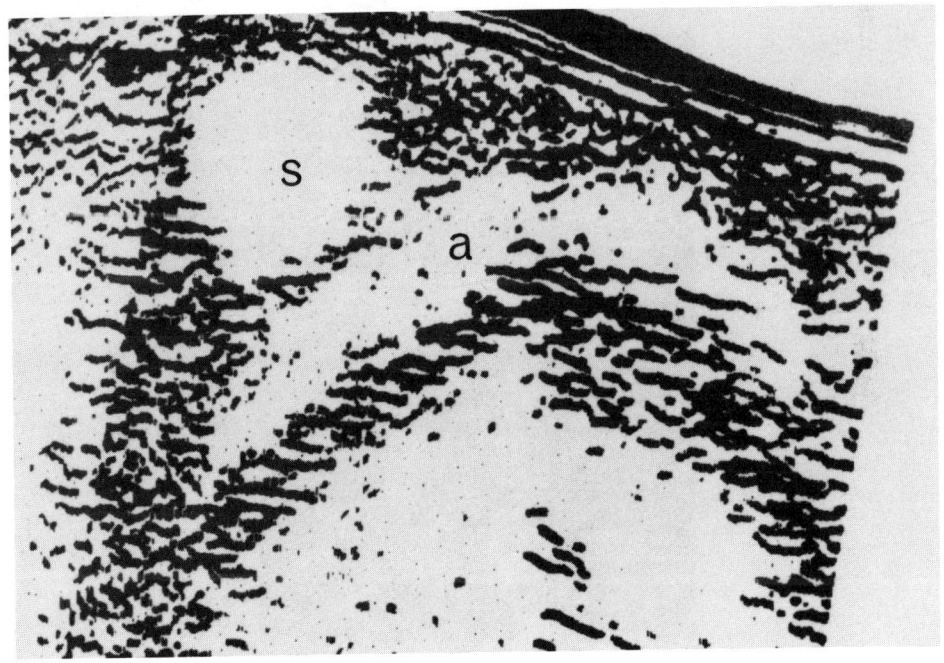

Fig. 6. Pt. N.Y. Iliac artery (a). Seroma (s).

A ureteral obstruction can be suspected if dilated calyces are seen by ultrasound. In patient D.G., with suspected rejection and oliguria, the ultrasound scan showed a dilated collecting system (Fig. 7). His urine output improved following a retrograde catheter placement. Obstruction at the ureteral anastomosis was subsequently proven.

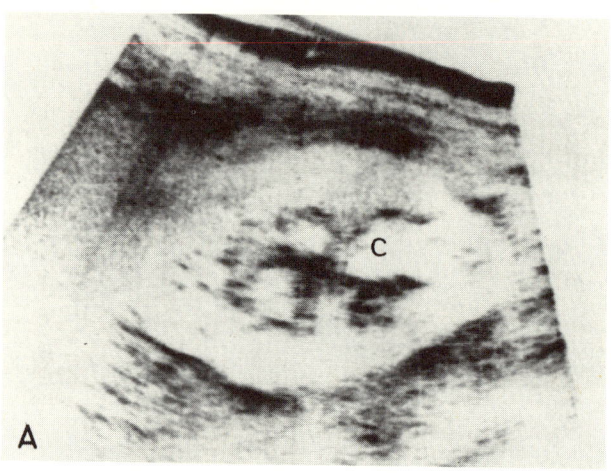

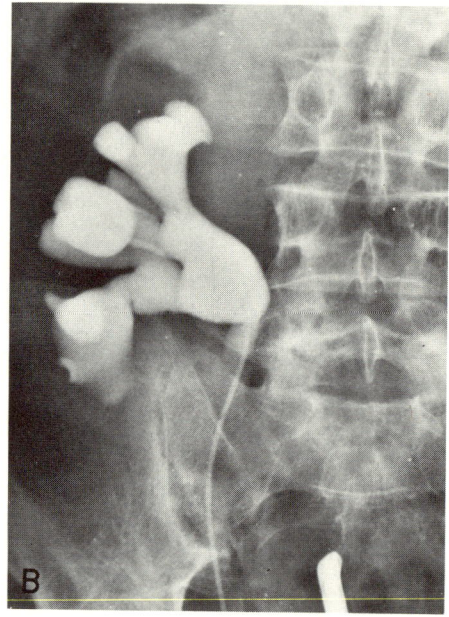

Fig. 7. Pt. D.G. (A) Allograft with dilated calyces (c). (B) Dilated calyces shown by retrograde pyelogram.

CONCLUSION

Ultrasound B-mode scanning provides a useful way of detecting a collection of abdominal fluid in the post-transplant period. Scans were done on 56 renal transplant patients, of whom 19 had positive findings, excluding rejection. While the scan is highly accurate in localizing an area of abnormality, the significance and etiology of the findings benefit from experience and a constant search for secondary clues.

Although abscess was usually suspected clinically, in this series of patients it was relatively uncommon. The various diagnoses discussed in this paper should therefore be considered.

REFERENCES

1. Leopold, G.: Renal transplant size measured by reflected ultrasound. Radiology 95:687-689, June 1970.

2. Sampson, D., Winterberger, A.R., Murphy, G.P.: The use of diagnostic ultrasound in renal transplantation. Review of Surgery 29:77-86, March-April 1972.

3. Winterberger, A.R., Palmer, L.D., Murphy, G.P.: Ultrasonic testing in human renal allografts. JAMA 219:475-479, Jan. 1972.

4. Maklad, N.F., Doust, B.D., Baum, J.K.: Ultrasonic diagnosis of postoperative intra-abdominal abscess. Radiology 113:417-422, Nov. 1974.

ULTRASOUND DIAGNOSIS OF LYMPHOCELES FOLLOWING RENAL TRANSPLANTATION

Avi Ben-Ora, M.D.; Nancy Sander, R.T.

Department of Diagnostic Ultrasound

Good Samaritan Hospital, Phoenix, Arizona

The encapsulated accumulation of lymphatic fluid in the pelvis, lymphocele, has been described previously as a rare complication of renal transplantation (1) (2) (3) (4). The incidence varies in different reported series from 2% (5), to 6.8%(6), to 18.1%(7).

Lymphoceles can impair renal function by producing obstruction to the urinary outflow tract. This must be differentiated from diminished renal function due to rejection, vascular occlusion or obstructive uropathy secondary to surgical complications.

Ultrasound examination has been found to be effective in the early diagnosis of lymphocele and in the evaluation of the response to therapy.

ETIOLOGY

At the time of the renal transplant procedure, the lymphatic vessels along the iliac artery and vein are stripped and severed. Lymphatic drainage normally continues via collateral channels, although at a reduced rate. Concomitantly, regeneration of lymphatic vessels begins, and can normally be completed in a period of seven to ten days(8). If the segment of resected lymphatic vessel is too long, however, regeneration will be hampered(9), contributing to the accumulation of lymphatic fluid. In addition, it has been shown that the proximal end of the severed lymphatic channel can remain open for up to 48 hours(8), thereby providing an additional pathway for transport of lymphatic fluid away from the wound.

An interesting recent development occurred in the renal transplant series at Good Samaritan Hospital, whereby a variation in surgical technique was associated with the development of lymphoceles in two consecutive transplant patients. The technique change consisted of a more careful and complete ligation of lymphatic vessels involving both proximal and distal channels. Although it has not been conclusively proven, it appears that there may be a greater accumulation of lymphatic fluid when a higher percentage of the vessels are ligated and so are prevented from transporting lymphatic fluid during the first 48 hour post-operative period. Excessive stagnation of lymphatic fluid may then interfere with regeneration of new lymphatic channels.

MATERIAL

The records of four patients who developed lymphoceles were reviewed. A fifth case, initially thought to be a lymphocele clinically and later found to be a seroma, is presented for comparison.

Case 1. A 20 year old female received a cadaver homo-transplantation on October 15, 1974. This was followed by routine immunosuppressant management and diuretics. An acute rejection reaction developed on October 21, 1974, and two days later clear fluid began to drain from the center of the skin incision which opened slightly. Although the rejection was suppressed, the drainage continued. On December 15, 1974 analysis of the draining fluid showed a urea nitrogen of 1 mg.% and total protein of 1.6 Gm%. On December 17, 1974 an ultrasound examination demonstrated an elongated cystic mass, measuring 6 cm. by 2 cm. immediately beneath and parallel to the skin incision(Fig. 1). A lymphangiogram the following day confirmed the presence of a lymphocele(Fig. 2). With this diagnosis the dose of diuretic was increased, using Lasix, with subsequent gradual cessation of the lymph drainage and reduction in size of the lymphocele(Fig. 3).

Case 2. On January 15, 1975 a cadaver renal transplant was placed into the right pelvis of this 20 year old female. Routine immunosuppressants and diuretics followed. A mild rejection developed on January 28, 1975 which was readily controlled. On March 3, 1975 she was admitted to the hospital with a right upper lobe pneumonia and a palpable firm slightly tender mass just medial to the transplant. An ultrasound examination demonstrated a cystic mass 8cm. by 4 cm. interposed between the transplanted kidney and the bladder(Fig. 4). A presumptive diagnosis of lymphocele was made, and the patient was treated with additional diuretics. Re-examination on May 9, 1975 showed almost complete resolution of the cyst(Fig. 5).

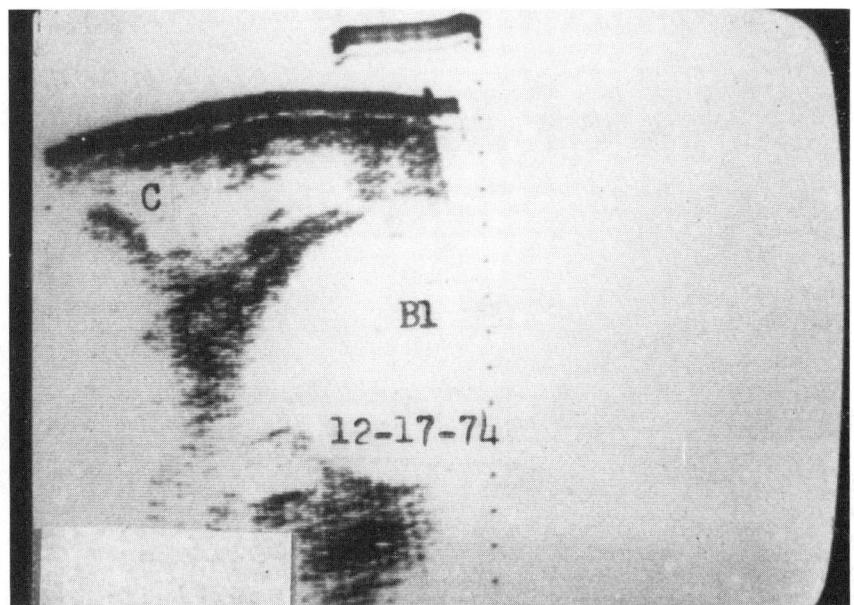

Figure 1. Transverse scan of lower right pelvis showing a lymphocele (C) to right of bladder (Bl).

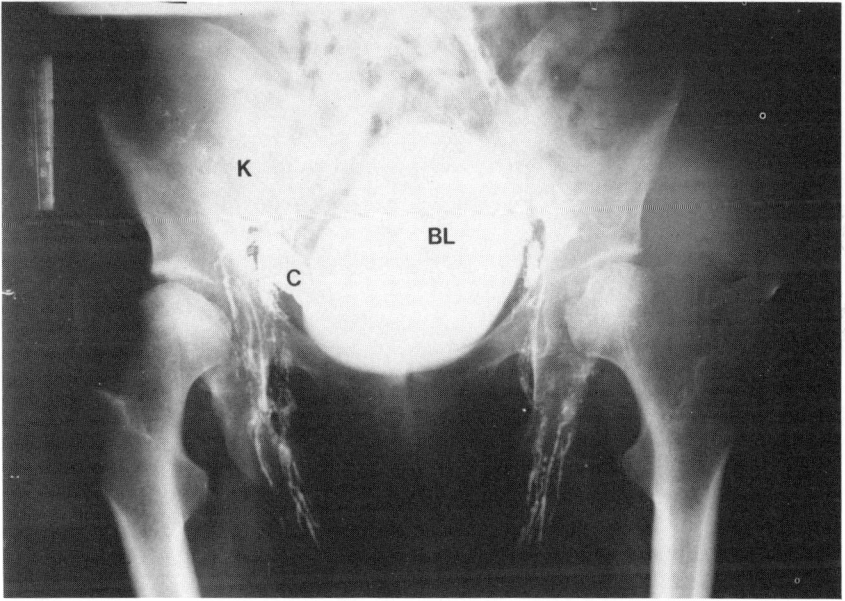

Figure 2. Lymphangiogram showing relationships of transplanted kidney (K), lymphocele (C) and bladder (Bl).

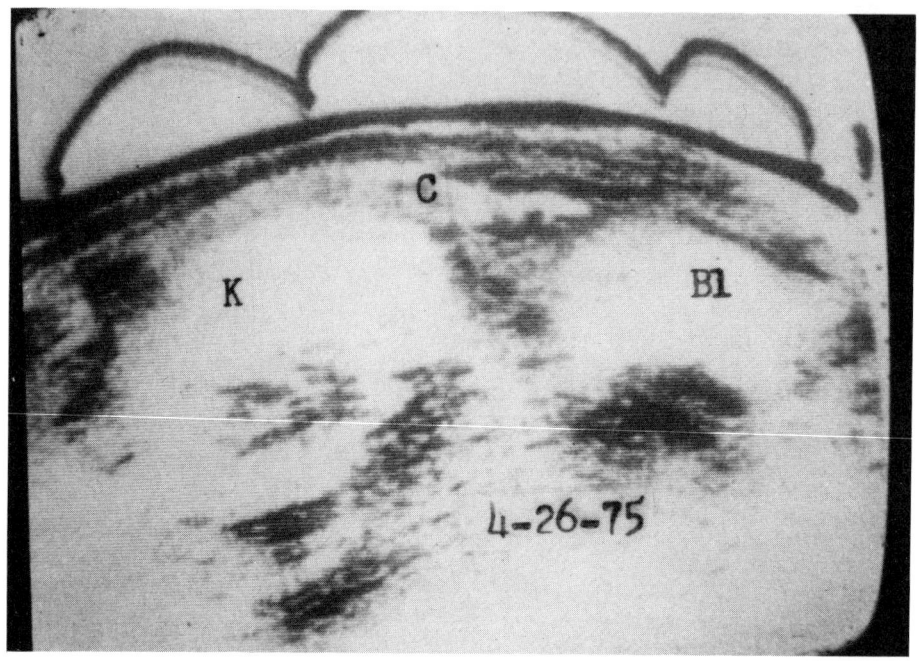

Figure 3. Lymphocele (C) has shown reduction is size following diuretic therapy.

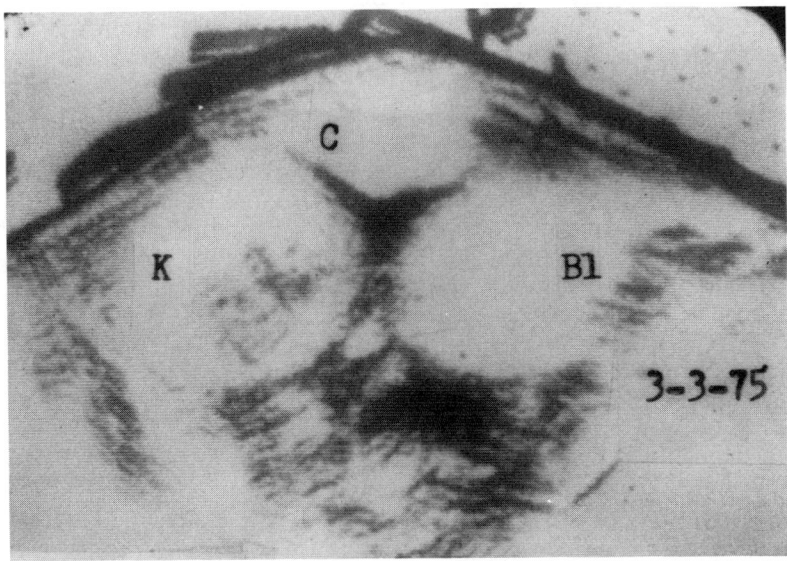

Figure 4. The lymphocele (C) is typically situated between the transplanted kidney (K) and the bladder (Bl).

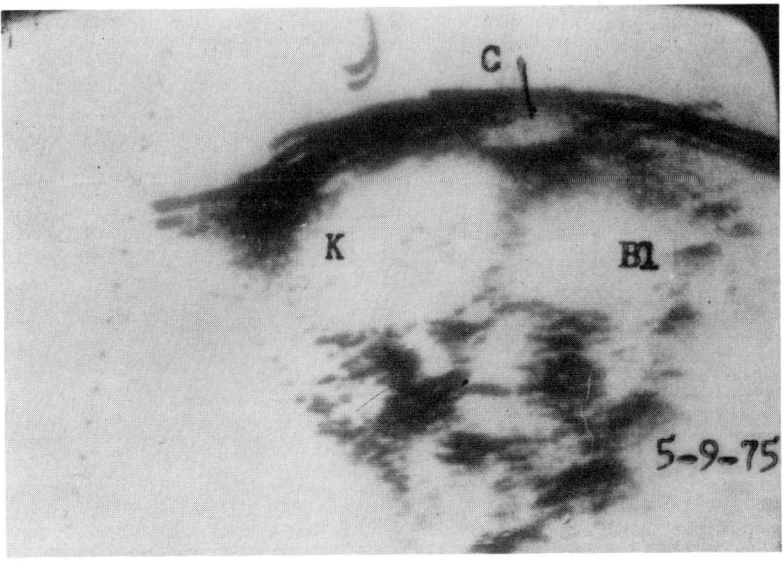

Figure 5. There has been nearly complete resolution of the lymphocele (C) with diuretic therapy.

Case 3. A cadaver renal transplant was placed into the left pelvis of a 29 year old male on January 15, 1975. Routine immunosuppressants and diuretics were utilized following surgery. Two mild acute rejection episodes followed, the first on January 17th and the second on February 10th, which were readily controlled. On March 20, 1975 the patient was found to have a decreasing urine output, urinary frequency and an easily palpable fluctuant suprapubic mass that was only minimally tender. An ultrasound examination demonstrated a 14 cm. by 10 cm. bi-locular cystic mass displacing and compressing the bladder (Fig. 6). A cystogram confirmed the displacement and compression of the bladder (Fig. 7). Aspiration of the cyst yielded 700 cc of clear yellowish fluid. Culture was sterile. Urea nitrogen of the fluid was 18 mg.%, indicating it was not urine. The cyst was therefore presumed to be a lymphocele and additional doses of a diuretic were prescribed. The patient has remained asymptomatic.

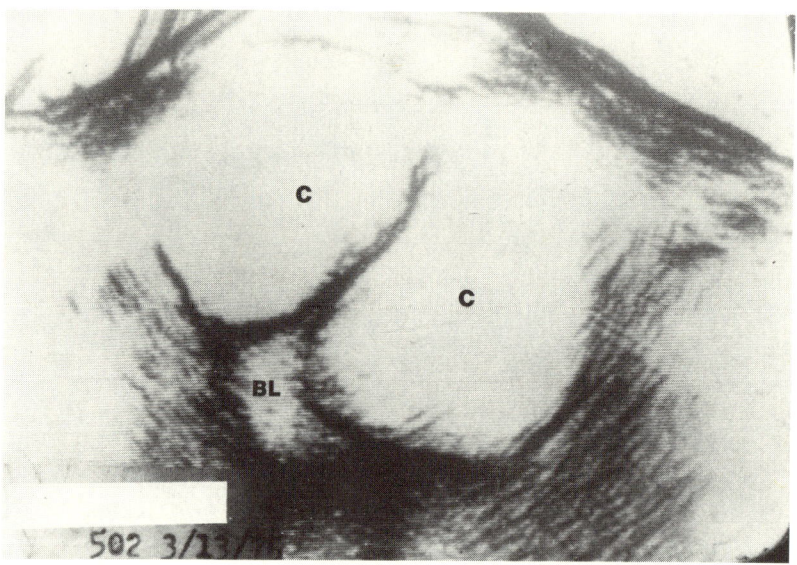

Figure 6a. Transverse scan across lower abdomen showing a bilocular cystic mass (C), the lymphocele, situated anteriorly to a compressed bladder (Bl).

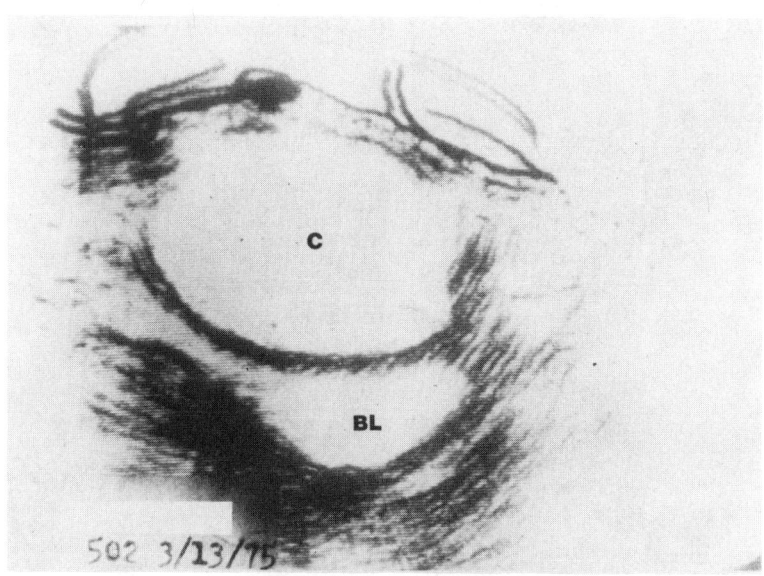

Figure 6b. Longitudinal scan 3 cm. to the right of mid-line showing the compression of the bladder (Bl) by the lymphocele (C).

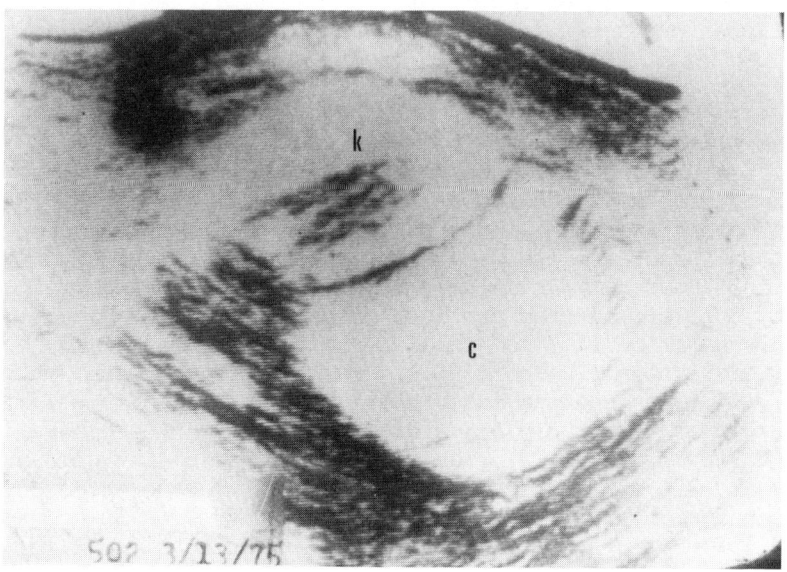

Figure 6c. Oblique scan of left iliac fossa showing relationship of renal transplant (K) to the lymphocele (C).

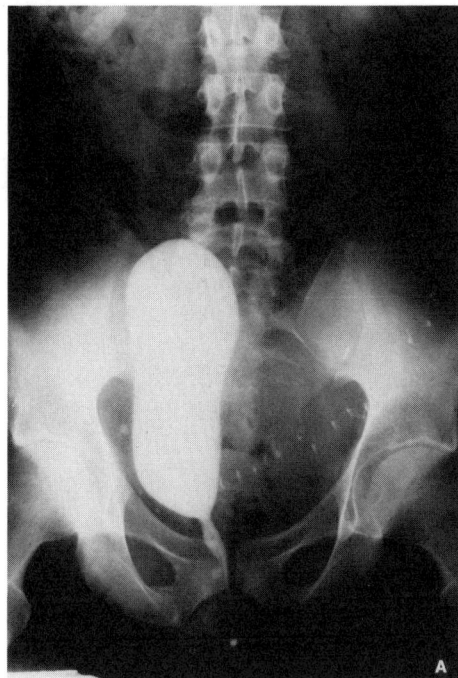 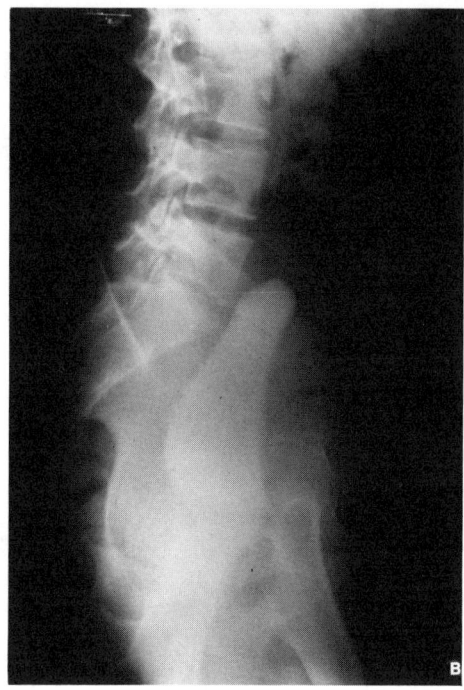

Figure 7. A cystogram in AP and Lateral projections. The bladder is compressed, elongated and displaced posteriorly and to the right by the large lymphocele.

Case 4. On April 14, 1971 a 19 year old female received a live related donor renal transplant from her Mother. This was followed by routine immunosuppressants and diuretics, however, two days post-operatively she began to manifest signs of rejection which became progressively more severe. On April 19, 1971 exploratory laparotomy revealed a rupture of the renal cortex secondary to swelling from acute rejection. The laceration was repaired, the associated hematoma removed and the rejection brought under control. She did quite well for four years, until July 31, 1975 when she was admitted to the hospital with pain and tenderness over the transplant area. She was 5 months pregnant at that time. Two days later an ultrasound examination demonstrated a 4.5 cm. by 3.5 cm. cystic mass adjacent to the lower pole of the transplanted kidney(Fig. 8). Cyst aspiration yielded 30 cc of clear yellowish fluid containing protein 3+, uric acid 5.1 mg.% and creatinine 1.3 mg.%. The cyst was presumed to be a lymphocele and the patient was placed on diuretics. Re-evaluation is pending.

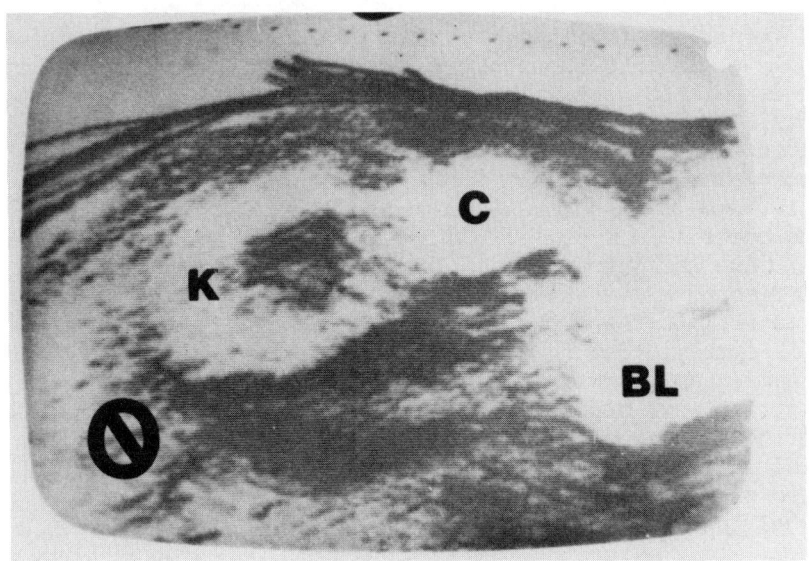

Figure 8a. An oblique scan across the right pelvis demonstrating the interposition of the lymphocele (C) between the transplanted kidney (K) and the bladder (Bl).

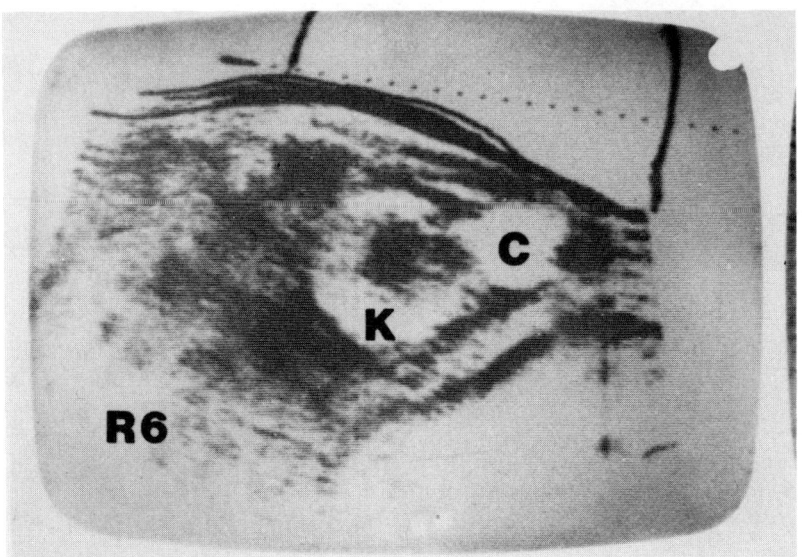

Figure 8b. A longitudinal scan 6 cm. to the right of mid-line showing the relationship between the lymphocele (C) and the kidney (K).

Case 5. A 17 year old male received a live related donor renal transplant from his Father on February 26, 1975. Routine management was instituted using Imuran, steroids, diuretics and local irradiation. A mild rejection occurred on March 8th, which was easily controlled. A second rejection episode developed on March 26, 1975, but treatment had to be limited because of leukopenia and thrombocytopenia. He then became persistently febrile, developed Herpes Zoster, and later was diagnosed as having coccidioidomycosis. On April 17, 1975 a soft slightly tender mass was palpable just lateral to the transplanted kidney. An ultrasound examination demonstrated a 4 cm. by 5 cm. cystic mass lateral to the upper pole of the kidney (Fig. 9). Aspiration of this cyst yielded 60 cc of clear yellowish fluid which clotted within minutes after aspiration. Cultures were sterile. No chemistries were ordered, but a presumptive diagnosis of seroma rather than lymphocele was made because of the rapid clotting and unusual lateral position of the cyst. The patient subsequently expired on May 14, 1975 and autopsy examination disclosed an overwhelming disseminated miliary coccidioidomycosis.

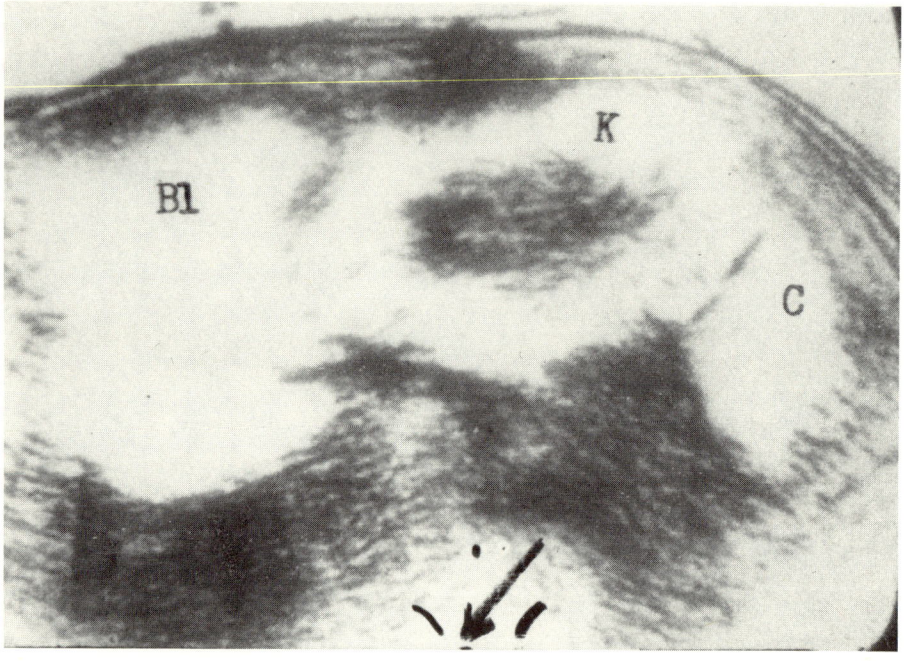

Figure 9. The oblique scan across the left lower abdomen shows the lateral position of the cyst (C), a seroma, in contrast to the usual medial location of a lymphocele.

ROENTGEN FINDINGS

In the past, roentgenographic procedures provided the only means of non-surgical diagnosis of a lymphocele. The intravenous urogram generally showed a flattened or deformed urinary bladder, with occasional dilatation of the ureter or collecting system. Unfortunately, if there was diminished renal function, the intravenous urogram was not helpful. A cystogram could show a characteristic deformity of the bladder if the lymphocele was large enough and contiguous with the bladder wall as in case 3.

A lymphangiogram would often show extravasation of contrast media from the lymphatic vessels of the pelvis into the fluid mass of the lymphocele as in case 1, however, the method can be cumbersome, time consuming, associated with morbidity and is not always helpful in evaluating the response to therapy.

ULTRASOUND FINDINGS

Lymphoceles generally have ultrasound features of a cystic mass. They are situated between the transplanted kidney and the bladder. When a cystic mass is located laterally to the kidney, as in case 5, it is probably not a lymphocele. The size of the lymphocele can vary, and if large enough can produce compression of the urinary outflow tract. A variety of shapes may be encountered. They may be thin and elongated, spherical or multi-loculated.

As shown in the preceding cases, the sonogram clearly demonstrates the variety of sizes and shapes that may be found. Ultrasound techniques provide a simple, non-invasive method of early diagnosis of a lymphocele. In addition, these techniques allow serial evaluation of the lymphocele as it changes in response to therapy.

DIAGNOSIS OF A LYMPHOCELE

In several of the reported cases in the literature (5)(6)(10), the mere presence of a cystic mass adjacent to the transplanted kidney led to a diagnosis of lymphocele. This was in part the case in our series as well. In case 5, however, where the aspirated fluid immediately clotted, a seroma was felt to be present. A more definitive diagnosis of lymphocele could have been made in those cases of our series that had been aspirated if more appropriate fluid analysis had been carried out.

When fluid can be aspirated it should be analyzed for those components that are most specific in differentiating lymph from serous fluid and urine (7). These parameters are summarized in Table 1.

TABLE 1

Composition of Lymphatic Fluid, Serum and Urine

	Lymph Mean ± SD	Serum Mean ± SD	Urine
Cholesterol (mg./100 ml.)	50.0 ± 42	168.0 ± 39	
Lactic Dehydrogenase (Wroblewski units)	74.0 ± 41	126.0 ± 43	
Alkaline Phosphatase (K. A. units)	4.0 ± 3	14.0 ± 5	
Total Protein (Gm./100 ml.)	2.2 ± 1.1	5.0 ± 0.6	
Albumin (Gm./100 ml.)	1.5 ± 0.8	3.2 ± 0.5	
Urea Nitrogen	46.0 ± 40	38.0 ± 27	4000
Clotting	Slow	Rapid	None

SUMMARY

The incidence of lymphocele formation following renal transplantation varies in different series from 2% to 18%. The reason for this wide variance may be related to surgical technique.

The most significant clinical finding associated with lymphocele formation is the reduction of renal function due to obstruction of the urinary outflow tract. It is most important to differentiate this finding from signs and symptoms of graft rejection as promptly as possible.

Diagnostic ultrasound has been found to be uniquely helpful in the early diagnosis of lymphocele formation, and provides a non-invasive means of following the response to therapy.

ACKNOWLEDGEMENTS

We wish to thank Dr. Marshall Lustgarten and Dr. Theodore Ditchek for their valuable assistance in the preparation of this manuscript.

REFERENCES

1. Koehler, P.R., Kyaw, M.M.: Lymphatic Complications Following Renal Transplantation. Radiol. 102:539-543, 1972.

2. Cockett, A.T.K., Netto, I.V.C.: Increased lymphatic Drainage from Renal Transplant. Urol. 11:571, 1973.

3. Kearney, G.P., Murray, J.E., Harrison, J.H.: Perinephric Pseudocyst: A Complication of Renal Transplantation. J. of Urol. 109:802-804, 1973.

4. Madura, J.A., Dunbar, J.D., Gerilli, G.J.: Perirenal Lymphocele as a Complication of Renal Homotransplantation. Surgery 68:310-313, 1970.

5. Schweitzer, R.T., et al: Lymphoceles Following Renal Transplantation. AMA Arch Surg 104:42-45, 1972.

6. Mott, C., Schreiber, M.H.: Lymphoceles Following Renal Transplantation. Am.J. Roentgenol. Rad. Therapy & Nuc. Med. 122:821-827, 1974.

7. Braun, W.E., et al: Lymphoceles Associated with Renal Transplantation. Am.J. of Med. 57:714-729, 1974.

8. McMaster, P.F.: Lymphatic Participation in Cutaneous Phenomena. The Harvey Lectures. 37:227-268, 1941-42.

9. Dodd, G.D., Rutledge, F., Wallace, S.: Post-operative Pelvic Lymphocysts. Am.J.Roentgenol. Rad. Therapy & Nuc. Med. 108:312-323, 1970.

10. Winterberger, A.R., Palma, L.D., Murphy, G.P.: Ultrasonic Testing in Human Renal Allografts. JAMA 219:475-479, 1972.

ROLE OF ULTRASOUND IN THE DIAGNOSIS AND THERAPY

OF PERIRENAL FLUID COLLECTIONS FOLLOWING RENAL TRANSPLANTATION

D.G. Spigos, M.D., V. Capek, M.D.

Department of Medical Radiology

University of Illinois, Chicago, Illinois   60612

ABSTRACT

Renal allografts are ideal organs for study by ultrasonic means because of their superficial position. It is well known that ultrasound can differentiate solid structures from fluid collections, a property which is very useful in the detection of perirenal fluid collection in patients with renal transplants. Examples of lymphoceles, urinomas, hematomas and abscesses are presented and a systematic approach for their differential diagnosis and treatment is discussed.

Kidney transplantation has become a standard treatment for patients with irreversible renal failure. (1). The successful outcome of this endeavor depends upon the proper selection and matching of donor and recipient, correct surgical technique, and prompt recognition and treatment of the various postoperative complications. (2). One common complication in the early, as well as late post-transplantation period, is fluid collection in the operative field and/or in the immediate vicinity of the transplanted kidney.

Most of these perirenal collections represent postoperative edema or lymph accumulation of little clinical significance and resolve spontaneously after a period of three to five days. The fluid collections that we found to be of clinical significance are large lymphoceles, hematomas, urinomas and abscesses. They always have a serious impact on the renal allograft's function and the patient's general status. (3-8).

INCIDENCE

We performed 320 ultrasonographic studies in 78 patients who received renal transplants. We discovered ten patients with large lymphoceles, four patients, who developed urinomas, three patients who developed hematomas, and one patient who developed an abscess. (Table 1).

Table 1

NUMBER OF PATIENTS WITH ECHO STUDY	78.	% incidence
NUMBER OF LYMPHOCELES:	10.	12.8 %
NUMBER OF URINOMAS:	4.	5.1 %
NUMBER OF HEMATOMAS:	3.	3.8 %
NUMBER OF ABSCESSES:	1.	1.3 %
TOTAL OF FLUID COLLECTION	18.	23.0 %

TECHNIQUE

The technique of examining renal transplants with pulsed ultrasound has been communicated in several reports. (9-12) In brief, several longitudinal and transverse sections are obtained over the area of the transplanted kidney, in relation to the axis of the body. The kidney's axis is found and then a second set is recorded in relation to the true axis of the transplanted kidney. We use polaroid films for permanent record of the B-mode presentations from the cathode ray tube.

In order to avoid confusing the urine-filled bladder with a low perirenal collection, the examination is performed with the bladder both full and empty.

FINDINGS

The renal allografts, because of their superficial location, resting on the muscular layer of the right or left iliac fossa, are ideal organs for study, using ultrasound. Fig. (1). The kidney is well delineated and its collecting system is well

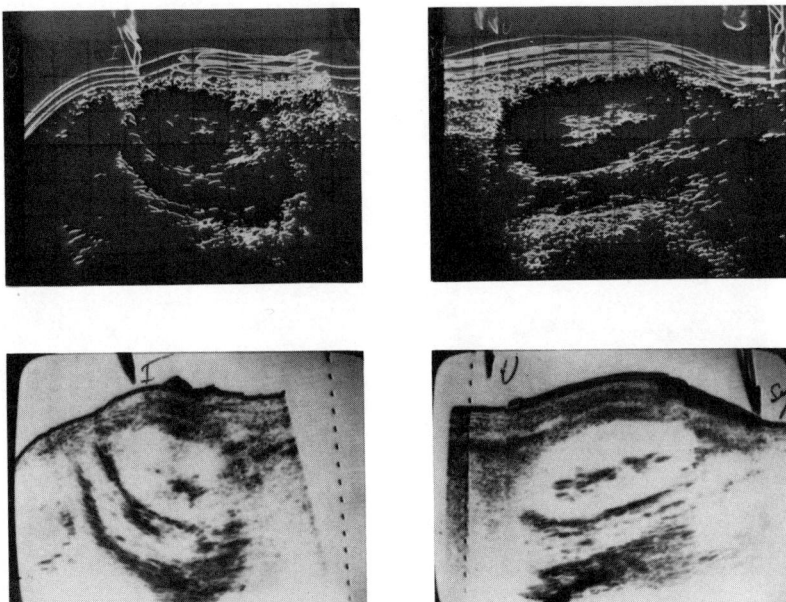

Figure 1: Transverse and longitudinal sections of renal transplants. Examples of normal studies using both conventional bistable equipment (upper row) and Gray scale (lower row). The kidney's outline, its collecting system and the underlying iliac and psoas muscles are well visualized.

identified. The underlying muscular layers can be easily visualized, and the possible perirenal collections are more easily detected than with any other technique.

One of the common fluid collections that is easily recognizable is the one in the incisional wound. Its ultrasonographic appearance is characteristic, having a triangular shape and being totally sonolucent. Fig. (2). Its location is also characteristic along the incisional wound. When it is found, it is always at its maximum size on the first postoperative day and then, gradually diminishes over a period of two to five days.

Another fluid collection seen relatively frequently, presents as a subcutaneous accumulation in the early postoperative period, Fig. (3). Like the fluid in the incisional wound, it gradually disappears without the need of any medical or surgical intervention. We believe that it represents either, post-operative edema, or a small lymphocele that disappears as soon as lymphatic collaterals develop.

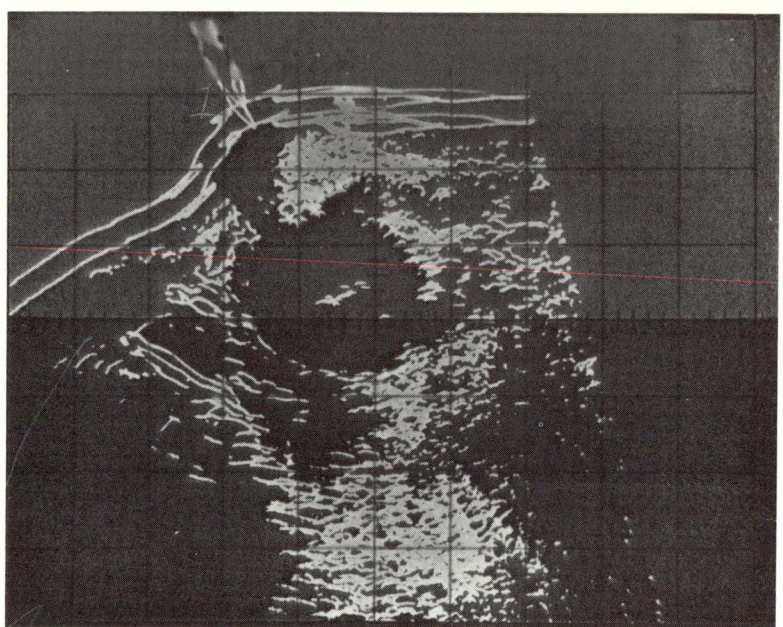

Figure 2: Transverse section of a renal transplant showing a triangular sonolucent area in the incision. This is the characteristic appearance of a local fluid collection.

Among the collections with clinical significance, the commonest are the lymphoceles. Their echographic appearance is that of a large anechoic area, next to the renal transplant, displacing adjacent organs, like intestines and urinary bladder. Figs. (4 and 5). They vary in their sizes from 100 to 1000 cc. One lymphocele of 1500 cc has been reported, which caused anuria. (13)

Lymphoceles occur early as well as late in the post transplant period. The small ones are asymptomatic, but the large ones might cause edema of the ipsilateral leg, and the genitalia. They also produce subjective feelings of heaviness over the area of the iliac fossa.

The general condition of patients with lymphoceles is good, a fact that helps to differentiate them from patients with urinomas, who are usually very sick.

We percutaneously aspirated the lymphoceles of five patients under ultrasonographic guidance with good therapeutic results. (14) More than one aspiration was needed in four patients. In

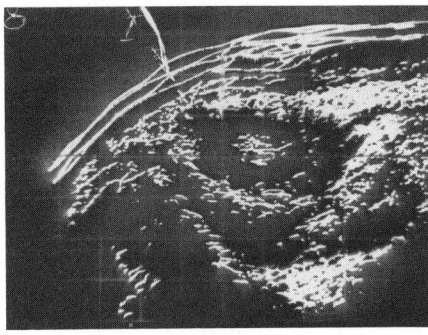 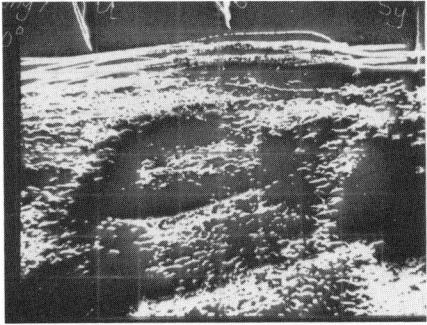

Figure 3: Transverse and longitudinal section of the renal transplant showing a small subcutaneous fluid collection superior and medial to the kidney. The urinary bladder is visualized on the longitudinal section.

one patient we used constant suction for a period of five days. The method failed in only one patient who had to be subsequently explored for drainage of the lymphocele. The perirenal fluid is totally aspirated and sent for biochemical and cytological studies, and microbiological cultures. Lymphoceles are sterile and contain no urea. Abundant lymphocytes are seen with cytologic study. This way, the aspiration serves a twofold purpose - a therapeutic one by evacuating the lymphocele, and a diagnostic one by identifying the nature of its content.

Urinomas occur mainly in the early post-transplant period. The patients are characteristically sick. This size is relatively small, and the fluid collection, as it is seen in the B-scan, is around the inferior pole of the kidney. Ultrasonographically, they present as completely sonolucent areas. (Fig. 6) If and when aspirated, the material is positive for urea, but negative for the presence of lymphocytes. Another finding that helps in differentiation between urinomas and lymphoceles is that the urinary bladder does not readily fill in the presence of the former.

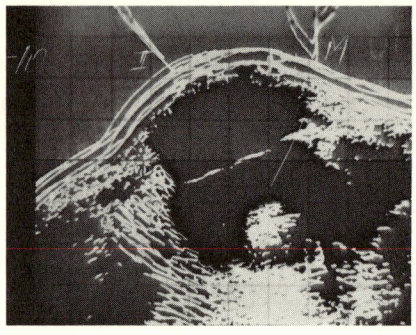 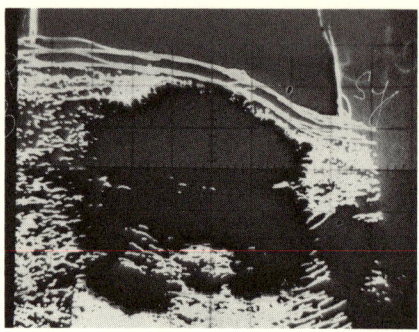

Figure 4: Transverse and longitudinal sections of the renal transplant. A large sonolucent area is present superior, to the kidney. It proved to be a large lymphocele.

Hematomas present in patients that are seriously ill, but their ultrasonographic appearance is quite characteristic readily distinguishing them from any other entity. The kidney is surrounded by a space, which is mainly sonolucent, however, very strong linear interrupted echoes are returned with high sensitivity settings (Fig. 7). We believe that the source of these echoes are blood clots, a finding that was observed in all of our patients that were subsequently surgically explored.

Abscesses are seen in patients, who are septic and critically ill. Their ultrasonographic appearance is mainly sonolucent; but, in high sensitivity setting, irregular echoes may be seen within the fluid collection probably due to the presence of debris. (Fig. 8)

DISCUSSION

In the study of the patients with perirenal collections, the ultrasonographic appearance of the fluid collections might be critical in establishing an early diagnosis, which then leads to the correct approach and treatment (Table 2).

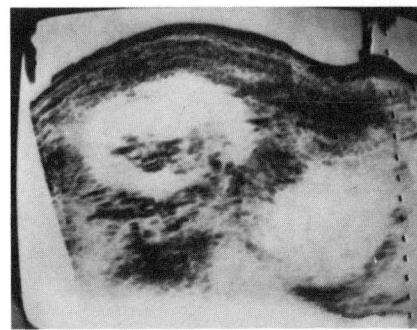 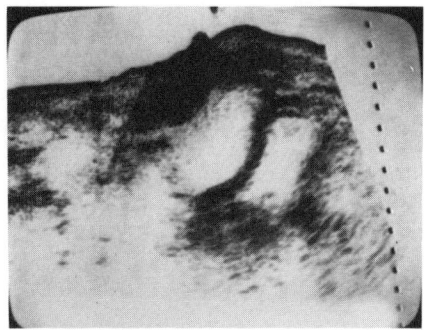

Figure 5: Longitudinal and transverse sections. In the longitudinal section, the lymphocele is shown medial to the inferior pole of the kidney. The displacement of the bladder by the lymphocele is well demonstrated on the transverse scan.

Table II

Perirenal collections
- a. Incisional wound fluid ... No intervention
- b. Lymphoceles .... Percutaneous aspiration.
- c. Urinomas .... Percutaneous aspiration plus
- d. Hematomas .... surgical exploration and repair.
- e. Abscess .... Percutaneous aspiration Surgical exploration and Antibiotics.

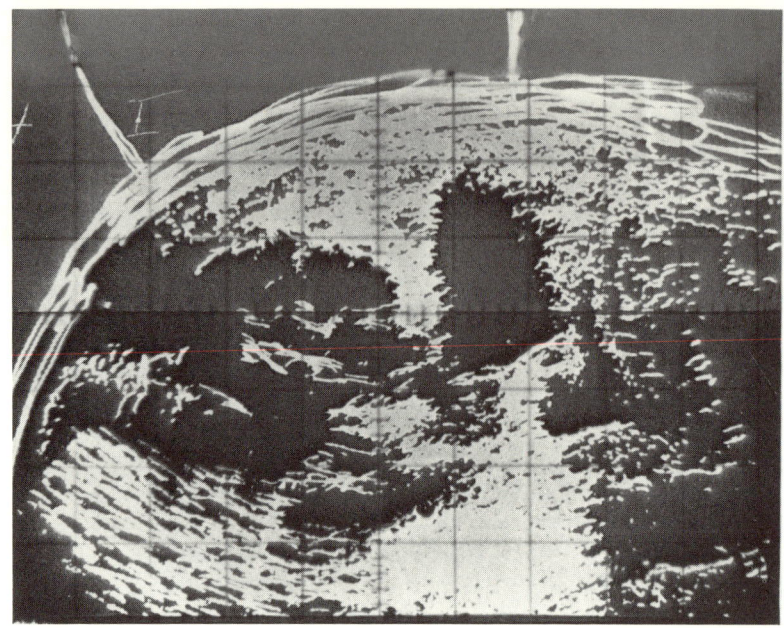

Figure 6: Transverse scan showing the kidney transplant and a sonolucent collection medial to it. This lesion, which was completely sonolucent, proved to be a urinoma.

In cases of lymphoceles and urinomas, the echographic appearance is more or less the same-that of a completely anechoic space. Some of the differences that help in the differentiation of these two entities are: (a). Most of the lymphoceles are larger than urinomas. (b). The urinary bladder is usually deformed by lymphoceles, (Fig. 9) but fails to fill readily in urinomas. (c). The aspiration fluid contains an abundance of lymphocytes in lymphoceles and is positive for urea in urinomas. (d). Radioisotope renal studies are also very helpful in identifying and localizing urine leaks.

We believe that lymphoceles should be percutaneously aspirated repeatedly until there is no reaccumulation. On the other hand, patients with urinomas should be explored as soon as the diagnosis is made. The point of urine leak should then be found and repaired.

Hematomas give quite characteristic internal echoes facilitating the diagnosis. Patients with hematomas should be immediately explored to evacuate the hematoma and find the source of bleeding.

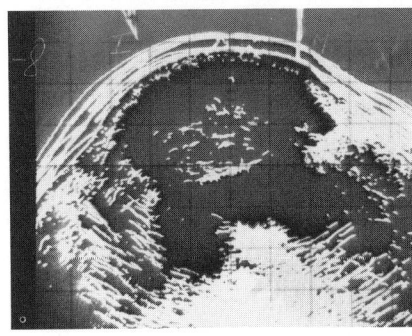 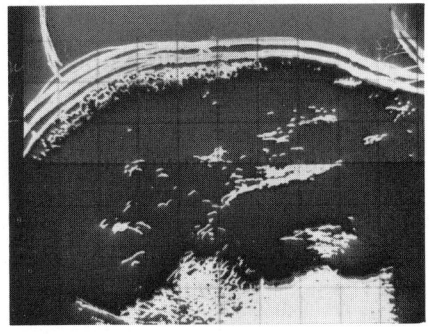

Figure 7: Transverse and longitudinal sections showing the renal transplant displaced posteriorly by a large fluid collection which at high sensitivity settings returns echoes. These echoes were from blood clots in a hematoma.

Abscesses might elicit some internal echoes. These patients who are septic should also be surgically explored to have their abscess evacuated.

An entity that can be confused with perirenal fluid collection especially in azotaemic patients is ascites. This can be avoided if the rest of the abdomen is examined. Then the diagnosis of ascites can readily be made. (Fig. 9)

CONCLUSION

Patients with renal transplants should be serially examined by ultrasound in their post transplant period. This innocuous method is highly sensitive in depicting perirenal collections and can serve as the primary diagnostic modality. Other studies, like intravenous pyelograms, cystograms, radionuclide renal studies and angiograms can be of complementary value. It is our experience that the ultrasonic examination is far superior to any other method in the early detection and differentiation of the perirenal collections in transplant recipients.

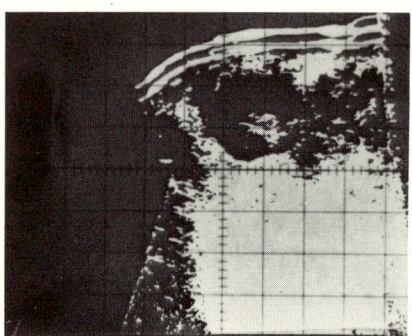 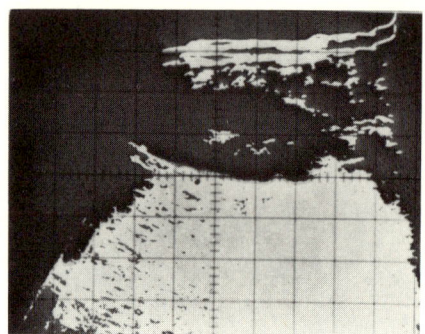

Figure 8: Transverse and longitudinal scans showing a fluid collection medial and inferior to the kidney which at high sensitivity returns internal echoes. This collection proved to be a pseudomonas abcess.

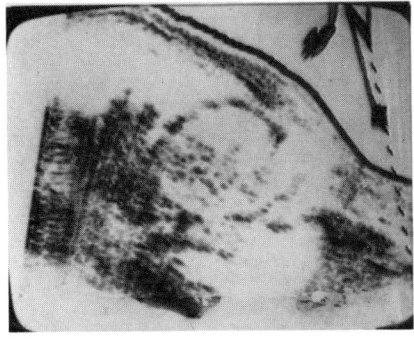 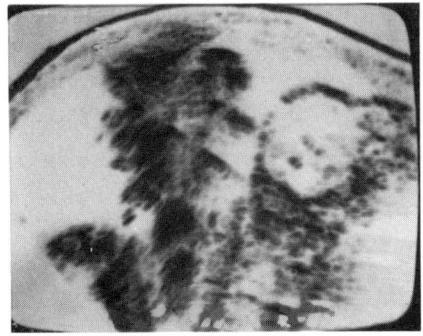

Figure 9: Transverse section over the area of the transplant showing a perirenal collection. 9B. When the entire abdomen was scanned, the presence of ascites was evident.

REFERENCES

1. Straffon R.A., Kiser W.S., Stewart B.H., Hewitt C.B., Gifford R.W., Nakamoto S.,: Four years of clinical experience with 138 Kidney Transplants. J. of Urol., 99,479-485,1968.

2. Woods, J.E., DeWeerd J.H., Johnson W.J., Anderson C.F., Shorter R.G.,: Experience in human renal allografts' transplantation. Surg. Gynecol. Obstert, 134,394-398,1972.

3. Koehler P.R., Kyaw A.M.,: Lymphatic complications following renal transplantation. Read 102,539-543,1972.

4. Mott C., Schreiber M.H.,: Lymphoceles following renal transplantation. Am. J. Roent. Rad. Ther. and Nucl. Med. 22:4, 821-827, Dec., 1974.

5. Anderson E.E., Glenn J.F., Seigler, H.F., Stickel D.L.,: Urologic complications in renal transplantation, J. Urol., 107,187-192, 1972.

6. Malek G.H., Vehling D.T., Dauk A.A., Kisen W.A.:
   Urologic complications of renal transplantation
   J. Urol., 109, 173-176, 1973.

7. Mackinnon K.Y., Oliver J.A., Morehouse D.D., Taguchi Y.,:
   Cadaver renal transplantation: emphasis on urological
   aspects: J. Urol., 99, 486-490, 1968.

8. Starzl T.E., Groth C.G., Putnam C.W., et al.: Urological
   complications in 216 human recipients of renal transplants.
   Ann.Surg., 172, 1-22, 1970.

9. Bartrum R.J., Smith E.H., D'orsi C.J., Dantonoy: Ultrasonic
   determination of renal transplant volume.: J. Clin. Ultrasound, 2, 281-285, 1974.

10. Leopold G.: Renal transplant size measured by reflected
    ultrasound. Rad., 95,687-689, 1970.

11. Winterberger A.R., Palma L.D., Murphy G.P.,: Ultrasonic
    testing in human renal allografts. JAMA 219:4,475-479,1972.

12. Capek V., Spigos D.: Ultrasound and angiographic techniques
    in renal transplant evaluation. Presented at the spring
    meeting of the central chapter of Society of Nuclear Medicine,
    March, 1975., Chicago. Submitted for publication in the
    J. of Nucl. Med.

13. Dielhelm A.G.: Anuria secondary to perirenal lymphocele:
    a complication of renal transplantarion. South Med. Y.,
    65,350-353, 1972.

14. Spigos D., Capek V.: Ultrasonically guided percutaneous
    aspiration of lymphoceles following renal transplantation.
    A diagnostic and therapeutic method. Accepted for
    publication in J. Clin. Ultrasound.

AORTOSONOGRAPHY - THE DIAGNOSTIC METHOD OF CHOICE

B. B. Goldberg, M.D.

Professor of Radiology
Temple University Health Sciences Center, Philadelphia
Head, Section of Diagnostic Ultrasound
Episcopal Hospital, Philadelphia, Pennsylvania

ABSTRACT: Ultrasonic aortography has been established in many institutions as the screening procedure of choice in patients suspected of having abdominal aortic aneurysms since it accurately displays the overall dimensions of the aneurysm. In several cases, a marked discrepancy has been observed between the internal lumen diameter as recorded by contrast aortography and by ultrasound. The ultrasonic measurements are generally larger and conform more closely to the actual overall dimensions than do those obtained by contrast aortography (roentgenographic or nuclear). It was hypothesized that this discrepancy was due to the presence of internal clot. Indocyanine green injections into the aortic lumen, while simultaneous ultrasonic scanning was performed, confirmed this hypothesis. By utilizing grey scale B-scan equipment, echoes were often recorded from the clot helping to differentiate it from the lumen. These clinical experiments suggest that aortosonography is a more accurate method of evaluating the overall dimensions of the abdominal aorta than either nuclear or roentgenographic aortography.

Introduction: The importance of ultrasound as the initial study in the evaluation for abdominal aortic aneurysms has been established. (1,2,3,4) Ultrasound should be considered the study of choice when a clinician palpates a pulsatile abdominal mass. The accuracy of ultrasound in differentiating the normal aorta from an aneurysm has been reported to be as high as 98.6 %. (5) Unlike other methods of examination, i.e. nuclear or roentgenographic aortography, ultrasonic aortography appears to record the overall dimensions of the abdominal aorta, including lumen and clot, preferentially. However, nuclear or

roentgenographic contrast aortography tends to demonstrate only
the lumen, with only secondary signs indicating the extent of
internal clot, which has resulted in false-negative diagnoses.
(6,7,8) In order to test the hypothesis that aortosonography is
a more accurate method of evaluating the abdominal aorta than
either nuclear or roentgenographic aortography, clinical
investigations were performed in which indocyanine green was
injected into the aortic lumen during ultrasonic examinations.

Technique: Studies were performed with commercially
available ultrasonic equipment capable of producing two-
dimensional B-scan images in both standard bi-stable and grey
scale modes of display. Standard internally focused 2 1/4
megaHertz transducers were used. In the evaluation of the
abdominal aorta, all four types of pulsed ultrasound as described
below were utilized. With the A-mode type of display, the
returning echoes were displayed as vertical spikes arising from a
horizontal baseline. The height of the spike was related to the
strength of the returning echo. The horizontal baseline was
electronically calibrated allowing for easy determination of the
depth and dimensions of the vessel being evaluated. With the
M-mode type of display, the returning echoes were displayed as
dots rather than as spikes. These dots were swept in a vertical
direction allowing for the recording of any motion toward or away
from the transducer. This type of display was used in
distinguishing expansile vascular motion from transmitted motion.
The B-scan mode of display was utilized to produce a two-
dimensional image. The dots representing the returning echoes
were recorded on a bi-stable oscilloscope so that they were of the
same relative intensity. Although the dots did vary in size, the
difference was not readily apparent. In the grey scale B-scan
mode of display, however, this problem was overcome since
variations in the amplitude of the returning echoes were displayed
as shades of grey. In effect, grey scale B-scan combines the
features of the bi-stable B-scan with the amplitude modulation of
the A-mode display resulting in improvement in the resolution of
the two-dimensional images produced.

After application of mineral oil to the skin surface, both
longitudinal and transverse B-scans were obtained by moving the
transducer over the area of interest. If the abdominal aorta was
tortuous, additional ultrasonograms were obtained at varying
degrees of obliquity. The scanning technique was usually linear
due to the nature of the vessel being examined. For maximum
detail, respiration was suspended during each sweep of the
transducer. The images obtained were recorded on instant
developing film as well as video-tape.

In this article, all transverse images are displayed as if

one is looking at the cross section of the body from the feet towards the patient's head. The longitudinal scans are displayed as if looking from the patient's right side toward the left.

Results: In two patients undergoing contrast aortography prior to having resections of aortic aneurysms, ultrasonic B-scan and M-mode examinations were performed during the simultaneous injection of indocyanine green into the lumen of the aorta. The catheter was positioned with its tip very near the proximal end of the aneurysm. Once baseline ultrasonic readings were recorded, a second series was obtained in the same positions during the hand injection of four milliliters of indocyanine green (Fig. 1).

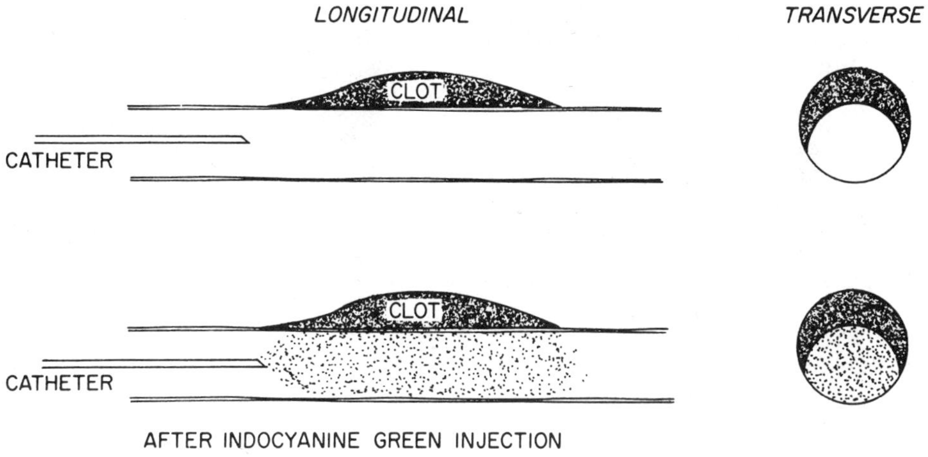

Figure 1. Diagrammatic representation of an aortic aneurysm containing clot with a catheter in position proximal to the aneurysm. Upper diagram shows lumen before and lower diagram after the injection of indocyanine green.

This material has been shown to contain microbubbles of air which go back into solution rapidly. (9,10) These microbubbles produced strong reflections resulting in multiple echoes, suggestive of a snow-storm which filled portions of the previously echo-free lumen (Fig. 2). Measurement of the now echo-filled lumen compared favorably with the contrast-filled aorta taking into account x-ray magnification (Fig. 3).

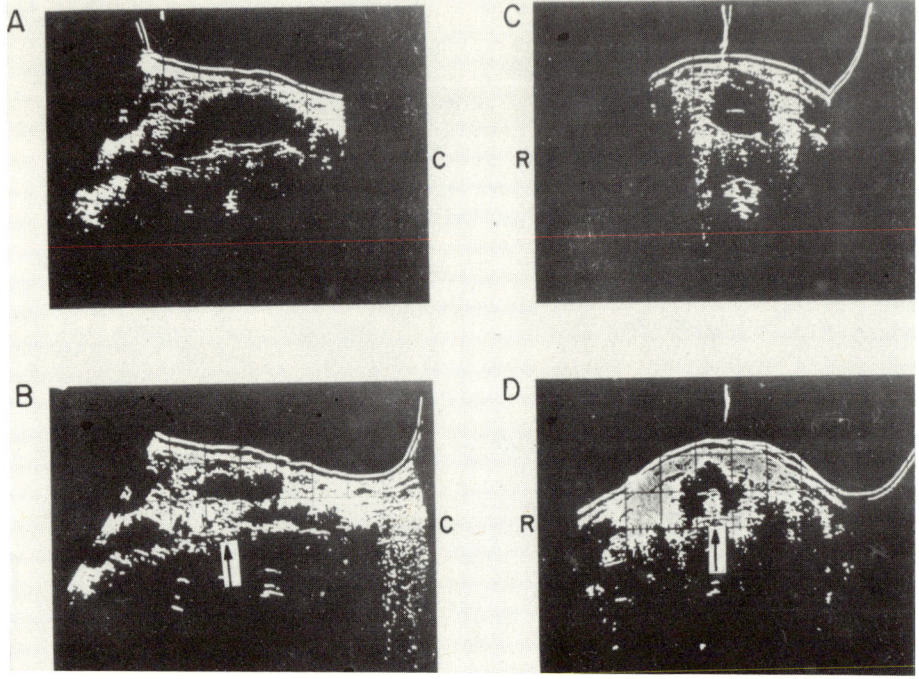

Figure 2. B-scan ultrasonograms (longitudinal A,B and transverse C,D) of a distally located aortic aneurysm. Upper tracings (A,C) were obtained before and lower tracings (B,D) after the injection of indocyanine green. Note the multiple echoes filling the non-clot portion of the aorta after the injection of the indocyanine green (arrows).

The discrepancy between the two (remaining echo-free zone) was thus due to clot, which was confirmed at surgery in both cases. In these cases the grey scale B-scan mode of display recorded echoes from a significant portion of the clot (Fig. 4). The blood-filled lumen remained essentially echo-free.

Discussion: It has been noted that, when roentgenographic or nuclear contrast aortography is performed on patients having an aortic aneurysm, the lumen demonstrated is sometimes much smaller than that demonstrated by the ultrasonic examination. In most cases, secondary signs of aneurysm are shown on the contrast aortogram; that is, draping of vessels, such as the superior mesenteric artery, around the aneurysm. The question has been raised as to the reason for this discrepancy.

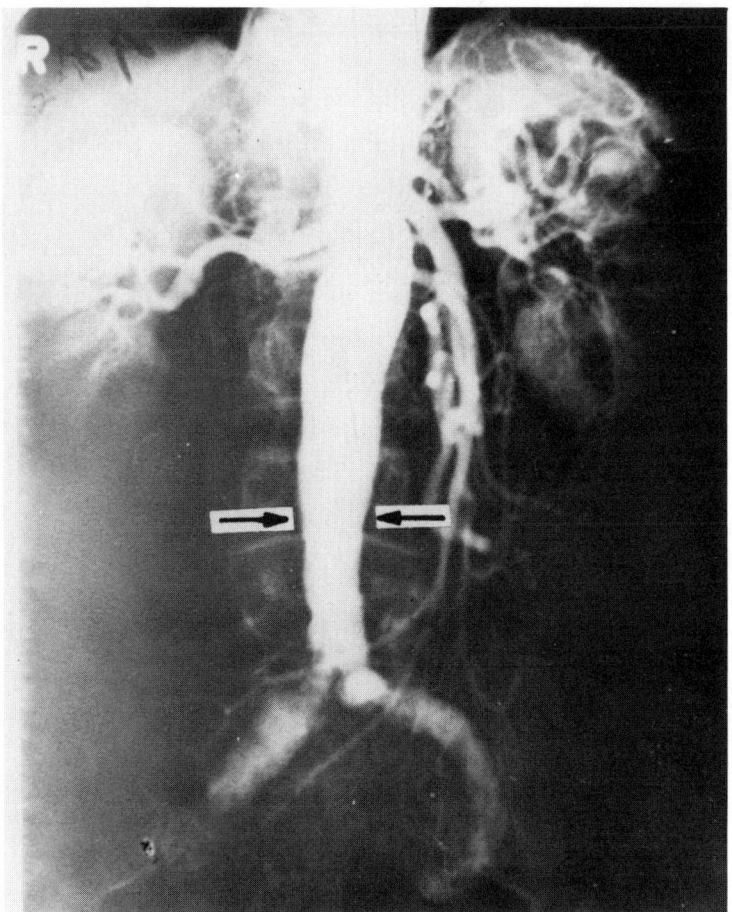

Figure 3. Roentgenogram shows contrast filling the aortic lumen. except for minor stretching of the superior mesenteric artery, the extensive aneurysm is not demonstrated due to the presence of the clot. The diameter of the contrast filled portion compares favorably to the multiple echoes produced by the indocyanine green injection on Figure 2 (arrows).

The most logical explanation is that this discrepancy is due to the presence of internal clot. In some of these cases, internal echoes are recorded from the region where aortography

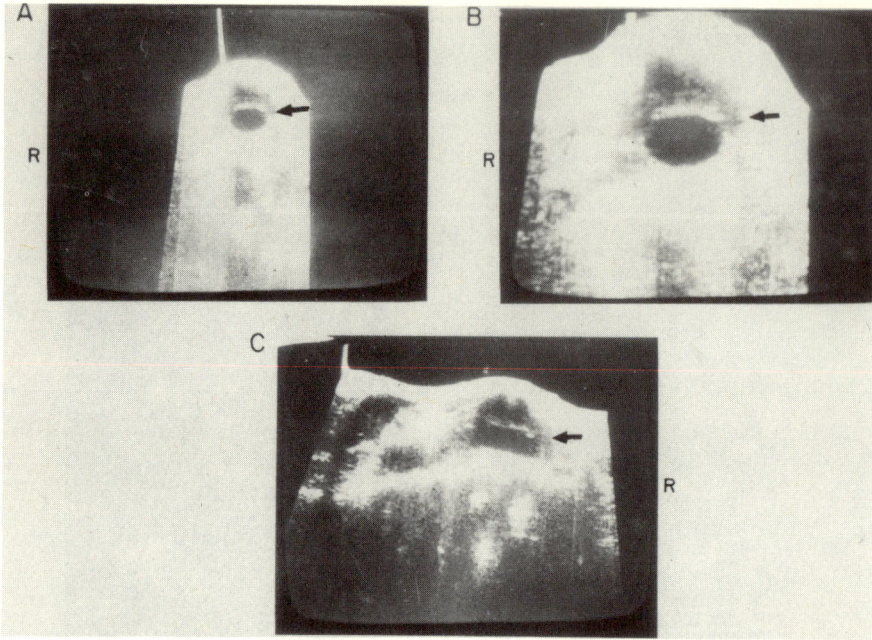

Figure 4. Grey scale B-scan ultrasonograms (transverse A, magnified B, and longitudinal C) demonstrate the separation (arrows) between the relatively echo-free inferiorly located blood filled lumen and the superiorly located clot.

shows lack of filling by the contrast material. However, these echoes are often not well defined nor do they account for the entire space.

In order to confirm the hypothesis that the discrepancy between the internal lumen diameter as recorded by contrast aortography and by ultrasound is due to clot, ultrasonic B-scan examinations were obtained during the simultaneous injection of indocyanine green into the lumen of the aortic aneurysm. These experiments were performed during the routine contrast aortographic examination of patients for ultrasonically detected aortic aneurysm prior to surgery. As a result of these experiments, typical snow-storm patterns characteristic of indocyanine green were demonstrated in both longitudinal and transverse planes conforming in dimensions and position to the lumen detected by contrast aortography. The remainder of the

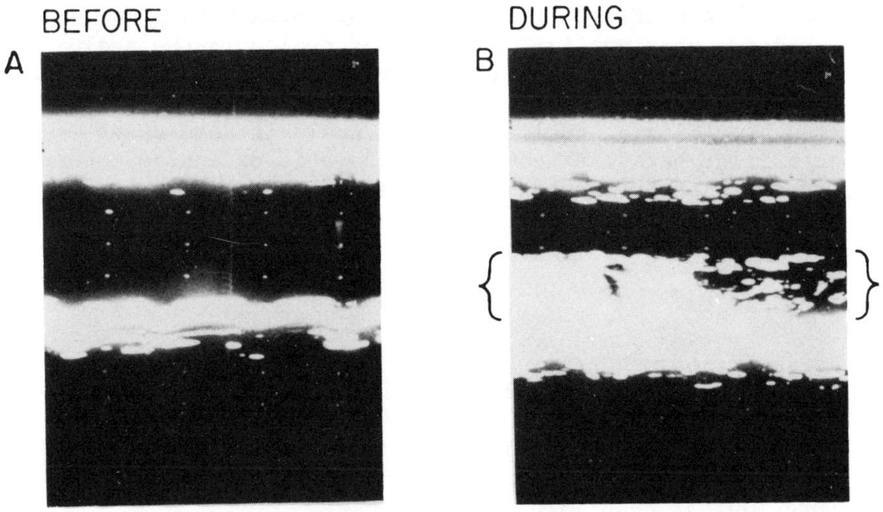

BEFORE   DURING

A   B

Figure 5. M-mode ultrasonograms obtained before (A) and after (B) the injection of indocyanine green resulting in multiple echoes filling the inferior portion of the previously echo-free lumen (brackets). Note the expansile motion of the aortic walls

echo-free area was thus filled with clot. In addition to the B-scan ultrasonograms obtained, M-mode ultrasonic displays were also recorded to confirm the expansile motion of the aortic walls. As with the B-scan ultrasonograms, the snow-storm appearance was seen to fill only that portion of the previously echo-free area not filled by clot (Fig. 5).

It is suggested that a uniform gel-like clot, similar to the vitreous of the eye, will have poor internal reflecting interfaces and thus will produce very weak or no echoes. When internal echoes are easily recorded, a more organized, vascularized clot is generally present. Grey scale B-scan ultrasonography does show promise in its ability to detect echoes from minimal reflecting interfaces. Thus, with this technique, differentiation between the blood filled lumen and clot appears to be more easily recorded.

It has been suggested that nuclear scanning should be considered the non-invasive procedure of choice in the evaluation for aneurysm. However, experiments conducted in this laboratory with injection of indocyanine green, indicate that aortography performed by utilizing nuclear imaging could in some cases produce a false-negative result when there is extensive internal clot, as can also be the case with roentgenographic contrast aortography.

REFERENCES:

1. Goldberg, BB., Ostrum, BJ., Isard, HH.: Ultrasonic aortography. JAMA 198:353-358,1966

2. Goldberg, BB., Lehman, JS.: Aortosonography: Ultrasound measurement of the abdominal and thoracic aorta. Arch Surg 100:652-655, 1970

3. Leopold, GR.: Ultrasonic abdominal aortography. Radiology 96:9-14, 1970

4. Leopold GR., Goldberger, LE., Bernstein EF.: Ultrasonic detection and evaluation of abdominal aortic aneurysms. Surgery 72:939-945, 1972

5. Nusbaum JW., Freimanis, AK., Thomford, NR.: Echography in the diagnosis of abdominal aortic aneurysm. Arch Surg 102:385-388, 1971

6. Crawford, ES., DeBakey, ME., Morris GC., Garrett, HE., Howell JF,: Aneurysm of the abdominal aorta. Surg Clin North Am 46:963-978, 1966

7. Robicsck, F., Daugherty, HK., Mullen, DC., Tam, W., Scott, WP.: The value of angiography in the diagnosis of unruptured aneurysms of the abdominal aorta. Ann Thorac Surg 2:538-550, 1971

8. Bergan JJ., Yao, JST., Henkin, RE., Quinn, JL.: Radionuclide aortography in detection of arterial aneurysms. Arch Surg 109:80-83, 1974

9. Gramiak, R., Shah, PM., Kramer, DH.: Ultrasound cardiography; contrast studies in anatomy and function. Radiology 92:939-948, 1969

10. Goldberg, BB: Suprasternal ultrasonography. JAMA 215:245-250, 1971

RADIATION THERAPY PLANNING USING ULTRASOUND

Saar Porrath, M.D.; Leopold T.Avallone,M.D.

Department of Radiology and Radiation Therapy
Santa Monica Hospital Medical Center
Santa Monica, California 90404

Ultrasound is playing an increasingly important role in radiation therapy planning. It now becomes possible through the use of ultrasound to visualize tumors, which were previously only partially felt and at times incompletely managed. Not only can a better estimate of the extent of the tumors be made, but because of this a change in radiation therapy planning has come about as well. It is possible through contour scanning to get a better appreciation for the actual tumor dose and the dose to the underlying organs.

Contour scanning is done on all radiation therapy patients. The resultant ultrasound scan is then projected life size on to a piece of tracing paper. (Figure 1 - Transverse scan of the pelvis with carcinoma of the vagina - post-vaginectomy).

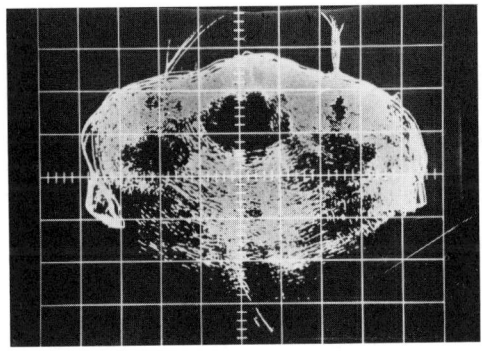

Figure 1.

The patient's contour is then drawn and the location of the vital organs and tumor is put in proper perspective. The radiation therapy portals are drawn in as well. This is then computerized and accurate dose measurement can be ascertained to both the tumor and vital structures. (Figure 2 shows the computerized scan).

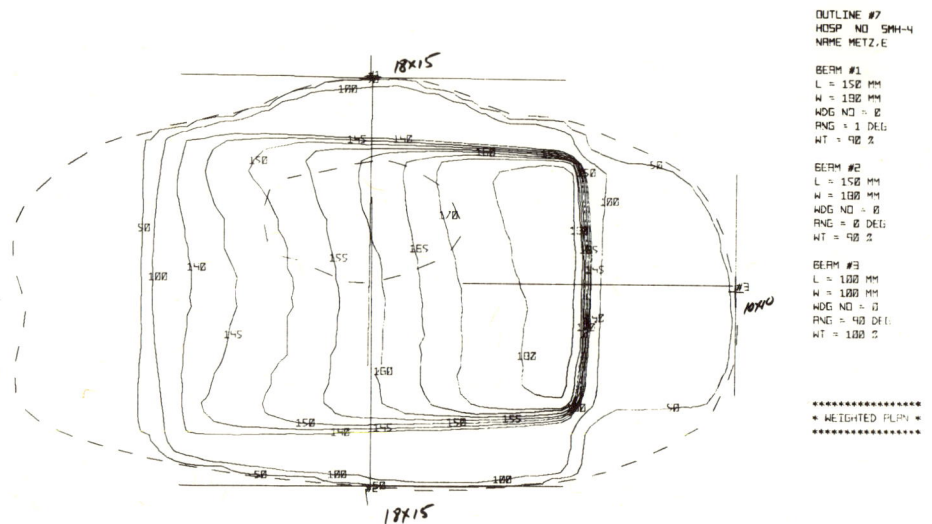

Figure 2.

Contours are obtained on all abdominal and pelvic radiation therapy cases, and they are extremely useful in breast cases for determination of the size of the chestwall, as well as for head and neck tumors with irregular contours. It is possible with ultrasound to get an accurate measurement of the true depth of the spinal cord so that the dose to the spinal cord can be known. When treating pancreatic lesions the pancreas can be scanned by ultrasound, and the area in question, as with other tumors, can be adequately included in the radiation therapy portals.

We have found ultrasound to be more accurate than nuclear medicine in marking out the kidney's so that they can be blocked from further radiation. (Figure 3 shows a longitudinal scan of the kidney). (Figure 4 shows transverse scans with the kidney marked out.)

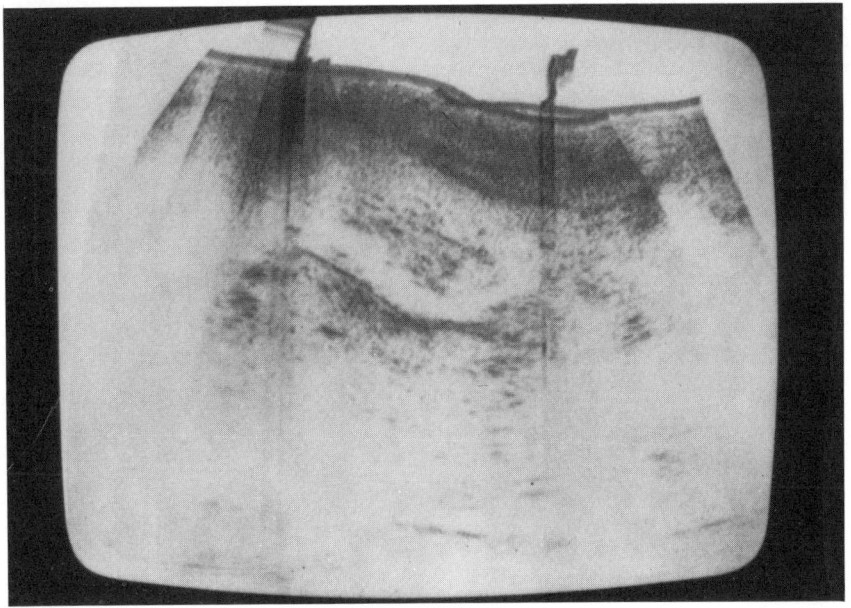

Figure 3.

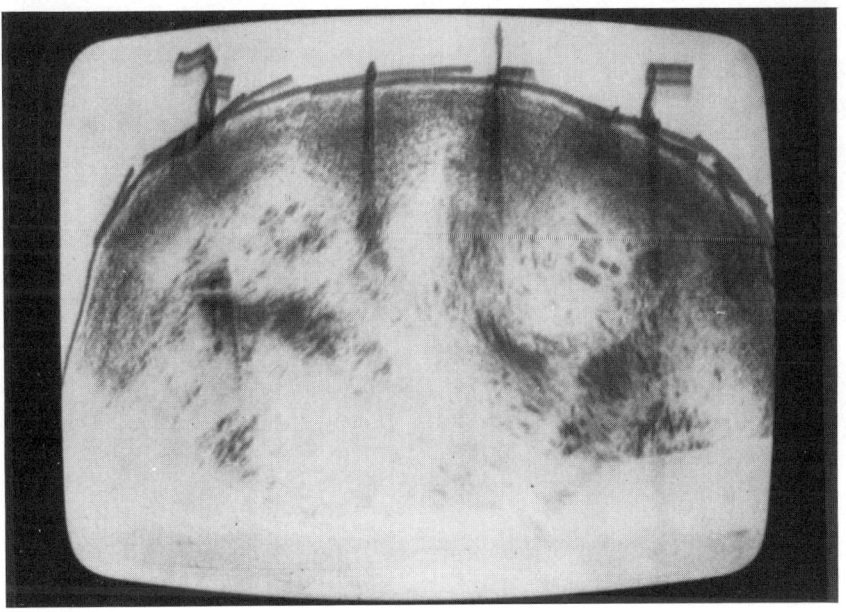

Figure 4.

A very commonly used radiation therapy port for pelvic disease is a 15 x 15 anterior-posterior and posterior-anterior portal. Many radiation therapists like to treat the pelvis with the bladder at least partially distended so as to push the small bowel out of the pelvis to allow for as much small bowel sparing from radiation as possible. We have found that approximately one third of the patients examined for pelvic portals do not have the entire uterus included in the pelvic portal with even a slight degree of distension of the bladder. (Figure 5 shows a longitudinal scan of a patient with carcinoma of the cervix. The patient has a slightly enlarged uterus which extends slightly beyond the upper edge of the radiation therapy portal as delineated by the small line extending of the skin above the uterus). (Figure 6 shows a transverse scan with the uterus far to the right on the same patient as figure 5. The uterus extends almost to the pelvic wall).

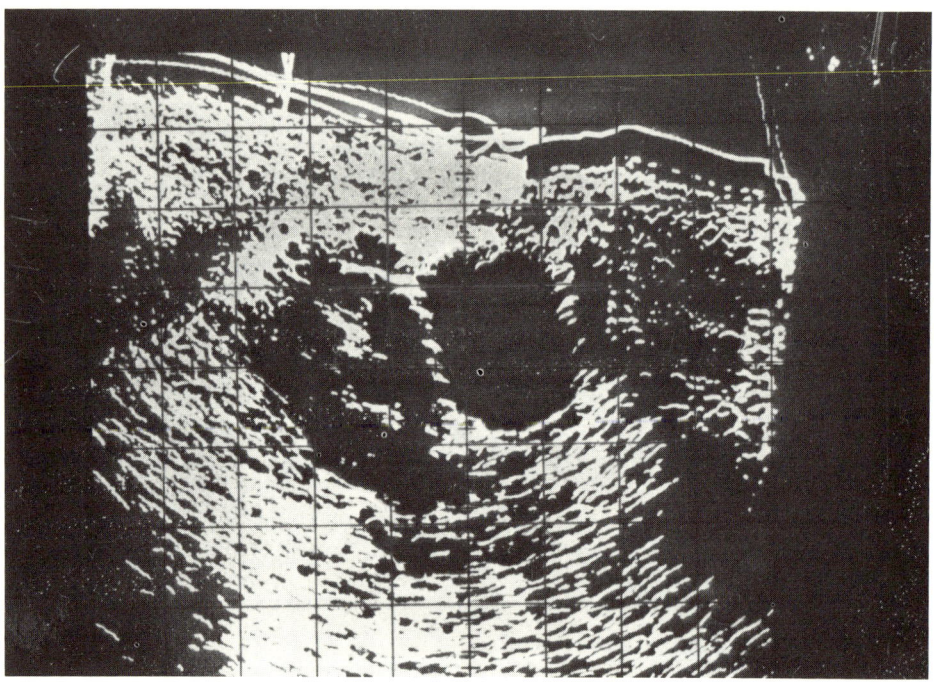

Figure 5.

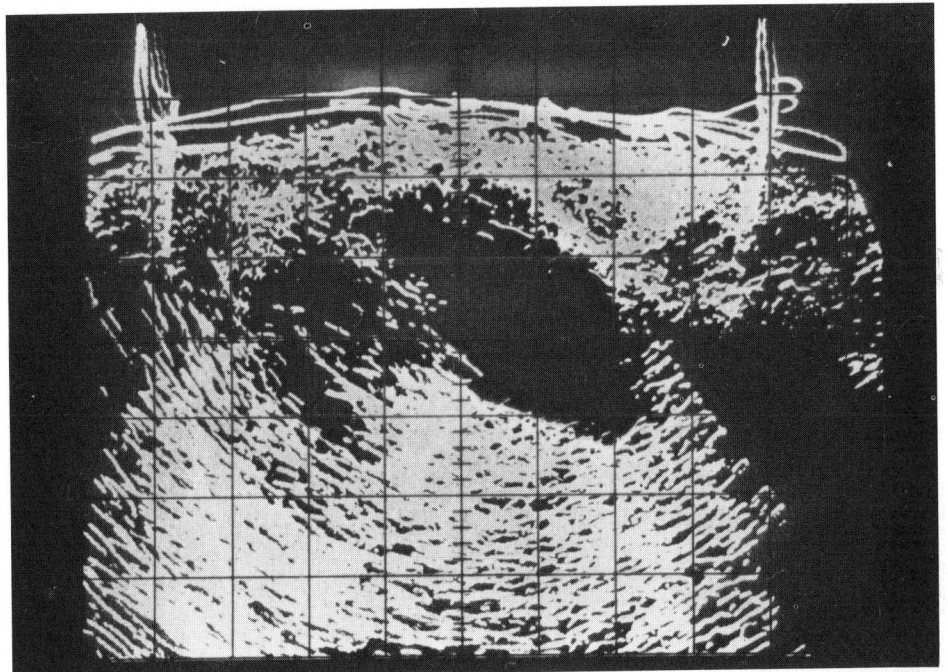

Figure 6.

The uterus as well is seldom a midline structure and is very commonly off to one side. Eccentricity of the uterine position, as well as the fact that the uterus on many patients extends beyond the radiation therapy portal with an even partially filled bladder, has made it necessary for us to change our radiation therapy planning to fit the individual case. Many patients must be treated with an empty bladder or the radiation portal extended.

Ultrasound is also extremely helpful for checking position of radium tandems within the uterus to get a true depth dose measurement. This should not be done however with the radium in the patient, and therefore is useful only with the afterloading systems.

We have also found that in some cases of bladder tumors the bladder is eccentric enough that ultrasound is extremely helpful in setting up adequate radiation therapy portals.

Ultrasound is also useful in the work up of radiation therapy portals. It is an excellent way to evaluate nodes and to note a response during the course of radiation therapy. It is extremely helpful for following patients with chemotherapy as well. It has been found to be useful in the evaluation of adrenal metastases as well as other metastatic lesions within the abdomen.

Figure 7 shows a longitudinal scan on a patient with diffuse malignant lymphoma. There is an extremely large retroperitoneal mass present. Figure 8 shows a follow up scan on the same patient with marked reduction in the amount of nodal mass present. Figure 9 is a longitudinal scan on the patient approximately 6 months later following the onset of abdominal pain. The patient's HGB was extremely low. It is felt that the upper mass represents the tumor and the lower of the two masses represents a retroperitoneal bleed which cleared rapidly.

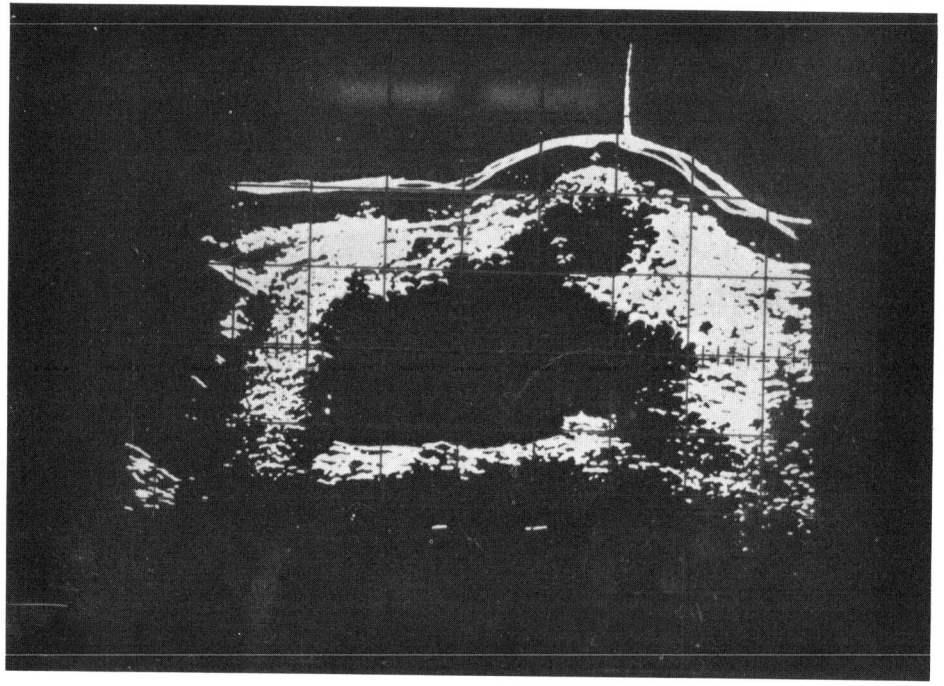

Figure 7.

RADIATION THERAPY PLANNING USING ULTRASOUND

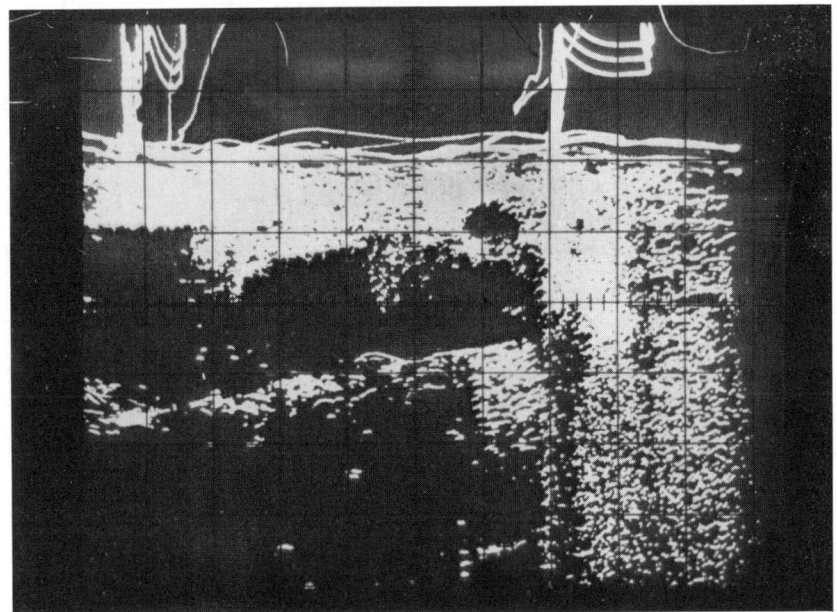

Figure 8.

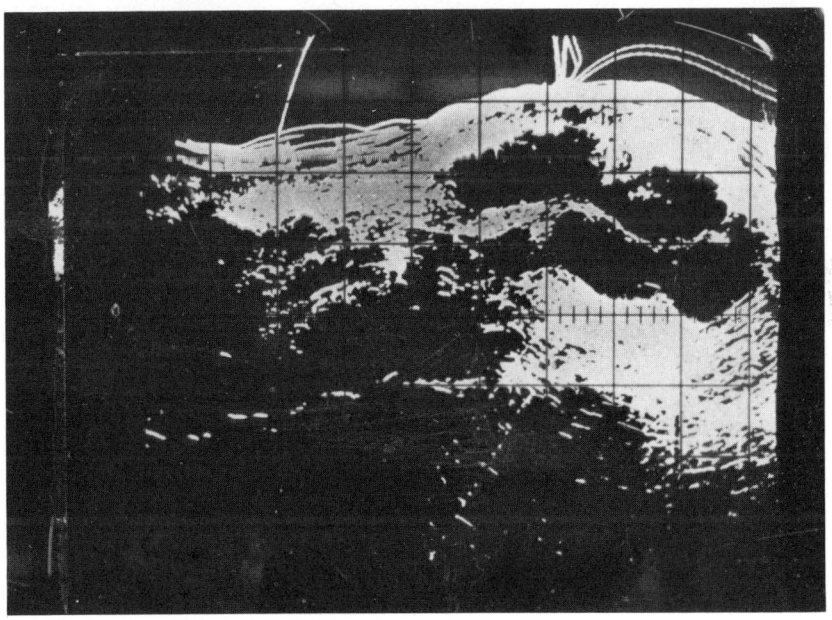

Figure 9.

In summary, ultrasound is an extremely useful addition to radiation therapy, which gives us the "eyes" to go along with the "hands" in evaluating and treating tumors.

ACCURACY OF GREY-SCALE ULTRASONIC EXAMINATION OF THE LIVER

1.K.J.W.Taylor;2.J.P.Glees; 3.I.A.Smith; 4.D.A.Carpenter
1.Department of Radiology, Yale University, New Haven.Conn;2.Dept.of Radiotherapy and 3. Dept. of Medicine, Royal Marsden Hospital,Sutton, Surrey, UK; 4. N.A.L.,5 Hickson Road,Millers Point, NSW 2001, Australia

Liver examination by grey-scale ultrasonography has been under extensive clinical evaluation on over 4000 patients over the past two years at the Royal Marsden Hospital. The results have been followed up by independent physicians, the accuracy assessed and compared with other investigative techniques.

Seventy patients with carcinoma of the breast developed metastases during the period of study. Ultrasound was found to be superior to all other techniques in excluding liver involvement and only equalled by the results of acid phosphatase estimation in detecting liver involvement when it was present.

Fiftytwo patients came to a staging laparotomy for Hodgkins' disease or a lymphoma. Again, ultrasound was found to be superior to clinical examination, isotope examination or acid phosphatase estimation in excluding liver involvement. Both isotope and ultrasound examination were superior to multiple needle biopsies for detecting liver involvement.

In a series of patients with carcinoma of the bronchus, hepatomegaly associated with cor pumonale could be distinguished from malignant involvement. The ability to accurately display liver metastases permits the response to therapy to be assessed both by change in size and consistency.

In patients with various liver pathologies, different types of space-occupying lesions could be differentiated while diffuse liver disease can be recognised by the pattern of the liver parenchyma. Thus cirrhosis, fatty infiltration, lymphocyte infiltration, cholangitis and other inflammatory states produce recognisably different ultrasonic appearances.

The most accurate results were found in patients with cholestatic jaundice - a difficult diagnostic problem with other non-invasive techniques. A series of 104 consecutive patients with cholestatic jaundice were followed up. Of these, 66 had an extrahepatic cause for biliary obstruction and this was correctly predicted in 64 cases. In some it was possible to demonstrate the site of the obstruction but once the surgical nature of the pathology had been established, percutaneous cholangiography and laparotomy were indicated. Of the remaining 40 patients with intrahepatic causes of jaundice, all were correctly predicted as such and in some, a precise diagnosis was possible.

The equipment used was custom-built and results in fine resolution. The machine was also specifically designed for liver, rather than obstetric scanning. Considerable experience has been accumulated in the interpretation of scans but these results justify an adequate period of training in the method. Scans will be shown of the diagnostic criteria that were used in the diagnosis of each group of patients.

CORRELATIVE STUDIES BETWEEN MULTI-PLANE TOMOGRAPHIC NUCLEAR IMAGING

AND GREY SCALE ULTRASOUND IN EXTRA AND INTRAHEPATIC ABNORMALITIES

W. F. Sample, M.D.; Jonathan B. Po, M.D.; Norman D. Poe,
M.D.; L. Stephen Graham, Ph.D.; Leslie R. Bennett, M.D.
Department of Radiological Sciences
University of California, Los Angeles, CA 90024

Differentiating between intra and extrahepatic abnormalities by conventional nuclear imaging has often been difficult particularly in the transitional and left lobe regions of the liver. The development of a commercially available multi-plane tomographic scanner has provided a means of better visualizing these difficult regions in three dimensions. In addition, the improved resolution and intra-organ detail now possible with commercially available second generation grey scale ultrasound has provided a rapid way of further localizing and characterizing the isotope defects.

With the multi-plane nuclear imaging system, six equidistant planes are obtained from each of the anterior and posterior scintillation probes. The normal regions of diminished isotope uptake in the hepatic vein, gallbladder, and portal regions have been better localized in the anteroposterior dimension. Normal variations in the location and size of gallbladder and portal regions are more clearly discernible. Lesions presenting anterior or posterior to these normal areas of decreased uptake are more readily distinguished. By more accurately visualizing the regions of normal liver uptake around the abnormal areas of diminished isotope accumulation, the intra and extrahepatic differentiation is more easily made.

Although the localization of isotope defects has been improved by tomographic nuclear imaging, a rapid means of confirming the intra or extrahepatic location as well as characterizing the nature of the defect has been required. The improved resolution and new intra-organ grey tone patterns now available with second generation grey scale ultrasound has fulfilled this need.

The almost routine visualization of the portal vein and its

first order tributaries, the hepatic veins and their junction with the inferior vena cava, the variations in size of the left lobe of the liver, and the variety of gallbladder configurations with grey scale ultrasound has clarified the nature of unusual isotope defects resulting from anatomic normal variations. Prominent isotope defects in the portal region secondary to a dilated biliary system have been better localized by the tomographic nuclear imaging and distinguished from prominent portal veins by closely following the tubular structures with grey scale ultrasound and demonstrating lack of continuity with the inferior vena cava and portal venous system.

The improved ability to localize prominent normal or abnormal isotope defects in the anteroposterior dimension as well as to distinguish various types of intra and extrahepatic abnormalities by means of their grey tone patterns have led to more specific and accurate diagnoses. Isotope defects of similar size and configuration but in maximal focus at different levels in the A-P dimension on the tomographic nuclear images resulting from normal anatomic variants and intra or extrahepatic pathology have been found. Grey scale ultrasonic evaluation of these defects have distinguished different types of intrahepatic metastases, abscesses, cysts, and unusual portal vein configurations or extrahepatic pancreatic and nodal abnormalities.

From over 50 cases examined by both modalities, examples of the various principles and entities outlined above will be shown.

ULTRASONIC EVALUATION OF THE COMMON BILE DUCT

G.S. Perlmutter, B.B. Goldberg

The Reading Hospital, Reading Pennsylvania and
Episcopal Hospital
Philadelphia, Pennsylvania

While early reports in the literature suggest that grey scale B-scan ultrasound is capable of delineating the common bile duct, there has been no anatomical confirmation. This report will deal with in vivo experiments that establish beyond doubt the fact that grey scale B-scan ultrasound is able to delineate the common bile duct especially when it is dilated. Patients with jaundice were examined ultrasonically utilizing commercially available grey scale equipment. Portions of the bile duct were visualized consistently in the presence of extrahepatic obstruction. It was often possible to demonstrate the cause of the duct dilatation, i.e. choledocholithiasis. Transhepatic cholangiography as well as surgery confirmed the initial ultrasonic impressions. The common bile duct was localized after surgery in those patients in which a T-tube had been inserted. By injection of contrast material the exact course of the common bile duct could be marked on the skin surface, thus allowing for maximum visualization by grey scale ultrasound. Experiments were then performed in vivo with injection initially of contrast material followed by indocyanine green, both of which contained micro-air bubbles. These micro-air bubbles produced strong reflections of the ultrasonic beam resulting in a snowstorm type appearance filling in the previously echo-free area representing the dilated common bile duct. Injections of air into the duct through the T-tube resulted in disappearance of the posterior wall due to reflection of the beam almost totally by the air which rose to the anterior surface of the duct. Serial ultrasonograms demonstrated regression in duct size. Those obtained before and after removal of stones showed disappearance of the strong intraluminal echoes after removal of the stones. Thus by the injection into the common bile duct of indocyanine green containing micro-air bubbles through previously inserted T-tubes, the initial reports that grey scale ultrasound could record the common bile duct was confirmed.

NORMAL AND ABNORMAL PANCREATIC ECHOGRAPHY

D. B. Rosenberg[1]; K. Haber[1]; W. M. Asher[2]

[1]University of Arizona Medical Center, Tucson, AZ
[2]San Diego Regional Medical Center, San Diego, CA

   Prior to ultrasonic B-scanning, imaging of the pancreas had been both difficult and lacking in diagnostic accuracy. Conventional radiology, including barium studies, and radionuclide imaging of the pancreas are often suboptimal. The diagnostic accuracy of selective angiography is approximately 80 percent. Furthermore, this is an invasive procedure with definite incidences of patient morbidity, precluding its use as a screening procedure.
   In the recent literature, echography of the pancreas has received increasing attention. Its usefulness has been well shown. It has become a familiar tool at this institution in the routine, early work-up of patients suspected of pancreatic disease. Our experience with this study will be reviewed.
   Before the commercial availability of the latest generation of persistent Gray-scale display equipment, the normal pancreas could not be identified. The expected area of the pancreas was seen to be an amorphous cluster of echoes, inseparable from vessels, fascial planes and other retroperitoneal structures. The highly complex acoustic nature of the pancreas is most probably due to its histological inhomogeneity and fibrous nature. The increasing sensitivity and superior video display of Gray-scale ultrasonography has allowed visualization of the normal pancreas in the vast majority of cases. This was demonstrated by comparison with images obtained during retrograde cannulations of the pancreatic duct and pancreatic arteriography. The technique and results have been described by us elsewhere.
   The pancreas is a highly variable organ in size, shape and position within the upper abdomen. One of the few constant features about its location is that it lies directly in front of the aorta and vena cava near the midline. Therefore, all of our pancreatic scans are begun by scanning at or near the midline in

longitudinal direction. The left lobe of the liver serves as a sounding tank for beam transmission to and from the expected retroperitoneal location of the pancreas. In the normal case, this allows visualization of a separate, ovoid structure lying just anterior to the great vessels. This represents the body or medial portion of the head of the pancreas. Once this structure is identified, the cephalocaudad boundaries can be marked on the patient's skin. Repeating this procedure at 1 cm increments both to the right and to the left of the midline usually allows mapping of the majority of the pancreas, even in the normal. Some difficulty is, however, frequently encountered in the region of the tail of the pancreas due to overlying gas within the intestinal tract. Transverse scanning is carried out in a usually oblique orientation over the long axis of the pancreas which had previously been marked out from the images of the longitudinal sections.

Of the more than 70 patients with suspected pancreatic pathology, good visualization of the majority of the pancreas was obtained in 84%. The main reasons for non-visualization were intestinal gas, barium within the bowel, patient obesity or unusually small size or unusually high position of the left lobe of the liver.

The size of the normal pancreas was, of course, quite variable from patient to patient. In addition, there is an area of overlap between the upper limits of normal in size and pathologic enlargement. An analysis of pancreatic size in patients in this study, as well as in previously reported studies, indicates that the body or tail of the pancreas is abnormal if it is greater than 2.9 cm in AP dimension or 3.6 cm in cranio-caudad dimension ($p < 0.05$). Most of the normal patients showed dimensions less than 2.4 cm and 3.0 cm in AP and cranio-caudad dimensions, respectively. The head of the pancreas is somewhat more variable in size and the upper limits of normal is 3.4 cm in AP dimension.

Acute pancreatitis could usually be differentiated from either chronic pancreatitis or tumor. The typical echographic picture of acute pancreatitis consists of enlargement of the pancreas and a more sonolucent pattern than normal. In those cases in which acute pancreatitis could not be differentiated from other pancreatic pathology, many patients had been studied during the healing stage of the disease process. Serial scanning was often helpful in further differentiation.

Unless marked enlargement in the region of the pancreas could be demonstrated, definite differentiation between chronic pancreatitis and carcinoma of the pancreas could not be reliably made. However, when carcinoma of the pancreas involves the Ampulla of Vater, obstruction of the biliary system could often be visualized. This was seen by actual visualization of the dilated common bile duct or intrahepatic biliary radicals. Furthermore, a dilated gall bladder which does not contract upon administration of a fatty meal was frequently present.

Utilizing Gray-scale imaging and a knowledge of normal anatomy, most of the normal pancreas can almost always be identified.

Utilizing echographic morphologic data and clinical information, a reasonable impression of pathologic processes within the pancreas can be obtained. Although there is some overlap in size between the normal and the diseased pancreas, size information can be quite helpful.

GREY SCALE ULTRASONOGRAPHY IN THE DIFFERENTIAL DIAGNOSIS OF CHRONIC SPLENOMEGALY

K. J. W. Taylor

Department of Radiology
Yale University School of Medicine
New Haven, CT   06510

Grey scale ultrasonography involves the selective amplification of very low-level echoes which emanate from the internal structure of organs. Diffuse pathology may be apparent both by an abnormal echo pattern and/or abnormal echo amplitudes.

In 60 patients presenting with chronic splenomegaly, it was noted that the echo amplitude seemed to be strongly related to the pathology. Three groups of diseases could be differentiated: very low-level echoes are characteristic of untreated malignant infiltration of the spleen, for example, in the lymphomas and leukemias. However, energetic treatment may increase the echo amplitude returned. In contrast, inflammatory causes of splenomegaly produce very high-level echoes, which permitted successful differentiation from malignancy in 90 per cent of cases.

An intermediate group exists returning medium-level echoes; and these are found in predominantly benign conditions, most commonly in splenomegaly secondarily to portal hypertension. In particular, 18 vinyl chloride workers were examined, some of whom had induced portal hypertension with splenomegaly; and both the size and the typical consistency of the spleen were of value in the non-intrusive display of pathology induced by industrial exposure to a hepatotoxic agent. Digital A-scan analysis confirmed three different groups of splenic pathology.

Ultrasonic display of spleen to date has merely recorded the organ contour, while the grey scale modification strongly suggests successful differential diagnosis may be made from the displayed consistency.

SOLID RENAL LESIONS: ULTRASONIC AND ANGIOGRAPHIC CORRELATION

N. F. Maklad, V. P. Chuang, B.D. Doust and
J. E. Curran
Department of Radiology, University of Michigan
at Wayne County General Hospital
Eloise, Michigan 48132

Over a period of two years, 52 solid (non-cystic) renal lesions were evaluated by renal echography and angiography. The echographic analysis was done after a possible or definite space-occupying lesion was discovered on intravenous uorgraphy. All cystic lesions were excluded. The solid lesions were analyzed echographically for distortion of renal outline or calyceal echoes, identifiable mass lesions, and homogeneity as compared with the normal kidney tissue. Using these criteria, 21 tumors were diagnosed echographically, and were divided into two groups. In the first group (13 patients) the tumor showed more echoes than the surrounding and adjacent normal kidney tissue. In the second group (8 patients) the tumors showed less echoes.

The renal masses were classified angiographically into two broad categories - hypervascular and hypovascular, according to the over all density of the mass lesion in the nephrographic phase and the presence and number of pathologic vessels.

The echographic pattern of the tumor was correlated with the vascularity as revealed on angiography. The first group of 13 patients showing more echoes, proved to be hypervascular renal cell carcinoma in nine patients, and hypovascular renal cell carcinoma in four patients angiographically. In the second group of eight patients with less echoes, four were hypovascular renal cell carcinoma, two transitional cell carcinoma, and two metastases. All 21 cases were proven by surgery and pathology.

Of the 31 cases with normal echograms, only one proved to be a hypovascular renal cell carcinoma. In the remaining 30 patients,

19 had normal angiography, and two negative exploration. The other nine patients had a subsequent clinical course denoting absence of a tumor.

The study indicates that all hypervascular renal cell carcinomas showed more echoes than surrounding normal and adjacent renal tissue. Four hypovascular renal cell carcinomas showed more echoes, and four showed less echoes than the normal kidney tissue. Transitional cell carcinomas showed less echoes as did metastases.

The most important contribution of echograms in evaluating solid renal masses is in those cases that show hypovascular lesions on angiography and more echoes on ultrasound (4 cases). These are difficult to interpret angiographically. However, on echographic analysis, if more echoes are found, then these all prove to be renal cell carcinomas. In cases which show lesions that are more homogeneous on the echogram, angiography plays an important role in demonstrating pathologic vessels.

The role of echography in evaluating suspected renal masses should not be limited to differentiating cystic from non-cystic masses only. Every effort should be made to delineate the echoing characteristics of the lesion seen on the intravenous urogram. In those patients who have a questionable renal mass on intravenous urograms and a normal echogram, angiography is not required. Follow-up with intravenous urography or echography is recommended. Angiography is indicated in symptomatic patients or in those in whom a definite renal mass on intravenous urography is seen.

THE PLACE OF B-SCAN ULTRASOUND IN THE EXAMINATION OF

KIDNEYS NOT SEEN ON INTRAVENOUS PYELOGRAPHY

R.C. Sanders, B.M., M.R.C.P., F.F.R.

Department of Radiology, The Johns Hopkins Medical
Institutions
Baltimore, Maryland 21205

If radiological visualization of the kidneys at intravenous pyelography with tomography fails, further radiological techniques for the evaluation of the kidneys have included retrograde pyelography, angiography, and anterograde pyelography. All of these procedures carry risks and we have found that B-scan abdominal ultrasound represents a superior technique for the initial evaluation of nonvisualizing kidneys since it is harmless, safe, rapid and easy. In most instances, the nonvisualizing kidney has a characteristic ultrasonic pattern.

A series of 64 patients with unilateral or bilateral nonvisualizing kidneys have been examined by ultrasound. Twenty-eight patients with previously unknown diagnoses were in severe renal failure with high blood urea nitrogens. Of these, 16 had small end-stage kidneys, six had bilateral hydronephrosis, one had polycystic kidney, two hydronephrosis and a small kidney, two subacute glomerulonephritis, and one prerenal azotemia. One example of small end-stage kidneys was missed at ultrasonography because it was so small and subsequently diagnosed by retrograde pyelogram. The remainder were diagnosed ultrasonically on the basis of the finding of a small kidney which had normal pelvic echoes. The six examples of bilateral hydronephrosis were all correctly diagnosed on the basis of sonolucent center to the usual pelvic echo pattern or the development of a sonolucent lubulated sac. The single example of polycystic kidney was recognized by the presence of numerous irregularly walled cysts of differing sizes. Correct diagnoses were made of the two examples of unilateral hydronephrosis and contralateral small kidney and three cases with normal sonograms in patients who were suffering from prerenal azotemia or subacute glomerulonephritis.

Of the 36 patients with unilateral renal failure, 20 patients with unilateral hydronephrosis were recognized ultrasonically, eight patients with multicystic kidney were correctly diagnosed preoperatively by the presence of multiple cysts and absence of a pelvicalyceal pattern. In three out of six patients with apparent absence of the kidney at intravenous pyelography, small kidneys were found at sonography. Individual examples of patients with pyonephrosis and perirenal abscess, renal vein thrombosis, renal artery occlusion, tumor, and trauma with nonvisualizing intravenous pyelograms were seen. Either a characteristic ultrasonic pattern was found or the diagnosis could be made taking the findings at intravenous pyelography along with the sonogram.

LONG-TERM RESULTS OF ULTRASONICALLY GUIDED PERCUTANEOUS ASPIRATION OF RENAL CYSTS

Fl. Jensen; J. Kvist Kristensen; H. H. Holm

Ultrasonic Laboratory

Gentofte Hospital, DK-2900 Hellerup Denmark

In 1969 Westby reported shrinkage or disappearence of solitary renal cysts, after injection of an oil soluble contrast-medium, pantopaque ®. In the Ultrasonic Laboratory Gentofte Hospital we often diagnose renal cysts and simultaneously carry out an ultrasonically guided puncture to achieve material for cytological examination. It is always attempted to empty the cyst completely. In this report the results of injection of pantopaque shall be given in a series of 25 patients chosen at random with solitary renal cysts without tumor cells and with a size more than 3 cm in diameter.

In half of the patients only simple emptying was attempted but in the rest a mixture of pantopaque® and isopaque® (a water-soluble contrast medium) was injected through the puncture needle. Moreover the cyst was filled up with carbondioxide and an X-rays taken. This was done to ensure a smooth outline of the cyst wall to exclude a possible solid tumor in the wall. This was not found in any of these cases.

One yearlater, the patients were followed-up by ultrasonic scanning to see if the cysts had reappeared. In about 5o% of cases the cysts had disappeared or diminished. In the remainder of the patients they had regained their previous size. We found no difference between the patients where only emptying was done and the patients where emptying was combined with injection of contrast media. It is concluded that ultrasonically guided renal cyst puncture is a safe and sometimes curable procedure, while we consider the injection of contrast medium superfluous.

ULTRASONIC IMAGING OF THE ABDOMINAL AORTA

WITH REAL - TIME MULTIELEMENT SYSTEMS

Shane H. Abowitt, Edward B. Diethrich, M.D.,
Vincent E. Friedewald, Jr., M.D., Fuad Ibrahim, M.D.,
and Betty J. Phillips
Arizona Heart Institute, St. Joseph's Hospital and
Medical Center, Phoenix, Arizona 85013

Assessment of the abdominal aorta utilizing conventional B-mode ultrasound with static format display provides, in nearly all cases, delineation of aneurysmal pathology. The advent of ultrasonic real-time imaging details aortic dimensions, spatial relationship, displacement, intravascular echoes, and additionally demonstrates the aorta throughout the cardiac cycle. The significant advantage to real-time imaging is the ability to monitor the aorta continuously through the diastolic and systolic intervals.

One hundred patients have undergone real-time ultrasonic scanning for evaluation of the abdominal aorta. The aorta was visualized in all but six (6) patients in which overlying bowel gas or contrast agents interfered with sound propagation. All examinations were accomplished with a 2.25 MHz and 3.5 MHz, free-moving, multielement linear-array transducer with an acoustic power output lower than conventional single-beam imaging systems. Specific acoustical power output will be analyzed by an independent laboratory, and the results of that study will be presented.

The diagnosis of aortic pathology by ultrasonic real-time imaging is based on five parameters: (1) lateral and anterior--posterior dimensions, (2) arterial wall thickness, (3) displacement, (4) intraluminal dimensions, and (5) characteristics of pulsations. This study demonstrates the feasibility of real-time imaging in assessing the abdominal aorta. All ultrasound scans have been compared with clinical findings, plane roentgenograms, and aortograms. Of the 38 surgical cases, the diagnosis was confirmed in every instance at the time of operation. Further, a comparative result with single-beam static display lends credence to the value of real-time imaging in differential diagnosis of abdominal aortic pathology and intra-abdominal pathology.

NORMAL UPPER ABDOMINAL VASCULATURE - A STUDY CORRELATING

CONTACT B SCANNING WITH ARTERIOGRAPHY AND GROSS ANATOMY

M. Leon Skolnick, M.D. and David R. Royal, M.D.
Department of Radiology
School of Medicine - University of Pittsburgh
Pittsburgh, Pennsylvania   15213

A major problem in studying the pancreas by ultrasound B scanning results from the difficulty in precisely identifying the margins of the gland with non-grey scale contact scanners.
Since the pancreas is intimately related to multiple abdominal vessels, some of which partly outline its margins, the ultrasonic imaging of these vessels will improve our ability to determine panreatic size and detect focal mass lesions.
This paper will describe and illustrate with contact scans the normal peripancreatic vasculature in subjects without pancreatic enlargement, correlate these images with arteriograms of the same subjects, and with cross-sectional cadavar photographs and anatomic drawings. The vessels we have visualized include: aorta, the superior mesenteric artery, celiac axis with proximal splenic and hepatic branches, superior mesenteric, splenic and portal veins, inferior vena cava and left renal vein. As one result of our studies, we realized that what several authors have identified as the normal pancreas is really the normal splenic vein arching over the spine.
The Picker Echoview VI system was used. Vessels were initially identified by setting the traverse table moving the scanner arm in continuous scan mode and rapidly scanning first in saggital and then in transverse planes across the upper abdomen. During this procedure the ultrasound images were transiently visualized on the storage oscilloscope in non-storage mode. The operator mentally integrated these images to produce a three dimensional conception of the normal vascular anatomy. Besides distinguishing arteries from veins by their anatomic relationships, arteries can be identified in the T/M mode by their pulsatile motion and veins by the absence of these pulsations, and also often also by their

changing caliber with different phases of respiration.

For permanent recordings, serial single sweep scans at 1 - 5 mm intervals during suspended respiration were performed and photographed from the storage oscilloscope in storage mode.

The key ingredient to photographing the smaller vessels was our performance of multiple closely spaced single sweep scans. A difference of even 1 - 2 mm between serial scans could result in visualizing or not visualizing a particular vessel.

PROSTATIC SCANNING WITH GRAY SCALE ULTRASOUND

Jonathan B. Po, M.D.; W. F. Sample, M.D.; Leonard Marks, M.D.; Rosemary Glenny, CRT
Department of Radiological Sciences and Department of Urology, University of California
Los Angeles, CA 90024

The evaluation of the prostate gland by ultrasonography has been described previously with both suprapubic and perineal scanning as well as transrectal and transurethral scanning. These studies have included evaluations of prostatic size as well as prostatic carcinomas. To our knowledge, the application of gray scale ultrasound to the evaluation of prostatic conditions has not been described. We have evaluated a series of patients with benign prostatic hyperplasia, prostatic malignancies and prostatitis.

The patients with benign prostatic hyperplasia have been evaluated pre-operatively as well as post-transurethral resection or prostatectomy. The clinical estimate of the weight of the gland has been compared with the ultrasonic estimate of the weight and with the weight of the operative specimen. The post-operative studies will be used to see the amount of adenomatous tissue removed at surgery and the correlation between the various methods of evaluation will be described.

The findings in prostatic carcinoma consist of distortion in the contour of the prostatic capsule with poor definition of its posterior margin and greater attenuation of the sound beam in the region of the carcinoma. This is in distinction to benign prostatic hypertrophy where the posterior margin is well visualized, the echogenicity is symmetrical and at times, the surgical capsule itself may be seen.

In prostatitis, the preliminary findings indicate an increased transmission of the sound beam due to the edematous nature of the prostate gland. Seminal vesiculitis is a frequent accompaniment of prostatitis and is difficult to diagnose clinically. The seminal vesicles are routinely seen with gray scale ultrasonography.

The method of examination consists entirely of contact scanning through the suprapubic route, preferably with a full bladder. This study takes less than 15 minutes and is totally atraumatic for the patient leading to ready acceptance by both the patient and the referring physician. The increased resolution with gray scale ultrasound and the simplicity of the study, we feel, outweighs the improved contact and accessibility of the transrectal and transurethral route.

MEASUREMENT OF SIZE AND WEIGHT OF PROSTATE BY MEANS OF TRANSRECTAL ULTRASONOTOMOGRAPHY

Hiroki Watanabe

Department of Urology, Tohoku University
School of Medicine, Sendai, Japan 980

Size and weight of prostates were measured in 95 cases by means of transrectal ultrasonotomography. The error at this measurement likely to be caused by direction of insertion of the transducer and differences in sonic velocity inside the prostate was originally estimated at 5%. This estimation was later confirmed over 5 cases where radical prostatectomy was performed.

The measured prostatic sizes in normal subjects (20 cases) were 20-40 mm (mean, 28.0 ± 5.2) at the supero-inferior (S-I) diameter, 21-34 mm (mean, 27.6 ± 3.7) at the antero-posterior (A-P) diameter and 39-53 mm (mean, 48.1 ± 4.0) at the lateral diameter. The estimated prostatic weight was 12.9-37.1 g (mean, 21.0 ± 5.6).

The sizes in Klinefelter's syndrome (5 cases) were 10-30 mm (mean, 21.0 ± 7.4) at the S-I diameter, 15-30 mm (mean, 20.0 ± 5.9) at the A-P diameter and 28-50 mm (mean, 40.2 ± 8.2) at the lateral diameter. The weight was 2.9-20.2 g (mean, 9.6 ± 6.8).

The sizes in prostatic hypertrophy (50 cases) were 13-60 mm (mean, 38.8 ± 8.5) at S-I diameter, 17-50 mm (mean, 33.8 ± 7.2) at the A-P diameter and 40-79 mm (mean, 54.7 ± 8.2) at the lateral diameter. The weight was 19.6-99.3 g (mean, 45.8 ± 20.9).

The sizes in prostatic cancer (20 cases) was 25-45 mm (mean, 35.5 ± 5.8) at the S-I diameter, 26-48 mm (mean, 34.3 ± 5.9) at the A-P diameter and 42-67 mm (mean, 53.7 ± 6.3) at the lateral diameter. The weight was 14.9-52.3 g (mean, 32.7 ± 9.8). A remarkable reduction of the prostate was recognized in these cases of cancer after hormone treatment.

It was not always possible, however, to decide whether the prostate was normal only from these measurements.

ABDOMINAL ULTRASOUND AND COMPUTERIZED AXIAL RADIOGRAPHIC TOMOGRAPHY

L. Gonzalez, M.D., J. Haaga, M.D., R.J. Alfidi, M.D.

Cleveland Clinic

Cleveland, Ohio 44106

The recent development of Computerized Radiography for total body examination (Delta Scanner, Ohio Nuclear, Inc., Solon, Ohio) has opened a new field of diagnostic imaging with great repercussions in medicine. The predecesor, the EMI Scanner has already proven its great value in the examination of the brain.

Thirty patients with a variety of abdominal conditions have been examined with Ultrasound and with Computerized Radiographic Tomography: renal tumors and cysts, pancreatitis, pancreatic tumors, gastric carcinoma, retroperitoneal tumor, retroperitoneal hematoma, ovarian carcinoma, aneurysm of the aorta.

Pancreatic lesions were equally demonstrated with both modalities. The differentiation between the lesion and the normal pancreas was possible only morphologically and not on the basis of tissue density with either modality. The dilated pancreatic duct has been demonstrated with the Delta Scan which still remains to be done with ultrasonography.

Rather large tumors of the liver, primary and metastatic, have been seen with both modalities, better defined with the radiographic method. Dilated biliary ducts could be seen distinctly in the Delta Scan.

Evaluation of the abdominal aorta could be done advantageously with Ultrasound. In particular, the longitudinal scan offers an overall view of the structure not possible to be done with the Delta Scan.

Retroperitoneal tumors could be equally shown with either modality.

Economic considerations also are presented. The high cost of the Delta Scan will be an important factor to keep in mind in selecting a modality in an institution. The scanning time with the

Delta Unit is prolonged and comparable to the Ultrasound.

Another consideration is the high doses of radiation delivered to the patient during the radiographic tomography which will preclude the use of the Delta Scanner in obstetrics.

To this point the modality of choice for the examination of the abdomen is Ultrasound. The Delta Scan is a modality for the examination of the brain and mediastinum.

USE OF SIMETHICONE IN ABDOMINAL ECHOTOMOGRAPHY

H. Walter Pepper, M.D. and Joan Keene, R.T.,
ASUTS
Downey Park Radiology Medical Group
1213 Coffee Road, Modesto, Calif.

The presence of air in the stomach and the small bowel continuously interferes with abdominal echotomography. Excessive and even small amounts of gaseous accumulations in these organs, virtually precludes obtaining an acceptable scan. Patients with pancreatitis, chronic or active, may frequently have excessive amounts of air in their stomach and small bowel. Gastric intubation has been suggested to eliminate some of this unwanted air but is ineffectual in regard to small bowel accumulation. External abdominal compression, elevation of the feet or head of the patient, in lateral decubitus views may be helpful in displacing the unwanted air but these methods are time consuming and often in vain. When these methods fail, the examination is generally attempted 24- to 78-hours later. Improvement during the subsequent examination is generally unpredictable regardless of any dietary adjustments which have been made.

It has been our practice to administer Simethicone when excessive air interferes with abdominal echotomography. We have had favorable results by administering Mylicon tablets (Simethicone, 80 mg) four times daily for the period preceding repeat echotomography. This period has varied between 24- and 72-hours depending upon the clinical setting and necessity for echotomography. Definite improvement in penetration is evident after Simethicone has been administered.

When re-examination is desired before 24-hours, a small bowel Simethicone cocktail may be helpful. This cocktail contains two to four ml of Mylicon drops, 15 ounces of water and 10 ml of Gastrografin. The ability of Gastrografin to traverse the small bowel within a relatively short time may help the Simethicone to exert its effect rapidly. Re-examination may often be possible within two hours with definite improvement in penetration.

When possible Mylicon (Simethicone) may be administered routinely prior to echotomography, 40 to 80 mg, Q.I.D. for one to three days prior to examination has been quite helpful and may alleviate the need for repeat examination. This method, by no means does away with all problems of non-penetration due to gaseous accumulation but may salvage a sufficient number of otherwise non-diagnostic studies.

Obstetrics and Gynecology

REAL-TIME SCANNING IN THE MANAGEMENT OF

EARLY PREGNANCY COMPLICATIONS

> Donald Ziehm, M.D., Lawrence Findleton,
> Jacklyn Ellis
>
> Ultrasound Diagnostic Services, Arizona Medical Plaza
> 1728 W. Glendale Avenue, Phoenix, Arizona 85021

The management of complications in early pregnancy can be difficult for the physician as well as emotionally trying for the patient. Objective evidence for determining viability of a pregnancy is difficult to obtain. When faced with a threatened or missed abortion, most patients are generally unable to tolerate prolonged conservative therapy. The use of real-time ultrasound scanning is a valuable adjunct in the management of this problem. Fetal movement and/or cardiac activity can be noted as early as 8-9 weeks of gestation. If present, these findings are very reassuring to the patient and helps the physician to more confidently suggest continuation of conservative therapy. In the absence of fetal activity surgical termination can be undertaken.

A series of patients is presented in whom therapeutic decisions have been greatly influenced by the results of real-time scanning. All cases of abnormal early gestation were correctly diagnosed by real-time scanning.

* * * * * * * * * * *

It is estimated that 10-15% of known pregnancies terminate in spontaneous abortions, most of them occurring in the first trimester. The majority of these patients present themselves to the obstetrician at various times in the first 12-14 weeks of pregnancy with vaginal spotting or bleeding and lower abdominal cramping. The diagnosis of threatened abortion is made and the patient is placed at bed rest. Unless the pregnancy aborts soon or the bleeding ceases, the average woman finds it difficult to continue prolonged bed rest. Unfortunately, few objective criteria exist which provide a satisfactory evaluation of the

status of the pregnancy. Positive pregnancy tests are not
always indicative of a normally progressing pregnancy since they
represent only the presence of some viable trophoblastic tissue.
Of particular concern to patients is that chromosomal anomalies
were detected in approximately 25% of analyzed aborted tissue
in some studies. In addition, a smaller number of patients may
develop a missed abortion in which the pregnancy is apparently
proceeding normally, only to have an intrauterine fetal death
occur with subsequent retention of the fetus. Early recognition
of this entity is extremely valuable to the intelligent and
symphathetic management of the patient.

The management of early pregnancy complications has been
greatly simplified with the development of real-time scanning.
For the first time, a dynamic, "real-life" image of the early
intrauterine pregnancy is possible. It's importance in the
management of early pregnancy problems has been well documented.[1,2]
Demonstration of active embryonic or fetal movements within
7-8 weeks of amenorrhea is indicative of a viable pregnancy at
the time of examination. Assuming an accurate menstrual history,
the absence of fetal activity or a gestational sac represents
either an aborted pregnancy or a missed abortion.

In the present study, pregnancies were evaluated with symptoms
of either threatened abortion (vaginal bleeding, cramping) or
missed abortion (decreasing uterine size after a normally
progressing pregnancy to approximately 16-18 weeks of amenorrhea).
In most of the threatened abortions the pregnancy test was
positive at the time of the scan, despite continued vaginal
bleeding. In almost all situations the patient was extremely
anxious, requesting a definitive evaluation of pregnancy well
being. A real-time scanner utilizing a 64 element transducer
array producing 40 images per second* was used employing the full
bladder technique. A viable pregnancy was determined by the
presence of a uterus enlarged consistant with menstrual dates,
with demonstration of active embryonic or fetal movement. In
the presence of this picture, conservative management was
continued and the patient felt greatly reassured. However,
several of these pregnancies proceeded to abortion, despite a
normal appearing scan. Location of the gestational sac within
the uterus was in no way indicative of impending abortion. If
fetal activity was not visualized a D & C was performed within
a few days of the scan.

---

* Advanced Diagnostic Research Corporation, 2202 South Priest Dr.,
Suite 102, Tempe, Arizona 85282.

Questionable scans were repeated in one or two weeks depending upon the individual case. In both incomplete and missed abortions no fetal activity was demonstrated, only scattered echoes being present. The pathological diagnosis confirmed the clinical impression in all cases of incomplete and missed abortions. One case of mole was correctly diagnosed on real-time scanning, confirmation being obtained on tissue examination.

Real-time scanning was found to be very valuable in the management of early pregnancy complications. This technique made it possible to distinquish a normal from a pathological pregnancy. An accurate, objective evaluation was possible to determine the intactness of the early pregnancy complicated by bleeding. Most patients were very appreciative of the opportunity to have an early diagnosis made of pregnancy adequacy, rather than subjecting them to "tincture of time" treatment.

REFERENCES

1. Stocker, J., Desjardins, P., Deleon, A.: Am, J. Obstet. Gynecol. 121: 1084, 1975

2. Hoffbauer, H.: Electromedica No. 3:227, 1970

REAL-TIME GRAY-SCALE B-SCAN ULTRASOUND RECORDING OF HUMAN FETAL

BREATHING MOVEMENTS IN UTERO

C. W. Hohler; H. E. Fox

Perinatal Center
University of Rochester School of Medicine and Dentistry
601 Elmwood Avenue, Rochester, New York 14642

There exists conflict in the obstetric literature as to the existence and significance of fetal respiratory movements in utero in the human. More than 30 years ago it was noted[1] that the then-current 8th edition of Williams Obstetrics stated that conclusions concerning the development of fetal respiratory movements had not been accepted and that there was doubt regarding the significance of some of the reported observations. In the current edition, the fourteenth[2] of the same text, uncertainty still remains regarding the time of onset of fetal respiratory movements and the ability of these movements to cause tidal flow of amniotic fluid.

Some investigators feel that the fetus does not normally make breathing-like movements in utero, yet may do so under conditions of distress.[3-5] The X-ray and Cr-51 tagged RBC studies of McClain[6] and Pritchard[7] are conflicting. Studies by Sadovsky and Yaffe[8] and Hems[9] have shown that assessment of maternally-perceived fetal movements (? gasps) may be a clinically useful tool for assessment of fetal well-being.

Professor Geoffrey Dawes, and his group at the Nuffield Institute in England now feel that fetal breathing movements are normal in human fetal life and may be of use clinically to monitor fetal well-being.[10] A parallel between human fetal breathing and neurological developmental patterns is becoming evident. The accurate documentation of normal breathing pattern development in the human fetus may lead to an indirect method for evaluating fetal brain function throughout gestation.[11]

Boddy and Robinson[12] have shown that fetal breathing movements can be recorded by A-scan ultrasound techniques with a time analog module built in to "gate" over the moving structure of interest, in this case the fetal chest wall. Simultaneous strain gauge records of fetal tracheal pressure changes and A-scan records of fetal chest wall movement have confirmed the validity of such A-scan measurements in sheep.

For the measurement of fetal breathing movements the A-scan ultrasound transducer is placed over the region of the fetal heart. The time "gate" module allows ranging on the thoracic wall. The output from the gated circuit is fed to a polygraph for permanent recording. The record can be calibrated as to amplitude and frequency (range of 30-70 per minute and excursions of 4-6 millimeters).

David Farman[13] and his colleagues at University College Hospital in London have demonstrated some difficulties of the application of A-scan principles to fetal chest wall movement. Maternal and fetal movements may interfere with the recordings from the chest wall. They have even shown that movements may be recorded from the non-pregnant uterus that could be mistaken for fetal chest wall movements. Correct orientation of the transducer in relation to the fetal chest wall is of primary importance and sometimes difficult to obtain.

As part of a major research effort into the presence and significance of human breathing movements in utero at the Rochester Regional Perinatal Center, in New York, we are using both the A-scan (Ekoline 20A Diagnostic Ultrasonoscope, Smith-Kline Instruments, Inc., Palo Alto, California) technique similar to that of Boddy and Robinson[12], as well as a real-time gray-scale B-scanner (Advanced Diagnostic Research, Inc., Phoenix, Arizona) to demonstrate fetal intrauterine chest wall movements.

Definite fetal breathing movements have been seen and recorded using A- and B-scan real-time ultrasound imaging, thus, documenting the existence of such movements in utero and allowing more sophisticated quantitative and qualitative analysis of them, which is in progress.

Limitations of A-scan chest wall movement recording, in our experience, have been as follows:
1. The technique is only qualitative at this point.
2. Proper orientation is difficult to find and maintain over the fetal chest wall.
3. The timing of onset and cessation of movement "episodes" is not always definite.
4. Other motions of maternal and/or fetal origin are not always easily separable, especially, at early gestational ages when the fetus has more room to move about in the amniotic cavity.

Advantages of real-time gray-scale B-scanning for recording fetal chest wall movements are:
1. Orientation is rapidly ascertained and maintained throughout the examination.
2. Timing of specific chest wall movements is sharply defined.
3. Other motions are quickly recognized and discounted.

4. The possibility of quantitation of fetal chest wall movements now exists.

In our experience, real-time gray-scale B-scanning is superior to the A-scan method of chest wall movement recording and may permit more intensive investigation of fetal chest wall movement in a more precise manner than has previously been possible, turning what has until now been a somewhat frustrating exercise into a potentially useful clinical tool.

A videotape of real-time gray-scale B-scan ultrasound fetal chest wall movement recordings is shown.

1. Bonar, B.E., Blumenfeld, C.M., and Fenning, C.: Studies of Fetal Respiratory Movements: Historical and Present Day Observations. Am. J. Dis. Child. 55:1, 1938.

2. Hellman, L.M., Pritchard, J.A., eds.: Williams Obstetrics Fourteenth Edition. Meredith Corporation, New York, 1971.

3. Adams, F.H.: Functional Development of the Fetal Lung. J. Pediat. 68:794, 1966.

4. Barcroft, J.: Researches on Prenatal Life. Oxford, Blackwells Scientific Publications, 1946.

5. Windle, W.F.: Physiology and Anatomy of the Respiratory System in the Fetus and Newborn Infants. J. Pediat. 19:437, 1941.

6. McClain, C.R., et al.: Amniographic Studies of Fetal Distress in Hypertensive Disorders of Pregnancy. Am. J. Obstet. Gynecol. 107:671, 1970.

7. Duenhöelter, J.H. and Pritchard, J.A.: Human Fetal Respiration. Obs. Gyn. 42:746, 1973.

8. Sadovsky, E. and Yaffe, H.: Daily Fetal Movement Recording and Fetal Prognosis. Obs. Gyn. 41:845, 1973.

9. Hems, D.A.: Palpable Regular Jerking Movements of the Human Fetus: A Possible Respiratory Sign of Fetal Distress. Biol. Neonate. 23:223, 1973.

10. Boddy, K., Dawes, G.S.: Fetal Breathing. Brit. Med. Bull. 31:3-7, 1975.

11. Fox, H.E.: Fetal Breathing Movements and Ultrasound. Amer. J. Dis. Child. (in press)

12. Boddy, K., and Robinson, J.S.: External Method for Detection

of Fetal Breathing In Utero. The Lancet. 2:1231-1233, 1971.

13. Farman, K.J. and Thomas, G.: The Use of Ultrasound for Monitoring Fetal Breathing Movements. Biomed. Eng. 10:172-174, May 1975.

DETECTION OF FETAL HEART BEATS USING THE TM-MODE

Sangarappillai Asokan, M. D.; David Premsagar, R. T.

Cook County Hospital - Department of Radiology Division of Ultrasound
1825 West Harrison, Chicago, Illinois 60612

We examined every obstetric patient of more than eight weeks gestation from February 27 to May 14, 1975. A total of 200 patients and 213 examinations. We were able to detect the heartbeat in 193 patients. Of the seven patients in whom we failed to detect the heartbeats, five delivered dead fetuses. One was a missed abortion. The seventh case was an obese patient, referred for fetal demise. The fetal heart tones were not heard with the Doppler. We were able to detect the presence of twins and record the heartbeats of one fetus. We failed to record the heart beats of the second fetus. A repeat examination was suggested to be done the following day, but the patient delivered two live fetuses that same night. We had two more cases of twins and one case of triplets in whom we were able to independently identify the heartbeats of the fetuses. The earliest fetal heartbeat detected was at 11 weeks.

Of the total examinations, 30 were from ten to 20 weeks, 24 were from 20 to 30 weeks, and 159 were from 30 to 42 weeks.

Twelve patients were referred for fetal demise. Five were diagnosed as fetal demise and proved to be correct. One failure was the case of twins described above. One patient was referred as a missed abortion and diagnosed as such. Subsequently we examined 27 patients who were referred for fetal demise: On the basis of absent fetal heartbeats we diagnosed fetal demise in 16 patients, all of whom delivered dead fetuses.

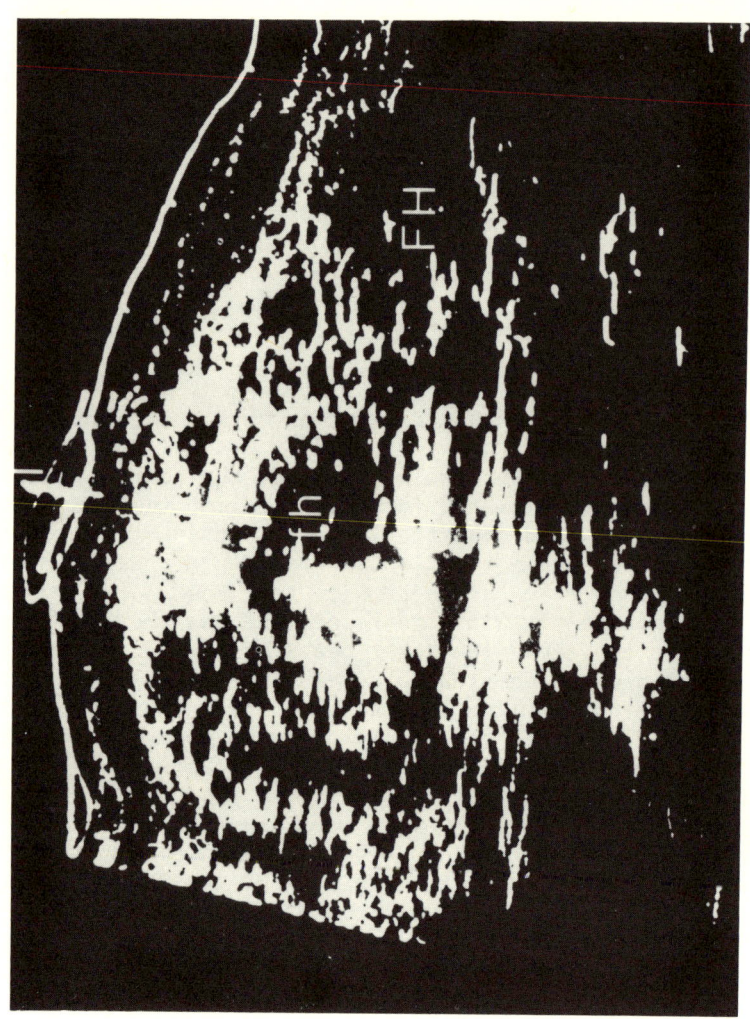

FIGURE - 1a (LONGITUDINAL SCAN) F.H. Fetal Head, FH-Fetal Heart
T-Transducer Position for Fetal Heart Recording (FIGURE 1b)

DETECTION OF FETAL HEART BEATS USING THE TM-MODE 209

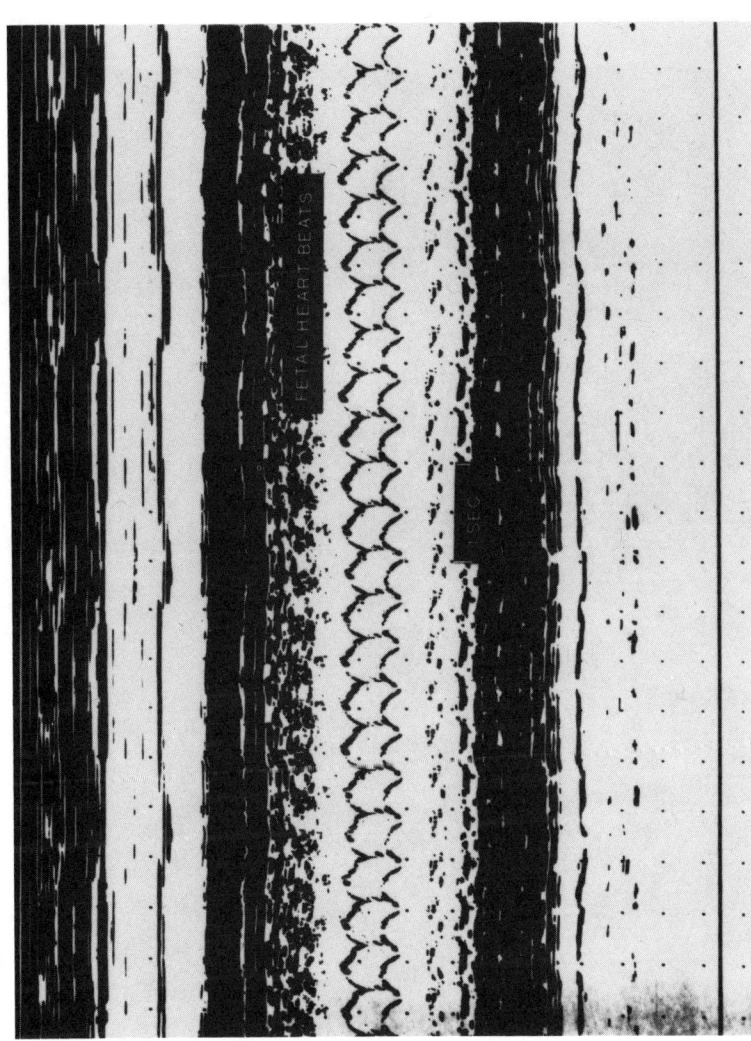

FIGURE 1b - Fetal Heartbeats on T-M Mode

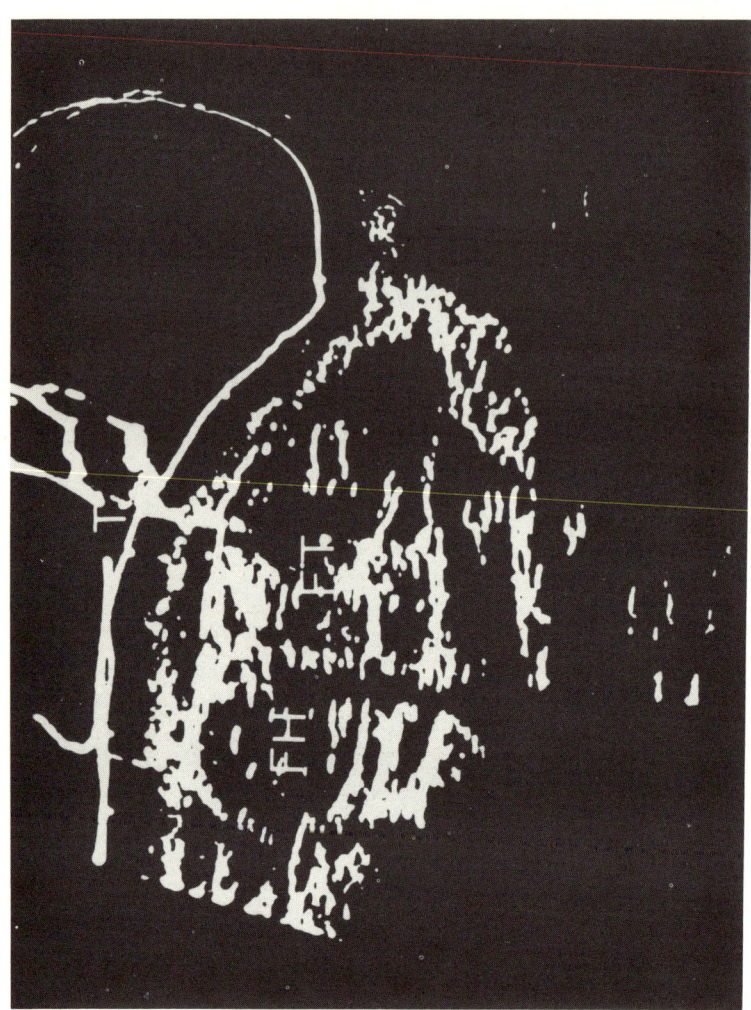

FIGURE - 2a (OBLIQUE SCAN) F.H. Fetal Head
FT - Fetal Thorax
T - Transducer Position for Fetal Heart Recording (FIGURE IIb)

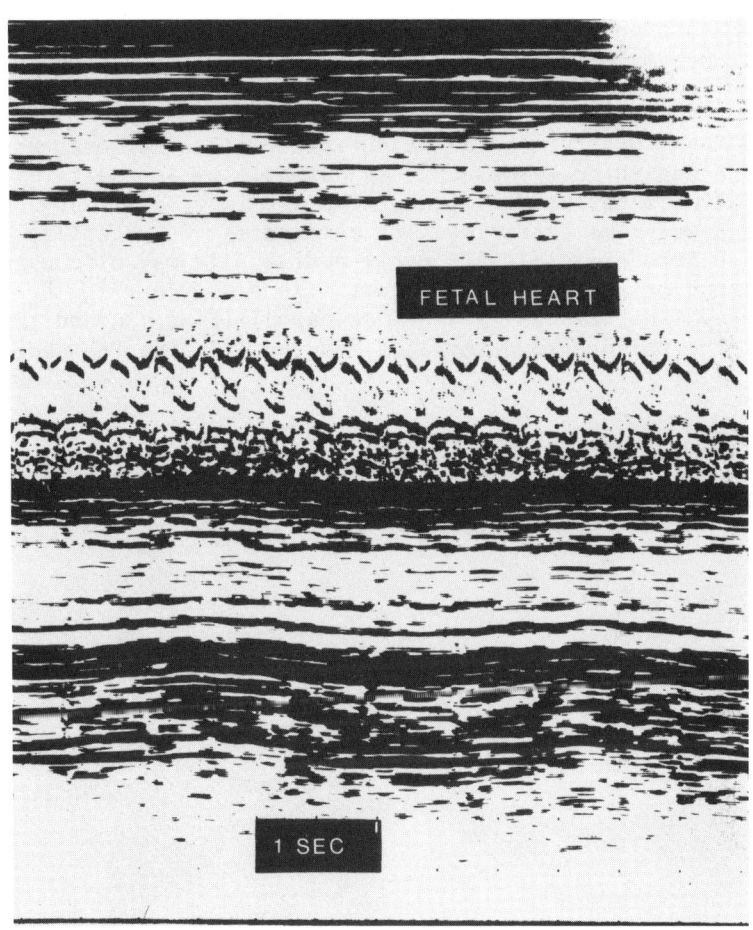

FIGURE- 2b - Fetal Heartbeats on T-M Mode

METHOD

The fetal thorax is located during a routine scan and the approximate position of the fetal heart located on a longitudinal scan, transverse scan or both. The instrument is then converted to the TM-Mode and the transducer placed on the maternal abdomen over the approximate position of the fetal heart. The fetal heartbeats are then identified both on the A-Mode and the M-Mode (FIGURE-1a, 1b, 2a, and 2b). A permanent record is made either on Polaroid or recording paper. Once an individual acquires some practice the fetal heart beats can be detected on the average in about three minutes.

The fetal heartbeats can be detected with great accuracy in the second and third trimester. Our experience in the first trimester patients has been limited. The examination is easy and simple and not time consuming. It eliminates the necessity for a repeat B-Scan especially in early demise. It may circumvent the purchase of additional equipment like a Doppler, to those who already have instruments with M-Mode capabilities, in addition to B-Mode. The failure to detect the heartbeats using T-M Mode is indicative of fetal demise.

USE OF GREY SCALE SONOGRAPHY IN THE MORPHOLOGIC DIAGNOSIS OF

SELECTED GYNECOLOGIC TUMORS

A.C. Fleischer;   M.D. Brown;   P.L. Wilds

Departments of Radiology and Ob/Gyn

Medical College of Georgia, Augusta, Georgia   30902

The recent widespread utilization of grey scale imaging has enabled the sonographer to obtain additional information concerning the internal consistency (echogenicity) of gynecologic tumors when compared to conventional B-mode leading edge techniques.[1,2] It has been our experience in 50 pathologically proven cases that the information obtained by grey scale imaging can be used to limit differential diagnoses of some gynecologic neoplasms.* Although grey scale sonography was only rarely sufficient to make a definitive diagnosis, it has great promise as a useful non-invasive method for establishing tumor morphology and extent of gross tumor invasion prior to surgical exploration or laparoscopy. Selected examples of cases in which grey scale sonography contributed to clinical diagnosis and management are represented here.

Uterine neoplasms presently amenable to sonographic inspection include carcinoma of the cervix and uterine leiomyomata. The extent of tumor invasion present in this patient with Stage IIB carcinoma of the cervix is suggested by the indistinct border of the posterior fornix (figure 1). Due to the technical difficulties of standardizing echoes received from the trans-abdominal approach however, sonography is only occasionally useful for the estimation of tumor invasion in this neoplasm. The solid uterine mass with numerous internal echoes seen in figure 2 exemplifies the findings seen in a subserousal leiomyoma.

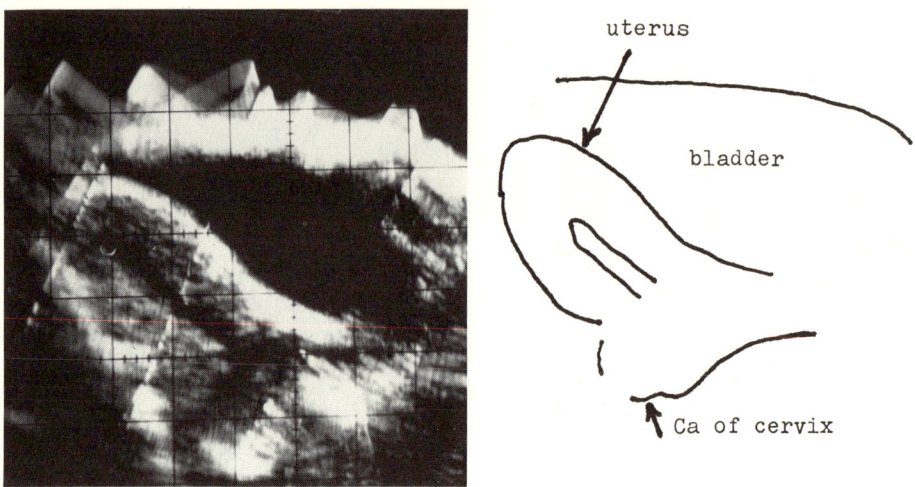

Figure 1—Stage IIB carcinoma of the cervix. Note evidence of tumor extension (midsaggital, 2 cm./division)

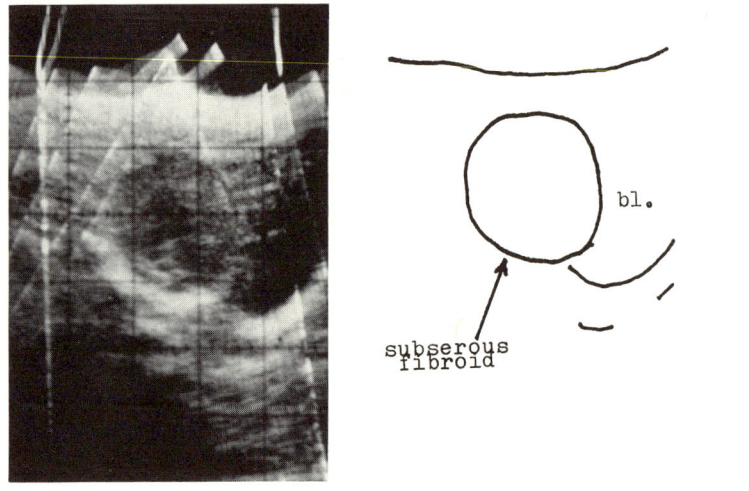

Figure 2—Subserousal leiomymomata. Note solid characteristics. (midsaggital, 3 cm./division)

The next series of figures illustrate the ability to differentiate the nature of adnexal tumors of similar size and location on the basis of their sonographic internal consistency. The homogeneously sonolucent ovarian cyst seen in figure 3 can be contrasted to the benign cystic teratoma seen in figure 4 because of the identifiable solid pole within the cyst. The solid consistency of an ovarian fibroma is revealed by its high degree of echogenicity when compared to cystic structures (figure 5). When compared to pelvic inflammatory disease, tumors in the pelvis usually have recognizable borders.

The internal consistency of large pelvo-abdominal masses can be similarly utilized to differentiate these tumors. For example, the endometriomas depicted in figure 6 do not contain the numerous thin septa seen in the large mucinous cystadenoma illustrated in figure 7. The thick, uneven septa seen within the mass in figure 8 suggested that this mass might be a granulosa cell carcinoma rather than a cystadenoma.

Although gynecologic tumors exist in wide morphological variety, certain neoplasms exhibit characteristically distinguishable grey scale sonographic findings. In our series, these include ovarian cysts, benign cystic teratomas, fibromas, leiomyomata, cystadenomas, and granulosa cell neoplasms. It seems possible that with further technical refinement and larger series, sonographic criteria could be established for specific pathological entities. Our experience suggests that grey scale sonography augments conventional methods of pre-operative evaluation of gynecologic tumors by limiting the differential diagnosis and by obtaining objective appreciation of the extent of the lesion.

*Unirad's Sonograf II was used in this study

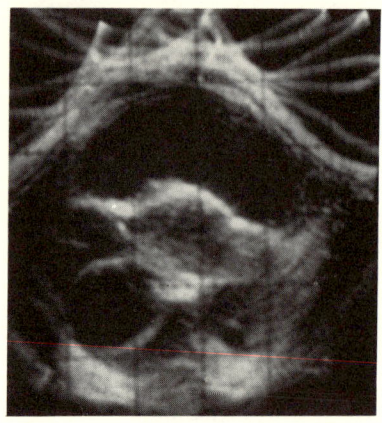 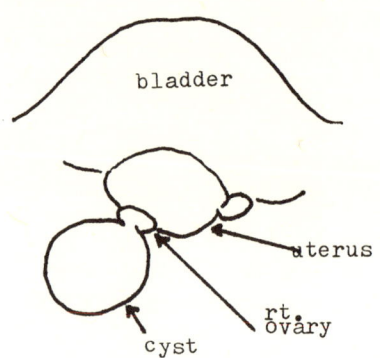

Figure 3-Right ovarian cyst. Note sonolucent character.
(transverse, 5 cm. above s.p., 3 cm./division)

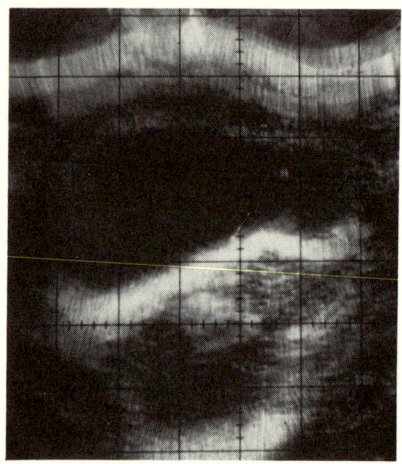 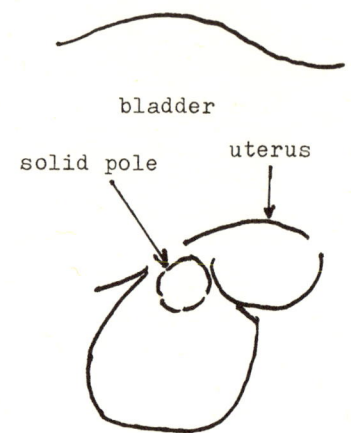

Figure 4-Benign cystic teratoma. Note solid pole within cyst.
(trans., 3 cm. above s.p., 2 cm/division)

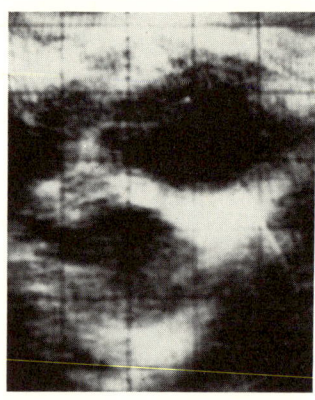 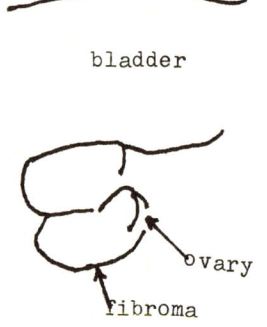

Figure 5-Right ovarian fibroma. Note solid character.(same as 4).

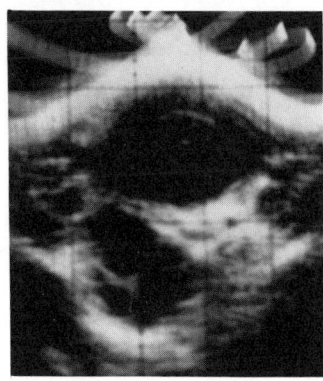 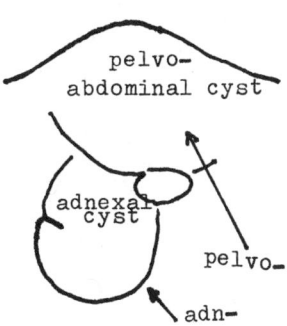

Figure 6—Multiple endometriomas, pelvo-abdominal (pelvo-) and adnexal (adn-). (trans., 6 cm. below umbilicus, 3 cm/div.)

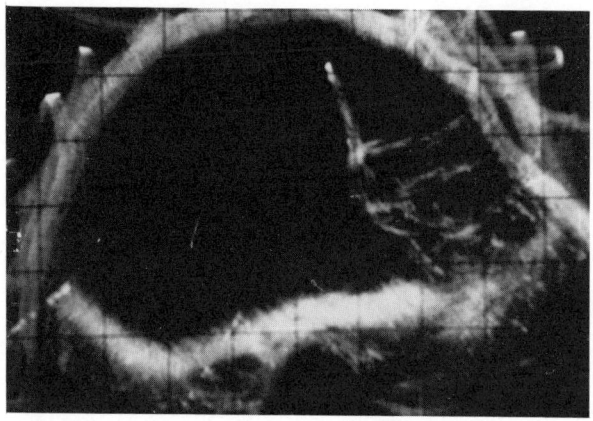

Figure 7 – Large cystadenocarcinoma. Note multiple thin septa. (trans., 2 cm. below umbilicus, 3 cm./division)

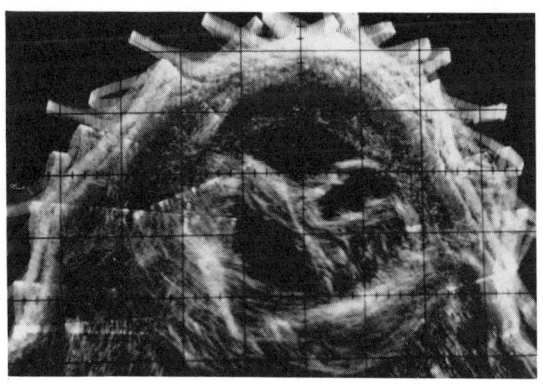 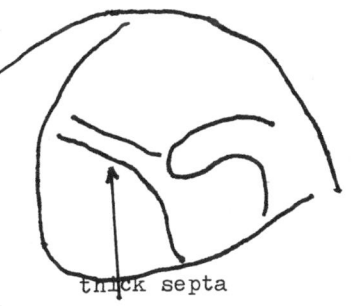

Figure 8—Granulosa cell tumor. Note thick, uneven septa. (trans., 4 cm. below umbilicus, 4 cm/division)

REFERENCES

[1] Morley, P and E. Barnett. The use of ultrasound in the diagnosis of pelvic masses. BR. J. RAD. 43:602, 1970.

[2] Novy, S., B. Samuels, J. Hevesi, J. Smith, S. Wallace, G. Dodd. Ultrasound in evaluation and diagnosis of ovarian tumors. ULTRASOUND IN MEDICINE, vol. 1, N.Y.: Plenum Pub., D. White, ed., pp. 219-228, 1975.

APPLICATION OF THE MULTIPLE HEAD TRANSDUCER

SCANNING DEVICE IN EARLY PREGNANCY

Lawrence Findleton, Donald Ziehm, M.D.,
Jacklyn Ellis

Ultrasound Diagnostic Services, Arizona Medical Plaza
1728 W. Glendale Avenue, Phoenix, Arizona 85021

Until the introduction of the real-time scanning device, the presence or absence of fetal life in early pregnancies has necessitated serial scans done with a B-mode scanner or the combined instrumentation of the B-mode, A-mode, M-mode and Doppler techniques. To assess the accuracy and facility of the multiple head transducer in evaluating early pregnancies, scans were performed on a series of patients with menstrual ages ranging from 7-14 weeks. In all cases, the real-time scanner allowed easy identification of intra-uterine pregnancies. Fetal motion and/or cardiac activity were demonstrated in all normal pregnancies from the 9th week on. Real-time scanning was shown to be a valuable aid in demonstrating early normal and abnormal gestations.

* * *

Since the studies of Donald, the use of ultrasound in early pregnancy has become an accepted technique. The presence, size and location of the gestational sac, as well as the uterine measurements can all be accurately determined by the sectional imaging technique in current use. The development of "real-time" B-scanning has added a new dimension to the use of ultrasound in early pregnancy. For the first time, a dynamic image can be presented with actual fetal and/or cardiac movement being seen.

The purpose of this study was to assess the accuracy and facility of the multiple head transducer in evaluating early pregnancies. A series of patients with periods of amenorrhea ranging from 7-14 weeks were examined. The equipment utilized consisted of an ADR scanner* with a linear array of 64 elements pulsed 4 at a time with a frame rate of 40 per second. A constant image 17cm wide x 20cm deep with the 2.25 MH_z transducer and 12cm with the 3.5 MH_z transducer is produced. Although the display is that of a B scan, the continuous image allows any motion to be detected. All patient studies were recorded on videotape for review by 2 examiners.

Employing the full bladder technique, satisfactory examinations were easily obtained on all patients. A gestational sac could be visualized at 5-6 weeks, with fetal and/or cardiac motion detectable at 7 weeks of amenorrhea. The gestational sac has a somewhat different appearance than with conventional scanning. A condensation of echoes is seen with active movement or cardiac activity being portrayed. The continuous imaging technique allows the uterus to be "scanned" much more rapidly than with conventional sectional imaging. Patient acceptance was excellent. With the expertise gained in evaluation of early pregnancies by "real-time" scanning, abnormal pregnancies were more easily identified.

---

* Advanced Diagnostic Research Corporation, 2202 South Priest Drive, Suite 102, Tempe, Arizona 85282

ROLE OF ULTRASOUND IN THE DETECTION AND MANAGEMENT OF INTRAUTERINE
GROWTH RETARDATION AND ASSOCIATED PLACENTAL ABNORMALITIES

H. R. Giles, M.D.; C. F. Anderson, ASUTS; D. B. Rosenberg,
ASUTS; C. D. Christian, M.D., Ph.D.
Department of Obstetrics and Gynecology
University of Arizona Medical Center, Tucson, Arizona 85724

In recent years, diagnostic ultrasound has been utilized extensively in the determination of gestational age through correlation with the biparietal diameter of the fetal head. This has been of immeasurable assistance in reconciling uterine size - menstrual date incompatibility or in projecting a delivery date when menstrual dates are unknown. Our experience has shown that single ultrasound evaluations are often confusing or inconclusive in such cases. Rather, serial examinations provide information regarding the general pattern of fetal growth. This trend may change from week to week, especially in high-risk patients at risk for intrauterine growth retardation. Poor fetal growth is especially common in patients with chronic hypertension, severe diabetes, or narcotic addiction.

Serial scanning is usually begun for the high risk patient between the 15th and 20th week of gestation, and is repeated at two to three week intervals until delivery. If fetal growth is suboptimal, scans are performed weekly. Biparietal measurements are obtained on bi-stable display for greater precision and are plotted on a "growth ladder" to demonstrate the general pattern of growth. Thoracic measurements are mandatory, especially when intrauterine growth retardation is suspected clinically. It has been noted that the thoracic diameter is a more sensitive indicator of fetal growth, since body mass in the growth retarded fetus is disproportionately compromised when compared to the fetal head. When plotted on the growth ladder, the average thoracic diameter curves to the left of the standard growth pattern. Although the biparietal diameter exhibits a similar curve, this trend does not become apparent as early as that of the thoracic diameter.

Gray scale processing is exceedingly useful in cases of intrauterine growth retardation in detecting abnormalities of placentation. Such problems as retroplacental hematoma, placental edema, low implantation and atrophic placentas are often easily recognized on gray scale display.

Patients with intrauterine growth retardation are managed by serial clinical examinations, tri-weekly serum estriol levels, oxytocin challenge tests and amniocentesis. Since these fetuses often exhibit precocious maturation, the optimal management consists of intensive observation, bed rest and delivery as soon as fetal maturity can be demonstrated.

FETAL AND NEONATAL HEART SIZE CORRELATION BY ULTRASONIC IMAGING

Fuad Ibrahim, Betty J. Phillips, Shane H. Abowitt,
Vincent E. Friedewald, Jr., M.D., Sam A. Kinard, M.D.,
Marilyn K. Laughead, M.D.
Arizona Heart Institute, St. Joseph's Hospital and Medical Center, Phoenix, Arizona 85013

Fetal heart movements have been demonstrated in the past by using the Doppler principle. Bang and Holm described the method for determining fetal heart movements by means of pulsating ultrasonics utilizing A-and B-mode scanning. The introduction of real-time ultrasonic scanning has now enabled visualization of the fetal heart.
The internal and external fetal heart dimensions will be measured in 25 pregnant women during the 24 hours prior to scheduled Caesarian-section delivery. An M-mode scan recording the left ventricle will be done on these neonates during the first 24 hours after delivery. Measurement of internal and external neonatal heart dimensions from the anterior wall of the right ventricle to the posterior wall of the left ventricle will also be accomplished. These pre-and post-delivery measurements will then be correlated and compared to normal neonatal heart size. Our inital studies on normal neonatal heart size utilizing ultrasound are in agreement with other investigative studies. To our knowledge, evaluation of the fetal heart for congenital abnormalitites has not been accomplished.

The purpose of this study is to determine normal fetal heart size, which can be easily distinguished from abnormal heart size. This information will form the basis for further ultrasonic real-time imaging studies in possible recognition of intrauterine congenital heart defects.

DIAGNOSTIC ULTRASOUND FOR DETECTION OF INTRAUTERINE GROWTH RETARDATION

>John T. Queenan, M.D., Sandra F. Kubarych, R.N.,
>Larry N. Cook, M.D., Garland D. Anderson, M.D.,
>Larry Griffin, M.D.
>Univ. of Louisville, Dept. OB/GYN, Louisville, KY
>Louisville General Hosp., 323 E. Chestnut, Louisville, KY

Intrauterine growth retardation (IUGR) has a markedly adverse affect on the outcome of pregnancy. The neonate has an increased incidence of asphyxia neonatorium, meconium aspiration syndrome, polycythemia and hypoglycemia. Although these problems are manifest in the nursery, the problem really begins in utero. Much evidence suggests that failure to grow in utero can be overcome by the pre-term delivery and proper care in the neonatal intensive care unit.

This study evaluates the use of diagnostic ultrasound fetal biparietal diameters (BPD) to detect IUGR. The detection of IUGR must be sufficiently accurate to detect most of the growth retarded fetuses and avoid the mistake of early delivery of a normal fetus.

Seven hundred and thirty eight fetal BPD were determined in 468 normal obstetrical patients between 16 and 43 weeks' gestation. Patients were included only if (1) the size of the uterus on initial examination corresponded to the duration of amenorrhea $\pm$ 1 week and (2) there were no complications during the pregnancy. The mean BPD $\pm$ 2 was determined for each week of gestation.

One hundred selected high risk obstetrical patients in whom the size of the uterus on initial examination corresponded to the weeks of amenorrhea were studied by serial BPD. Values in the 5th percentile or lower were considered presumptive of IUGR. At delivery additional newborns were identified who had growth retardation which could not be detected in utero by BPD measurements. These two groups were analyzed.

Retrospectively, a series of small for gestational age neonates having had fetal BPD determinations during pregnancy were studied. The growth retarded newborns that could be identified in utero by ultrasound and those that could not be identified were analyzed.

ULTRASONIC EVALUATION OF PELVIC MASSES IN PREGNANCY

A.A. Bezjian, M.M. Carretero

Dept. of Nuclear Med., and Dept. of Obstetrics and Gynecology, University of Miami, Miami, Florida

Diagnostic ultrasound has recently become a very useful tool in obstetrics and gynecology as it is a non-invasive and harmless procedure both to the patient and the fetus. Its usefulness in gynecology has somewhat lagged behind obstetrics since almost all persistent large pelvic masses are surgically removed and an additional diagnostic test with the additional cost and inconvenience to the patient is often felt to be unnecessary by the gynecologist.

The situation however is different in cases of pelvic masses associated with pregnancy as it is desirable to avoid surgery in pregnancy if the pelvic masses can definitely be shown to be benign.

We have reviewed all the cases (42 to date) of pelvic masses in pregnancy at Jackson Memorial Hospital who had a diagnostic ultrasound procedure performed, in an effort to evaluate the reliability of this procedure in diagnosing pelvic pathology in pregnancy.

16/42 were correctly diagnosed as having uterine myomas with pregnancy. 7/9 proven pathologically. 9/19 were clinically proven to be correct by post partum or post abortion follow up examination and 3 additional patients diagnosed sonographically as having myomas in pregnancy are undelivered and are being followed up conservatively. In 2 patients the diagnosis of ovarian cyst in pregnancy was erroneously made and on exploration were found to have large degenerating myomas.

9 cases of benign ovarian cysts in pregnancy were correctly diagnosed. 7/9 were proven pathologically and 2/9 diagnosed as corpus luteum cysts, clinically disappeared post abortion.

4/5 cases were correctly diagnosed as hydatidiform moles with theca lutein cysts. The fifth case had a similar diagnosis sonographically but was found to have a missed abortion with degenerating myomas.

3/4 cases were correctly diagnosed as having an ectopic pregnancy. The fourth patient with an ectopic pregnancy was erroneously diagnosed by sonogram as having a right pelvic mass.

2/2 cases were correctly diagnosed as bicornuate uteri with pregnancy in one horn.

AMNIOCENTESIS UNDER ULTRASOUND GUIDANCE WITH ASPIRATION TRANSDUCER

P. Barriga, M.D., G. Sarto, M.D., and J. Cassidy, R.T.

Center for Health Sciences, University of Wisconsin

Madison, Wisconsin 53706

Amniocentesis is now part of the work up of a large number of pregnant women. The value of compound ultrasound scanning in localizing the placenta and in selecting an optimal place for amniocentesis is well known and many reports concerning its usefulness have appeared in the last years. We want to report our experience with ultrasound-guided amniocentesis using the aspiration transducer. Even though the aspiration transducer has been widely used for renal cyst aspiration, there are very few reports on its use in amniocentesis. With preliminary longitudinal and transverse B-mode scanning of the lower abdomen, the uterus, the placenta and fetal parts are identified. Subsequently, a good place for amniocentesis with enough amniotic fluid and away from fetal parts and especially the head is located and marked on the patient's skin. Under sterile technique and monitoring with the aspiration transducer, amniocentesis is performed. Because of fetal movements, this is a much safer way to do this procedure since you are seeing the echo-free amniotic space in the actual moment of needle insertion. You can also easily measure the depth of the amniotic cavity from the skin. It has been reported that an additional advantage of aspiration transducer is the visualization of the spike that the needle produces in the A-mode as it enters the amniotic cavity, allowing you to know exactly where or how deep the needle is positioned. In our experience, the spike from the needle is seen only in about 50% of the cases. This is due probably to the fact that if we are obtaining amniotic fluid, we do not move slightly the transducer or increase the gains in an effort to visualize the needle spike as we would normally do if amniotic fluid is not seen coming from the needle. From 40 examinations done, we have successfully obtained amniotic fluid in 32 (80%); fluid could not be obtained in the remaining 8 (20%). Most of the 8 unsuccessful amniocentesis have been in patients that were too early along in their pregnancy (between 12 and 13 weeks). It is now our policy not to do amniocentesis too early along in pregnancy; also, we do not attempt it more than three times at one sitting. We prefer to call the patient back for a repeat study in one or two weeks, according to their estimated gestational age, rather than persist in obtaining amniotic fluid after the third attempt. All the repeated studies have been successful on the second time with the exception of two that had to come a third time. Although there is still a failure rate with ultrasound aspiration transducer in performing amniocentesis, we feel that this is a significant advantage and a much safer way to perform this study.

ULTRASONICALLY GUIDED FETAL INJECTION OF VITAMIN-K

(Phytomenadione)

Fl. Jensen; B. Jacobsen; J. Falck Larsen; J. Fog Pedersen
Ultrasonic Laboratory
Gentofte Hospital DK-2900 Hellerup, Denmark

One out of 2000 pregnancies is complicated with a thromboembolic disease, most often in the form of thrombi in the inferior extremities or pelvic veins with the possibility of dissemination of emboli to the pulmonary arteries. The cause for this is altered coagulability of blood as a result of hormonal changes in combination with compression of pelvic veins.

Since the delivery per viam naturalem causes increased intracranial pressure in the foetus, there is a risk of intracranial hemorrhage. This risk is even greater, when the mother and thereby the foetus is under anticoagulant therapy.

For that reason it has been common to stop anticoagulant medication to the mother some weeks before delivery to favour the foetus but not always without increasing the risk of further thrombo-embolic complications to the mother.

As phytomenadione relatively slowly equilibrates over the placental barrier, it would be advantageous to bring up the coagulability of the blood of the foetus to a normal level ante partum, without influencing the maternal blood. Efforts to do this have been made in some cases in Gentofte Hospital in a collaboration of the Coagulation Laboratory, the Obstetrical Department and the Ultrasonic Laboratory. It is the aim of this work to present the methods and results of these investigations with vitamin-K adminstered by different routes.

Initially 2 pregnant women received no vitamin-K before delivery and umbilical cord blood was taken from the baby shortly after delivery. The result was in both cases, P-P (prothrombin-proconvertin) values below 10% of normal range.

In 3 cases 3o mg of vitamin-K was given intravenously to the mothers 2 to 4 days before delivery. Still the P-P values of the babies were low: from 2o to 4o per cent of normal. In the next step vitamin-K was administered under ultrasonically guided amniocentesis into the amniotic fluid 4 days ante partum. The P-P values were 2o per cent shortly after delivery.We used a multitransducer (real time imaging) equipped with a special adaptor for guiding the cannula.

With the same equipment and a fine needle, 6 foetuses were given vitamin-K in utero by placing the needle intramuscularly in the rump or thigh. 24 hours after delivery the P-P values were as high as 6o to 8o per cent of normal values in cranial vein blood of the infants. No complications were registered and the mothers was continously treated with anticoagulants. We can hereby conclude that ultrasonically guided fine needle fetal injection of vitamin-K is a rational and safe procedure that should minimize the risk of hemorrhage subpartum, without influencing on a well indicated anticoagulant therapy to the mother.

GREY SCALE PATTERNS IN PELVIC INFLAMMATORY DISEASE

William F. Sample, M.D. and Jonathan B. Po, M.D.

Department of Radiological Sciences
University of California, Los Angeles, CA 90024

    The patient with pelvic inflammatory disease is often difficult to evaluate both from history and physical examination. Distinguishing clinically between the various forms of pelvic inflammatory disease, ectopic pregnancy, twisted or ruptured ovarian cyst, missed or impending abortion, ovarian carcinoma, and endometriosis, is sometimes impossible. By means of commercially available second generation grey scale ultrasound, a more precise set of criteria for distinguishing between these entities based on intra-organ internal echo patterns has been developed.
    Acute and at times, sub-acute pelvic inflammatory disease have presented with a unique triad of general findings: 1) Decreased echogenicity of all the pelvic tissues leading to lighter grey tones; 2) The difficulty in defining the pelvic organs and muscular landmarks; 3) The generalized increased transmission throughout the pelvis. All of these changes are felt to be related to the generalized edema which likely diminishes the subtle differences in acoustical impedance.
    The specific extra-uterine findings in pelvic inflammatory disease may vary from thickened, lighter (grey tones), but strongly transmitting adnexa to multiple thick-walled fluid collections. The multiloculated abscesses in pelvic inflammatory disease may at times be difficult to distinguish from endometriosis. However, in the latter, there tends to be more nodular and darker internal components to the cystic lesions and the triad of general findings is absent. In fact, the endometriomas have been most difficult to distinguish from benign cystic teratomas. An unruptured ectopic pregnancy has been characterized by the organized gestational configuration to the mixed adnexal mass as

well as the distinctive grey scale pattern of the surrounding decidual reaction. The extra-uterine findings in ovarian carcinoma may be similar to multiloculated pelvic inflammatory disease, but the triad of general findings is usually lacking.

Specific intra-uterine grey scale patterns have also been helpful in differentiating many of these entities. The uterus is not generally enlarged in pelvic inflammatory disease unless it is a pyometra in which case, the pattern is one of a fluid-filled expanded endometrial cavity. The decreased echogenicity and lighter grey tones of the uterine muscle distinguish this from a hematometra which usually has a normal uterine muscular grey tone and the blighted ovum which usually shows some residual decidua parietalis which has a different distinctive grey scale pattern.

When mild endometritis is associated with pelvic inflammatory disease, the normal sized uterus may show a linear dark endometrial pattern representing slight separation of the walls by exudate. However, the uterine muscle maintains a decreased lighter echogenic pattern. The latter finding distinguishes it from the more normal appearing grey tone uterine muscle pattern in adenomyosis associated with endometriosis and the normal uterus seen with twisted or ruptured ovarian cysts.

In ectopic pregnancy, the uterus often contains a linear dark echo in the endometrial cavity similar to the endometritis accompanying pelvic inflammatory disease. However, the uterus is usually larger and an increased darker echogenic pattern is seen throughout the uterine muscle reflecting the vascular engorgement and decidua parietalis engendered by the gestational hormone levels. A similar pattern may be seen in missed abortion, but the extra-uterine findings are absent.

The above concepts will be illustrated by case material. In addition, serial studies of patients with pelvic inflammatory disease will be shown to demonstrate the reversibility of these distinctive abnormalities as well as the sequela of this disease entity.

USE OF B-SCAN AND GRAY SCALE IMAGING IN THE DIAGNOSIS OF

BENIGN CYSTIC TERATOMA

> Caroline F. Anderson, ASUTS; H.R. Giles, M.D.;
> David Rosenberg, ASUTS; M.W. Heine, M.D.
> Department of Obstetrics and Gynecology
> University of Arizona Medical Center, Tucson, Arizona

One of the indications for diagnostic ultrasound is the clinical suspicion of an ovarian tumor on pelvic examination. Even when such masses are easily palpable beside the uterus, it is generally impossible to distinguish purely cystic ovarian neoplasms from those with either multiloculation or a solid component. B-scan ultrasound, especially when combined with gray-scale processing, affords excellent visualization of the internal structure of such masses and may allow pre-operative diagnosis of the lesion. For this presentation, the benign cystic teratoma, or dermoid, is discussed as an example of an ovarian neoplasm with both solid and cystic components which has a characteristic appearance on the ultrasound scan.

The benign cystic teratoma, or dermoid as it is commonly called, is an ovarian tumor comprised of multiple tissue types. It is not unusual to find skin, sebaceous glands, fat, hair, thyroid gland, and even teeth on cross-section of the tumor. Such tumors apparently arise from pleuripotential cells within the ovary which are capable of developing into any of a number of different tissue types. Dermoids are generally asymptomatic and range in size from several centimeters to tumors weighing ten pounds or more. They are most often seen in patients in their teens or early twenties, and such tumors are frequently bilateral.

Ultrasound diagnosis of a dermoid tumor rests on several criteria. First, because of the high fat content, such masses are usually noted in an extreme anterior location, generally resting atop the well-filled urinary bladder. Gray scale processing generally reveals a primarily cystic structure with sharply demarcated borders. Within the cyst cavity, linear echo activity is often noted representing septa or loculations. Calcified tissue is generally located near the periphery of the cyst and is evidenced by dense areas of echo activity. Calcification is the only dermoid element which can be seen on conventional x-ray, but this study should be used to complement the ultrasound examination when a dermoid is suspected.

Since dermoids are primarily encountered during the childbearing years and may in fact be associated with an early pregnancy, ultrasound provides non-invasive information which may allow pre-operative diagnosis of such tumors.

ULTRASONIC IDENTIFICATION OF THE POSITION OF CONTRACEPTIVE DEVICE
IN UTERO AND ITS RELATION TO SUBSEQUENT PERFORMANCE

T. Chow, M.D.;   B. Wittmann, M.D.

Department of Obstetrics and Gynaecology
University of British Columbia
Vancouver General Hospital, Vancouver, B.C., Canada

Two diagnostic methods are available for the identification of a contraceptive device in utero, radiology and ultrasound. Radiology involves two views, the placement of a sound, or a second intrauterine contraceptive device (IUCD), or dye into the uterine cavity. In contrast, ultrasound is a simple, safe and reliable method for the localization of the device, allowing also recognition of such details as thickness of myometrium, exact sites of insertion of the Fallopian tubes and the uterine fundus. The devices used in this study were Cu-T and Cu-7. The examination was performed with a bi-stable and grey scale B-scanner using the full bladder technique.

This study was undertaken not merely to localize the IUCD, but to determine the exact position of the device in the uterine cavity; correlation was made to subsequent complications - excessive cramps, bleeding, pregnancy, expulsion, etc. The more serious complications of partial or complete perforation can be identified immediately and appropriate measures instituted.

80 patients were scanned ultrasonically within 24 hours of insertion of IUCD, and asked to return for a recheck in 6-8 weeks. Those who developed complications were reassessed sooner.

At the initial scanning, a baseline was set as to the exact level of the transverse arm of the device in the uterine cavity. Immediate reinsertion was performed only in cases where the device was found to be well below mid-cavity. Additional contraceptive methods were advised to all patients until re-check was performed.

Improvement in design and efficacy of the IUCD has led to its increased use. The failure rate is low but increases if the device is not in proper position. This can be due to incorrect placement at insertion or to secondary dislodgment. Clinically, displacement is suspected if the string is absent or excessively long. Definite diagnosis is only possible by visualization of the device in relation to the uterine cavity.

Results show that ultrasound is an important adjunct to the management of patients with IUCD, and larger series and longer periods of follow-up are under way. Eventually, it is hoped that every woman who carries a foreign body in her uterus for contraceptive purposes undergoes periodic routine ultrasonic check-ups thus relieving her and her physician of the constant worry of IUCD failure.

Neurology

ULTRASOUND FOR IDENTIFICATION OF BRAIN DAMAGE IN INFANTS AND

YOUNG CHILDREN *

        R. F. Heimburger, F. J. Fry, T. D. Franklin, Jr.,
        R. C. Eggleton and E. Gresham

        Fortune-Fry Research Laboratory of the Indianapolis
        Center for Advanced Research, Neurological Surgery
        Section of the Department of Surgery, and Neonatology
        Section of the Department of Pediatrics, Indiana University School of Medicine, 1100 West Michigan Street,
        Indianapolis, Indiana 46202

    Infant skulls do not provide the severe barrier to ultrasound diagnosis that the adult skull does. Improved ultrasound instrumentation has made it possible to visualize the brains of infants and small children in detail, through the intact skull, non-invasively and non-accumulatively. This has decreased the hesitancy of physicians to request diagnostic brain studies on seriously ill babies, particularly premature and neonatal ones. The ability to provide considerable diagnostic information in children through age $3\frac{1}{2}$ or 4 years, when diploe start to appear in the parietal bones, adds to the usefulness of two-dimensional ultrasound brain visualization.

METHOD

    A prototype, portable, ultrasound scan instrument was used for this study. A 1.7 MHz transceiver, with a 5 cm. Lead Metaniobate element, ground spherically to focus the ultrasound beam at 20 cm., was passed in a linear path through a bath of warm degassed water. The bottom of a flexible plastic tank was applied to the child's parietal area with a coupling gel. The child was placed on a warming blanket which provided a soporific effect. Many of the children slept during the scan. The 3 - 4 cm. of water did not exert appreciable compression to even the loosely joined skull bones of severely hydrocephalic babies.

The ultrasound scans used to illustrate this paper are largely horizontal tomograms. Coronal tomograms were made to confirm abnormal findings in the horizontal scans, or to demonstrate additional aspects of pathology or structural anatomy. For maximally interpretable visualization, the patient's head was oriented precisely in relationship to the transceiver, so that the scan path was perpendicular to the midline plane of the brain and parallel to the canthomeatal plane. The break in the midline echo provided by the corpus callosum, impinging on it, was used to identify reference planes in horizontal and coronal scans. Using these reference planes, tomograms were made at either 5 mm. or 1 cm. intervals. These reference planes are often more difficult to identify in abnormal brains than in normal ones. The two-dimensional image was displayed on a 17-inch monitor. Selected tomograms were recorded permanently on polaroid film taken from a separate 9-inch monitor which recorded an identical image. It required 15 to 45 minutes to complete a study, depending on the detail needed.

RESULTS

A tomographic atlas was made very rapidly visualizing the entire brain (Fig. 1). The midline, lateral ventricles, including the temporal horns on the horizontal scans, the tentorial incisura and brain stem, (Fig. 2) were seen routinely in children younger than 1 year of age. A significant, but lesser amount of structural detail was seen in children up to 4 years. Fortunately, brain abnormalities could often be identified in older children even when anatomical structure could not be resolved. This is particularly true of hemorrhage, some margins of which reflect ultrasound more intensely than surrounding tissues with the exception of the bone (Fig. 3). Hemorrhage could usually be identified by using ultrasound sensitivity graded tomography as the reflections from its borders were visible at much lower gain settings than even strongly reflective midline structures.

Normal ventricles were often difficult to recognize because of their slit-like width. Dilated cerebral ventricles were more readily identified since both the superficial and deep ventricular walls produced linearly arranged echo patterns (Fig. 1). Tumors were reflective, particularly if they were surrounded by less dense ventricular fluid or cystic space (Fig. 4). Hemorrhage was more reflective than any of the tumors that were visualized. Cystic tumors were identified even through the thicker skulls of 3-4 year olds to aid in their differentiation from solid masses (Fig. 5).

The orientation of normal appearing anatomical structures provided a clue to dysfunction as in the case of a very slightly displaced and rotated brain stem (Fig. 2).

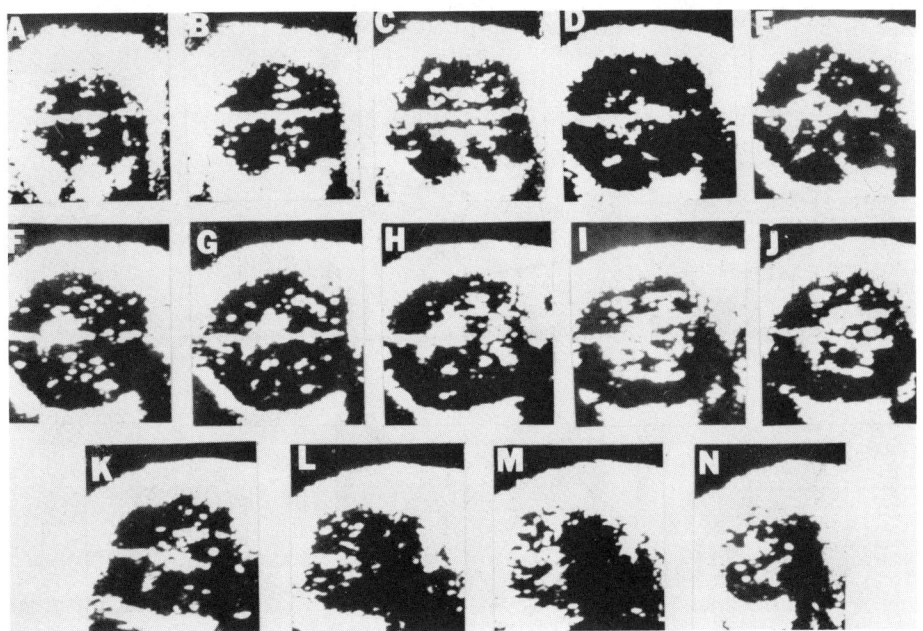

Figure 1.

Horizontal scans of 3 week old infant with convulsions and difficulty breathing and swallowing. The scans were made at 5 millimeter intervals from the superior plane where the lateral ventricle echoes (A) first appear to the cerebellum at the base (L, M and N). The child's head is oriented with the left side up face toward the right. Medial and lateral walls of the lateral ventricles are shown on either side of the midline in scan B. An abnormal echo appears to straddle the midline in scan E, and persists in the same location through scan H or possibly scan I. The brain stem is clearly outlined in scans I and J. The aqueduct of Sylvius, cerebral peduncles and quadrigeminate plate can be identified in scan J, and probably the basilar artery just anterior to the brain stem and bracketed by the tentorial incisura.

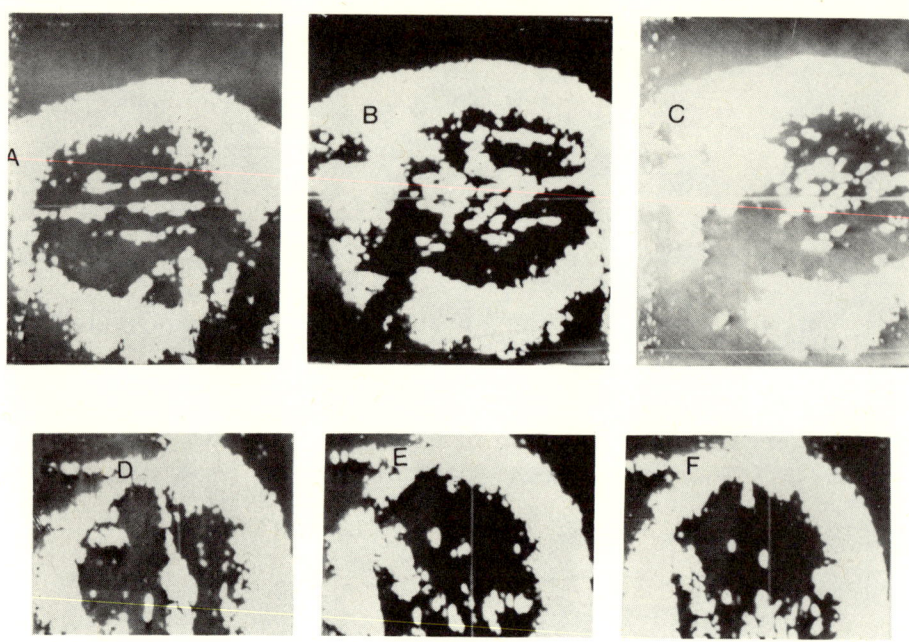

Figure 2.

Horizontal, (upper row) and coronal scans (lower row) of a 1 month old infant with right-sided convulsions. The right side of the head is at the top of the horizontal scans, face toward the left. The left side of the head is on the left of the coronal scans. Ventricular echoes are seen both horizontally and coronally, more easily identified in horizontal scans. The temporal horns bracket the tentorial incisura and brain stem in scan B, with more than the usual echo intensity in the chiasmatic and inter-peduncular cysterns just anterior to the brain stem. The brain stem appears slightly twisted in relationship to other structures in scan C. This twisting is confirmed by a slight shift of the brain stem toward the right in scan E. This shifting can be explained by abnormal echoes in the Sylvian fissure region, presumably a hemorrhage on the left in the other two coronal scans, D and F, in the superior left parietal area in scan A.

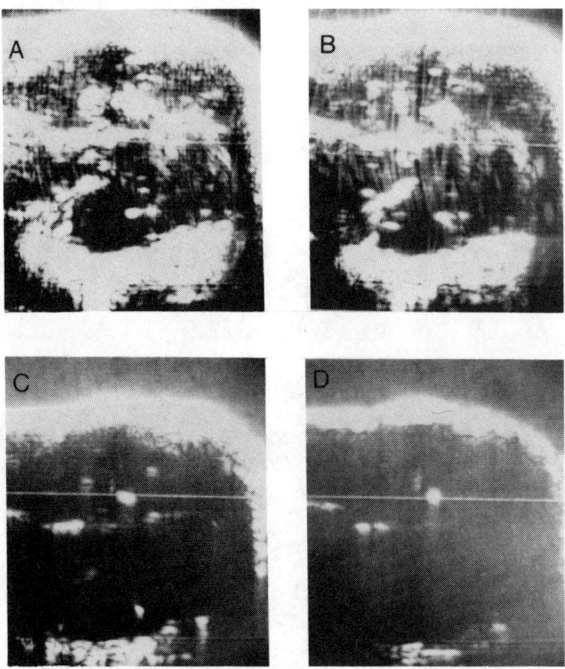

Figure 3.

Horizontal ultrasound scans were made on this 4 week old infant because of almost constant generalized seizure activity. The head is oriented left side up, face toward the right of the photographs. Small reflections from the medial and lateral walls of the right lateral ventricle can be seen below the midline, scan A. These are visible but not as distinctly in scan B and absent in scans C and D. Progressive decrease in instrument gain from an attenuation of 20 decibels in scan A, 25 db scan B, 40 db scan C and 50 db scan D was used. A linear reflection close to the inner table of the left (upper) parietal skull probably represents the lateral wall of the left lateral ventricle in scans A and B. The medial wall area of this ventricle is occupied by a dense reflection in the thalamic region. This dense reflection appears to be a continuation of an echo crossing the anterior portion of midline structures. The midline crossing echo disappeared with a slight gain decrease. Persistence of the left thalamus echo at progressively lower gains in B, C and D shows that it is different from the artifactual shadows which disappear. It undoubtedly represents contused or hemorrhaged brain tissue with an unusually highly reflective lateral (ventricular) edge.

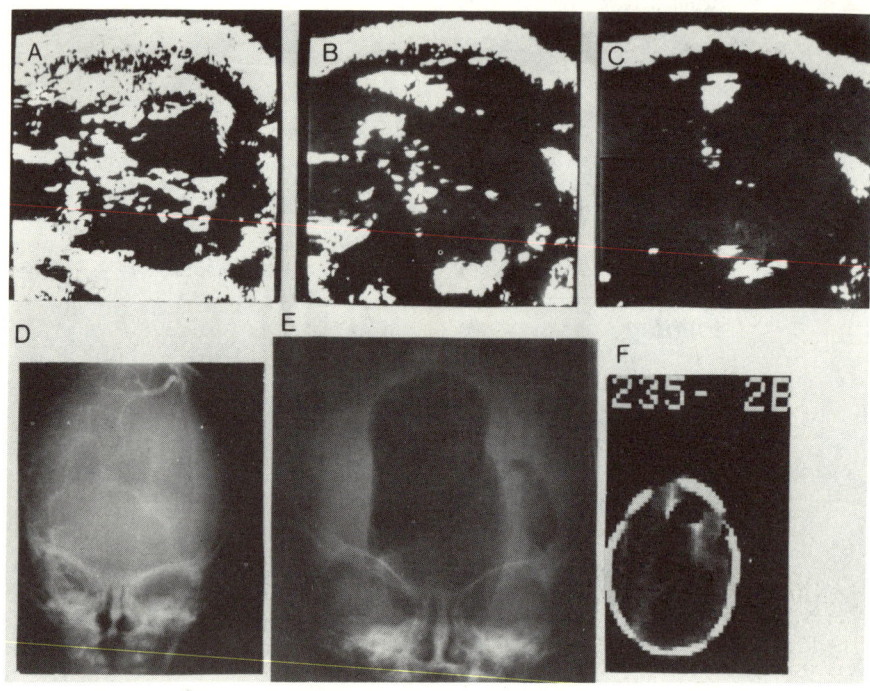

Figure 4.

A one year old unresponsive child with enlarging head had equivocal angiography D, air ventriculography E and computerized axial tomography F in two separate test "series". Because of the gross distortion of brain structure only a marked midline shift, left to right, is well demonstrated in scan A. The horizontal tomograms, left side up, face toward the right, show the medial and lateral walls of the left lateral ventricle, above the shifted midline structures. The linear echoes of the ventricular walls persist but less distinctly in scans B and C which show decreasing gain, attenuation 40 decibels A, 50 db B and 55 db C. The persistent heavy reflection hanging onto the lateral portion of the left (upper) lateral ventricle suggested a choroid plexus papilloma pre-operatively. A choroid plexus vascular malformation was removed at surgery. Many scans confirming the illustrated ultrasound displays were needed to make this diagnosis, with the added information from the three x-ray studies, without which the ultrasound scans above would have been even more difficult to interpret.

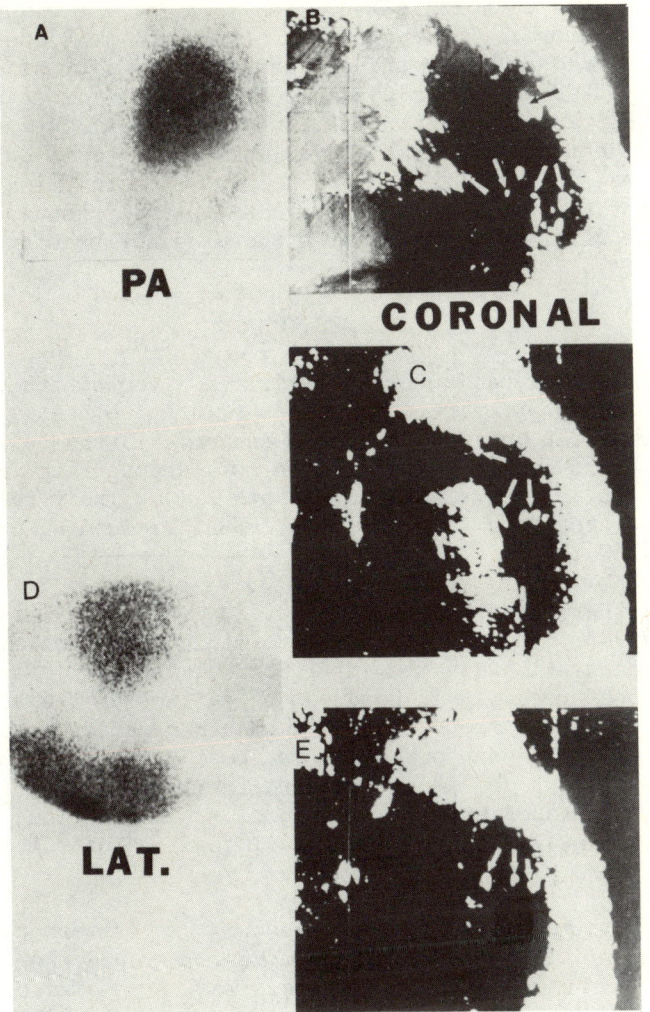

Figure 5.

Isotope scans, A and D, of this 3 year old with a recurrent right parietal ependymoma give the appearance of inoperability. A large cyst with heavily reflecting walls (white arrows) and small mural nodule (black arrow) was suspected from ultrasound scans made through the intact skull. Surgery proved this to be correct. Artifactual reflections provided the usual confusion in ultrasound scans through the intact skull, but the persistence and location of the cyst wall reflection provide enough confidence in the diagnosis to advise surgery.

Although the information provided seemed reliable, there were no anatomical or pathological confirmations of the diagnosis, except for the two tumors. The anatomical structures mentioned were accurately identified by using transparent overlays from atlases of excised brains cut as nearly as possible in the same planes as the two-dimensional ultrasound scans. Unfortunately, no atlases of the infant brain have been found, but the available adult brain outlines fit surprisingly well. This technic was helpful in confirming anatomical structures that appear reasonably certain on ultrasound tomograms, and also to point out additional structures not previously recognized.

DISCUSSION

Ability to visualize brain detail in infants with two-dimensional ultrasound was predicted by Kazner (17) and others. Kossoff and Garrett were able to identify gross anatomical structure of fetal brains in-utero in 1972 (18), and in 1974 demonstrated horizontal and coronal brain atlases of normal infants (19). Their technic has become an accepted screening test for infant brain diagnosis in Sydney, Australia (20).

Many other investigators (1-29), including the Dussiks (7,8) who were first to apply ultrasound to medical diagnosis, have reported two-dimensional brain imaging. Good diagnostic information has been developed recently in hundreds of patients. The scans recorded by these investigators provide valuable information to the trained eye, but have not been convincing to those less accustomed to reading ultrasound brain tomograms. The structural and pathological detail visualized increases each year. The clear information, possible to obtain in infants, should move this diagnostic instrumentation forward more rapidly in the near future.

The large aperture focus ultrasound transceivers used by Kossoff (19) and the authors of this report, have provided the clearest and most detailed brain scans in infants. The large size of the transceiver face makes it almost mandatory to use a water bath to provide adequate coupling, even though contact scanning would be more convenient both for the patient and the ultrasonographer. Somer's (16) phased array transceiver system is applied directly to the scalp and Freund (10) using the same instrument demonstrated most of the important diagnostic information available to the large aperture transceiver equipment. Whether the additional information available to the larger transceivers will be worth the additional trouble in application remains to be seen. The mild restraint, and soporific effect of the warm water bath may well offset the benefit derived from the ease of contact scanning, particularly in tiny infants with soft heads, or restless patients with head injuries. Additional exploration and imaginative innovation will undoubtedly bring about significant advance in the areas of patient handling as well as data acquisition and display.

Computerized axial tomography, using x-ray, has revolutionized the diagnosis of brain disorders. Whether ultrasound methods can provide additional useful information remains to be seen. Two-dimensional ultrasound brain tomography appears to have its place when dealing with very young infants, and possibly restless head injury victims. Rapid and continuous development of both computerized axial tomography and ultrasound instrumentation can only compliment each other, to benefit individuals seriously ill and disabled by brain pathology.

* This study was supported by the Fortune Behest, The Indianapolis Center for Advanced Research, and NIH Grant--R01-10983-RAD

BIBLIOGRAPHY

1. Adapon, B.D., Chase, I. I., Kricheff and Battista, F. F.: Cerebral ultrasound tomography. Radiology 84:115-21, 1965.
2. Brinker, R. A. and Taveras, J. M.: Ultrasound cross-sectional pictures of the head. Acta Radiol (Diagn) (Stockholm) 5:745-53, 1966.
3. Denier, von de Gon, Duinhouwer, J. J., Molin, G. E., de Vlieger, M.: Equipment for two-dimensional echoencephalography. Neurology 16:927-33, 1966.
4. de Vlieger, M., Denier, van der Gon, J. J. and Molin, C. E.: Two-dimensional echoencephalography of the third ventricle in hydrocephalus. Neurol 18:473-9, 1968.
5. de Vlieger, M., Sterke, A., Molin, C. E. and van der Ven, C.: Ultrasound for two-dimensional echoencephalography. Ultrasonice 1:148-51, 1963.
6. Dreese, M. J., McGee, F. E. and Harrelson, A. B.: Correlative aids in B-scan echoencephalography. Neurology . 16:766-70, 1966
7. Dussik, K. T.: Possibility of using mechanical high frequency vibrations (ultrasonic waves) as diagnostic aid. Ftschr. f. d. ges. Neurol u. Psychiat. 174:153-168, 1942.
8. Dussik, K. T.: Further experience in diagnosis of brain disease with ultrasound. Acta. neurochir. 2:379-396, 1952.
9. Erba, G. and Lambroso, C. T.: Detection of ventricular landmarks by two-dimensional ultrasonography. J. Neurol Neurosurg Psychiat 31:232-44, 1968
10. Freund, H. J. and Somer, J. C.: Electronic sector scanning in the diagnosis of cerebrovascular disease. Neurology 23:1147-59, 1973.

11. Galicich, J.H., Lombroso, C.T. and Matson, D.D.: Ultrasonic B-scanning of the brain. J. Neurosurg 22:499-510, 1965.
12. Heimburger, R.F., Fry, F.J. and Eggleton, R.C.: Ultrasound visualization in human brain: the internal capsule, a preliminary report. Surgical Neurology 1:56-58, 1973.
13. Heimburger, R.F., Eggleton, R.C. and Fry, F.J.: Ultrasonic visualization in determination of tumor growth rate. JAMA 224:497-501, 1973.
14. Heimburger, R.F., Fry, F.J., Franklin, T.D. and Eggleton, R.C.: Ultrasound visualization of intracranial hemorrhage. Ultrasound in Medicine edited by D. White, Plenum Press 1975 265-71.
15. Hovind, K.H., Galicich, J.H. and Matson, D.D.: Normal and pathological intracranial anatomy revealed by two dimensional echoencephalography. Neurology 17:253-62, 1967.
16. Kamphuisen, A.C., Somer, J.C. and Oosterbaan, W.A.: Two-dimensional echoencephalography with electronic sector scanning. Clinical experiences with a new method. J. Neurol Neurosurg Psychiat 35:912-8, 1972.
17. Kazner, E.: Echoencephalography with simultaneous A- and B-mode display. J. Neurol Neurosurg Psychiat 33:718, 1970.
18. Kossoff, G. and Garrett, W.J.: Intracranial detail in fetal echograms. Investigative Radiology 7:159-63, 1972.
19. Kossoff, G., Garrett, W.J. and Radavanovich, G.: Ultrasonic atlas of normal brain of infant. Ultrasound in Med. & Biol. 1:259-66, 1974.
20. Kossoff, G.: Letters to the Editor (Author's Reply) on Ultrasound atlas of normal brain of infant. Ultrasound in Med. & Biol. 1:412, 1975.
21. Lombroso, C.T., Erba, G., Yogo, T., Logowitz, N. and Hilaire, J.St.: Two-dimensional sonar scanning for detection of intracranial lesions. A comparison with isotope scans, electroencephalograms, and radiological studies in 97 cases. Arch Neurol 23:518-27, 1970.
22. McKinney, W.M.: The value of B-mode determination of midline in echoencephalography. (Abstract) Neurology 14:259, 1964.
23. Makow, D.M., Wyslouzil, W., White, D.N. and Blanchard, J.: Novel immersion scanner and display system for ultrasonic brain tomography.. Acta Radiol. Suppl. (Diagn.) 5:855-64, 1966.
24. Pendl, G. and Kratochwil, A.: Two-dimensional echoencephalography in the young child. Neuroradiol. 4:36-40, 1972.
25. Reese, C.L. 3d.: Two-dimensional echoencephalography: a clinical study. Neurology 20:417-8, 1970.
26. Tanaka, K., Kikuchi, S., Ito, K., Ishii, M., Katsumi, S. and Wagai, T.: Ultrasonic diagnosis of intracranial disease, J. Japan Surg. Soc. 61:761, 1960.

27. Wealthall, S. R. and Todd, J. N.: B-scope echoencephalography in the infant. Develop. Med. Child. Neurol. 15:338-47, 1973.
28. Wealthall, S. R. and Todd, J. H.: Ultrasonic B-scans in the diagnosis and assessment of hydrocephalus in infants (Letter). Br. J. Radiol 46:566, 1973.
29. White, D. N., et al.: Studies in ultrasonic echoencephalography. VII. General principles of recording information in ultrasonic B- and C- scanning and the effects of scatter, reflection and refraction by cadaver skull on this information. Med Biol Engin 5:3-14, 1967.

ULTRASOUND SCANNING OF EXCISED BRAINS TO LOCALIZE PATHOLOGY

R. F. Heimburger, M.D., F. J. Fry, T. D. Franklin, Jr.,
R. C. Eggleton and J. Muller*
Indianapolis Center for Advanced Research, Indiana University School of Medicine, Indianapolis, Indiana 46202
*Indiana University School of Medicine, Indianapolis, Indiana 46202 (Department of Pathology)

An "in vitro" study of human brains has been carried out to determine the accuracy of localizing and measuring pathological, as well as normal, structure. This type of careful correlation will aid in the interpretation of ultrasound images in living patients.

The excised, formalin-fixed brains were immersed in a water bath and visualized ultrasonically with transducers of various frequencies and focal lengths. Each brain was carefully aligned so that the mid-sagittal plane is parallel to the floor of the water bath, and the orbital surfaces of the frontal lobes are parallel to the scan path for horizontal scans, and perpendicular to it for coronal scans. Images are recorded at 5mm intervals. The planes of scanning can be accurately reproduced on subsequent occasions by careful alignment of the brains in relationship to the scan path and by utilization of readily identifiable reference points. These reference points are found where the corpus callosum starts to protrude into the falx anteriorly and posteriorly for coronal scans, or superiorly for horizontal scans. The posterior border of the corpus callosum is the most reliable of these reference points. Scans made by using this reference information conform closely to standard stereotaxic atlas reproductions. The posterior corpus callosum reference point can also be easily seen and used for the first coronal cut at the time that the brains are sliced for pathological study. When this plane has been established, the remainder of the brain can be accurately sliced at 5mm intervals on a mechanical slicing device. Photographs of the cut brain surfaces then conform to the planes of the ultrasound scans to provide accurate comparisons.

These studies suggest that the cerebral ventricles can be best appreciated with good grey scale image presentation, further implemented by logarithmic amplification. Subdural and epidural collections of blood appear more clearly outlined, and therefore more readily detected, with linear amplification. The internal capsule and other grey/white interfaces appear to be more clearly demonstrated with a sector scan sweep with appropriate transceiver focal position in the tissue. The method of sensitivity graded tomography helps to differentiate the reflections produced by hemorrhage from those of neoplasms. The portion of neoplasms that are grossly visible on cut brain sections are readily visible with the linear amplifier. The edematous areas around tumors are more easily delineated with appropriate grey scale presentation. Studies of this sort, although time consuming, are needed to continually improve the accuracy of clinical interpretations. Since transkull studies provide less information than is seen in brain scans after the skull has been removed, it is necessary to have the type of information available from correlated studies, like this one, to help in the identification of all the pertinent echoes that are recorded.

LATERAL VENTRICULAR MEASUREMENT DURING INFANCY

M. S. Tenner, M.D.; G. Wodraska; C. Montesinos, M.D.

Department of Radiology
State University of New York
Brooklyn, N. Y. 11203

In a previous communication with the society, we described our methods for establishing measurements of the width of the lateral ventricles at their superolateral corners. At that time a finding of 20 mm was accepted as normal. However, in infants and young children we have found that this value can normally be less than 20 mm and is related to the size of the head. A ratio has been established between the size of the lateral ventricles and the intracranial diameter.

TECHNIQUE

A 1 cm per division scale is used. Rather than the normal 1.0 MHz transducer used in adults, a 2.25 MHz transducer is used in infants as it is more sensitive and has sufficient penetration.

Step 1. A transmission is obtained at the ventricular level and placed on the top of the tracing.

Step 2. A second "search" tracing is then obtained using a low gain setting to "clean up" the far echo complex so that a triple echo complex corresponding to the inner and outer tables of the skull and air-skin interface is visible. The transducer is not moved between the first and second traces so that measuring the break between the transmission midline and the beginning of the far echo complex represents the diameter of the left or right hemicranium.

Step 3. With the transducer in the same position, the trace is reversed (spikes pointing downward), the gain

setting increased until the falx, superolateral
border of the lateral ventricle and possibly the
insula are sounded. The lateral ventricle is then
measured.

A ratio between the ventricle and hemicranium is made. Our findings in normal infants and young children is that the lateral ventricle will measure one-third or less of the hemicranial diameter and always 20 mm or less in size.

Ophthalmology

POWER SPECTRAL RESONANCE ANALYSIS IN THE EVALUATION OF VITREOUS PATHOLOGY

Mary E. Smith, Louise A. Franzen, Frederic L. Lizzi,
Eng. Sc. D., and D. Jackson Coleman, M.D.

Department of Ophthalmology, College of Physicians and
Surgeons, Columbia University
635 West 165th Street, New York, New York 10032
Riverside Research Institute (Dr. Lizzi)
80 West End Avenue, New York, New York 10023

The pre-operative evaluation of patients with vitreous opacifications has been greatly enhanced by ultrasonic examination. The location and extent of vitreous hemorrhage may now be ascertained with a high degree of confidence, but the differentiation of hemorrhage, vitreous membranes and retina is a difficult but essential distinction.

Conventional B-scan techniques of analysis will easily distinguish between diffuse hemorrhage and organized membranes, but this topographic categorization is inadequate in distinguishing organized membranes from retina at the posterior pole.

Implementation of more sophisticated ultrasonic techniques such as quantitative A-scan analysis, color coding and three-dimensional isometric viewing has greatly augmented the ability of the examiner to characterize membrane and retina on the basis of echo amplitude, but has not provided definitive diagnostic criteria. The use of kinetic B-scanning to demonstrate the comparative mobility of hemorrhage, membranes and retina has also proven of particular value, but is limited by the subjective nature of the evaluation.

In view of the critical nature of the pre-operative selection of patients, based upon their surgical suitability and prognosis, a more precise mode of differentiation of vitreous pathology is required.

A system using power spectral density curves to selectively distinguish these pathologic conditions has been utilized in our laboratory. A characterization of these differing vitreal abnormalities has been indicated by this method which will further assist the diagnostician. Distributed scattering structures, such as those within a diffuse hemorrhage, exhibit broad spectral density curves with no pronounced resonant peaks. Structures such as membrane and retina with discrete reflective interfaces, can produce distinct spectral resonances which vary according to factors such as thickness and organization.

The implementation of this ultrasonic diagnostic information and its correlative value to pathologic states expedites the surgeon's pre-operative assessment and permits him to proceed in a more knowledgeable manner.

ULTRASONOGRAPHIC DIAGNOSIS OF TUMORS OF THE ANTERIOR CHOROID AND CILIARY BODY

Louise A. Franzen, Mary E. Smith, D. Jackson Coleman, M.D. and Robert L. Jack, M.D.

Department of Ophthalmology, College of Physicians and Surgeons, Columbia University
635 West 165th Street, New York, New York 10032
Department of Ophthalmology, Stamford University School of Medicine, Stamford, California   (Dr. Jack)

Malignant melanomas of the ciliary body are often difficult to diagnose clinically, for they arise in a silent area of the eye not routinely examined. These lesions frequently cause cataracts, secondary retinal detachments, or pupillary blocks which make visualization difficult and unsatisfactory. Even ophthalmoscopically visible lesions may present a diagnostic problem.

Ultrasonographic evaluation of these lesions yields a morphologic description, a characterization of the cystic or solid nature of the mass, and the neoplastic potential.

Determination of the tumor type, size (i.e., posterior extent) and involvement of the adjacent structures is of great clinical significance in deciding the course of treatment, whether enucleation, radiation by cobalt plaque implant, corneo-scleral iridocyclectomy or observation. The decision to employ further more invasive types of diagnostic tests such as P32 can also be dictated by ultrasonic findings.

This paper describes the B-scan morphology and the A-scan acoustic profile of 35 cases of ciliary body and anterior choroid lesions confirmed by histologic examination or long-term followup. The series includes the following tissue types: malignant melanoma, metastatic carcinoma, epithelioma, cyst, and organized hemorrhage.

Acoustic examination of the anterior segment of the eye offers complexities not found in scanning lesions posterior to the equator. Acoustic differentiation of anteriorly located lesions on B-scan is made difficult by the absence of the choroidal excavation sign for malignant melanoma that is commonly found in tumors posterior to the equator. Furthermore, A-scan diagnosis of lesions less than 2 mm in thickness encounters masking of the tumor echoes by the high amplitude return from the preceding iris or sclera. We have found higher frequency transducers from 10 to 22 MHz to be useful in defining the extent and acoustic texture of these tumors of the ciliary region. Careful attention to angulation of the transducer beam in both the horizontal and vertical scan planes are important for obtaining a complete ultrasonic characterization.

The reliability of ultrasonic detection and characterization of anterior tumors is slightly less than that obtained in posterior segment examination due to the problems discussed above. Nevertheless, ultrasonography is the only examination method available for opaque eyes and is frequently necessary for determining the posterior extent and nature of visible lesions. The ultrasonic findings are thus pivotal in directing patient management

THE ULTRASONOGRAPHIC CHARACTERISTICS OF ORBITAL DERMOID CYSTS

Gwen Kunken Sterns, M.D. and D. Jackson Coleman, M.D.
Department of Ophthalmology, College of Physicians and Surgeons, Columbia University
635 West 165th Street, New York, New York 10032

Expanding lesions of the orbit are an important diagnostic problem frequently requiring a multidiscipline approach. The diagnosis is often made at the time of surgery. The radiologist is called upon to define the limits and extent of the mass radiographically. Many orbital lesions remain confined to the orbit with minimal if any bony disturbances. Ultrasonography is especially helpful in these cases in locating the mass, outlining the dimensions of the tumor, determining the extent of ocular involvement and in characterizing acoustically the tumor tissue to aid in the diagnosis of the lesion.

Dermoid cysts are classified as choristomas, i.e., normal tissue located in an abnormal site. They are congenital but frequently slow growing, and may not be appreciated until the patient is in his thirties. In one series of 504 consecutive cases of expanding lesions of the orbit, dermoid cysts comprise 4%. These lesions may or may not have associated radiographic findings.

By the use of high resolution A-, B- and M-scan ultrasound (5, 10 and 15 MHz transducer frequencies) we have examined several cases of pathologically proven dermoid cysts of the orbit. Some of these cases have had normal radiographic findings. One case was examined by the use of the EMI scanner (computerized axial tomography).

Ultrasonographically, these lesions demonstrate specific acoustic characteristics including boundary properties, internal reflectivity, acoustic absorption and location, which distinguish them from other expanding orbital lesions of a more malignant nature. Acoustically there may be evidence of associated orbital inflammatory changes which may represent rupture or leakage of the cyst with subsequent orbital inflammation.

The acoustic criteria seen with dermoid cysts of the orbit have been helpful in diagnosing these lesions and in providing important information to the surgeon in his pre-operative management and surgical approach to the patient.

POSTERIOR OCULAR CURVATURE BY B SCAN ULTRASONOGRAPHY

W.E. Cappaert; E.W. Purnell; K.E. Frank
Department of Surgery, Division of Ophthalmology
Case Western Reserve University
Cleveland, Ohio 44106

Analysis of the posterior curvature of the eye on B sector scan ultrasonography is an important parameter in the evaluation of normal and abnormal ocular conditions. In the normal eye, as sound waves pass through the crystalline lens they are refracted producing a well known artifactual change in its posterior curvature making it appear more concave and anteriorly displaced. The magnitude of this refractive effect is greatest as the distance from the crystalline lens increases and thus it is best studied in myopic eyes in which the axial length is greater.

When the beam is split by the peripheral portions of the crystalline lens, an artifactual projection into the vitreous is produced at the posterior pole of the eye. This tumor-like effect is again dependent upon the axial length of the eye as found in high myopia and congenital glaucoma. In these conditions the artifactual change is accentuated and may extend one or two millimeters into the vitreous cavity.

Horizontal rotation produces another change in the ultrasonic display due to lens refraction. Consequently the eye in rotation develops a square appearance posteriorly. This is again more prominent with increased axial length. Reversal of these curvature changes can be demonstrated following removal of the crystalline lens. Thus, the aphakic patient retains a more convex posterior curvature on the horizontal ocular rotation.

Changes in the cornea also accentuate the artifactual effect. With increased corneal curvature as found in keratoglobus the posterior artifact is again more prominent.

Involvement of the posterior layers of the eye with a pathological condition such as scleral shrinkage or edema may also produce posterior curvature changes. In this condition a flattening of the posterior aspect of the globe is produced which is not found with lenticular or corneal refractive changes.

ULTRASONIC FINDINGS IN DIABETIC VITREORETINOPATHY

K. E. Frank, M.D.; E. W. Purnell, M.D.;
W. E. Cappaert, M.D.
Division of Ophthalmology; Department of Surgery
Case Western Reserve University
Cleveland, Ohio 44106

   The purpose of this study is to demonstrate by serial ultrasonography the course of the vitreoretinal disease of diabetes, to determine what information may be obtained from ultrasonic evaluation and whether ultrasonic examination can predict remissions or exacerbations. The ultimate goals are to evaluate ultrasonography as a method for determining the advisability of vitrectomy in these eyes and to determine the role of ultrasound in the planning and execution of the vitrectomy procedure.

   Method: The authors are following a group of diabetic patients with varying degrees of diabetic vitreoretinal disease. All patients referred for evaluation are examined by the usual optical methods of eye examination, stereo fundus photographs are taken when the media permit, and the initial serial B-scan ultrasonography performed. Our technique of ultrasonic examination insures that each horizontal B-scan sonogram is separated from the previous one by a 0.5 mm vertical step. Each sonogram is recorded on film. Series of scans are done with the eye in primary position, nasal and lateral rotation.

   The patients are then re-examined at intervals by both optical methods and ultrasonography. The optical information is interpreted by one observer and the ultrasonic interpretation is performed by a second observer. The information is then correlated. In a few patients vitrectomy was performed and the findings at vitrectomy correlated with the sonograms.

   Results: Seventy-five eyes with diabetic retinopathy have been followed for three to eighteen months. In three-quarters of the eyes the media cleared sufficiently (spontaneously or by vitrectomy) to correlate optical and ultrasonic findings.

Thirteen characteristic patterns were found. These were classified into two groups: hemorrhagic and fibroproliferative. The earliest hemorrhagic ultrasonic pattern was that of a pre-retinal hemorrhage which presented on the sonogram as a smooth solid density just anterior to the retina. If the pre-retinal hemorrhage began to break through into the vitreous, the ultrasonic pattern showed the same localized density anterior to the retina but with an irregular anterior border instead a smooth one. With further diffusion of the hemorrhage into the vitreous body, there was frequently little evidence of the hemorrhage on the B-scan sonograms. If the poor ultrasonic visualization persisted, this was a good prognostic sign for spontaneous clearing.

Older vitreous hemorrhage showed two patterns. Either the blood was posterior to a detached posterior vitreous face and appeared as a density in the posterior vitreous cavity or the blood was within the contracted vitreous body itself and appeared as a density in the anterior vitreous cavity.

Several fibroproliferative patterns were detected by ultrasonography. The most common pattern was enhancement of the posterior vitreous face with single or multiple attachments to retina or disc. On the sonogram this was seen as an irregular linear density usually in the posterior one-third of the vitreous cavity with fine linear attachments to the posterior pole. Another pattern was that of single or multiple vitreous membranes within the contracted vitreous body. These membranes presented on the sonogram as multiple linear densities paralleling the retracted posterior vitreous face. A rare pattern in diabetics was amorphous organization of the entire vitreous which was seen on the sonogram as a diffuse density filling the entire vitreous cavity.

A pattern unique in diabetic eyes was that of pre-retinal membrane formation. Three types were identified. The first was a pre-retinal membrane without evidence of vitreous attachments, which was seen as a dense, flat, highly reflective surface just anterior to the retina. The second was a pre-retinal membrane with vitreous attachments. In this pattern one or more linear densities were anterior to the flat surface found in the previous pattern. These densities would merge with the membrane at the points of attachment. The third pattern was commonly associated with a traction retinal detachment. In this pattern there was sharp angulation of the membrane at the points of attachment or a solid "mass" pattern posterior to the membrane. Both of these patterns were secondary to reflections from sharply tented retina in a localized detachment.

Other Organs

Evaluation of Solitary Cold Thyroid Nodules by Echography and Thermography

GC Coggs, OH Clark, FS Greenspan, L Goldman

Department of Radiology, University of Calif., S.F.

M-380, San Francisco, CA 94143

Thyroid operations are an effective form of treatment for thyroid nodules and are associated with minimal morbidity and rare mortality. The major indication for thyroidectomy in non-toxic goiter is the suspicion of thyroid malignancy. Despite the excellent therapeutic effectiveness of thyroid operations, the diagnostic accuracy in differentiating benign from malignant thyroid neoplasms without operation is low. Most medical centers report that the incidence of thyroid cancer in patients having thyroid operations varies from between 5 and 35 percent. Obviously, if only 5 percent of patients who have thyroid operations have cancer of the thyroid, too many people are having thyroid operations and if 50 percent are found to have cancer, too few patients with thyroid disease are having operations and many patients are being followed without definitive treatment.

Because of the difficulty in predicting the presence of thyroid cancer in solitary thyroid nodules that are nonfunctioning by 131^I scan and because thyroid cancer is rare in cystic thyroid nodules less than 4 cm in diameter, we initiated a prospective study using echography, ultrasound, and thermography in our preoperative evaluation of thyroid nodules. This was undertaken first to try to improve our diagnostic accuracy in differentiating between benign and malignant thyroid nodules and secondly to determine the reliability of echography and thermography in distinguishing between solid and cystic thyroid nodules.

From February, 1973, through December, 1974, at the University of California Hospitals in San Francisco, sixty-one patients with solitary cold thyroid nodules, as determined by clinical examination and 131^I scan, were evaluated by echography and thirty-one by thermography. Twenty-seven of the sixty-one patients had their thyroid lesions confirmed by histological examination. Two additional patients were successfully treated by aspiration. In all cases, where a lesion was thought to be solid or cystic by both echography and thermography, this was the finding at operation or aspiration. The overall diagnostic accuracy of echography alone was eighty-two percent and thermography fifty-seven percent. The combined use of these tests is valuable in differentiating between solid and cystic thyroid nodules. If cystic, thyroid nodules may be safely treated by aspiration, thus avoiding unnecessary operations.

A LARGE APERTURE REAL-TIME EQUIPMENT FOR IMAGING THE CAROTID ARTERY*

Anant K. Nigam, Ph.D.
NYIT Science & Technology Center, Ft. Lauderdale, Fla.
and
Charles P. Olinger, M.D.
Stroke Clinic, Univ. of Cincinnati, Cincinnati, Ohio

This talk outlines the design and performance of a portable, real-time, high resolution ultrasound imaging system. The basic design consists of an imaging probe containing a large aperture transducer and a reflective scanning mechanism sealed in a water chamber with a transparent membrane at one end. The entire probe is portable. High resolutions are attained by the use of the large aperture transducer which may be dynamically focussed in depth and real-time operation is provided by the scanning mechanism which is capable of operation in excess of 30 frames/sec. For preliminary testing, a prototype system of this design employing mechanical focussing was built and evaluated for applications in imaging the human carotid artery in-vivo. In this system the transducer aperture was F/4 to provide better than 0.5mm resolution in depth and about 1mm resolution in the transverse directions, and the scan rate was 4 frames/sec. The entire probe, together with the mechanical focussing arrangement for the transducer, weighed less than 9 lbs. and provides a field of view of about 5cm x 7cm. The probe weight may be further reduced by employing dynamic focussing. The equipment displays B-section views in sequences of four via commercially available gray scale storage display. Preliminary in-vivo images obtained by the prototype equipment are presented and discussed. The carotid artery appears well resolved, however, in some cases, some loss in detail is observed at interfaces which are parallel to the ultrasound direction. This is minimized by employing (a) larger aperture transducers which provide better sensitivity for the scattered echo field, and (b) better sidelobe suppression in the transmitted ultrasound beam which permits expansion of equipment dynamic range without introducing artifacts due to ringing within the portable probe. The non-linear compression of the gray scale also appears to be a critical parameter in optimizing image quality.

The image quality is also discussed in relation to other equipment parameters. These indicate directions for further equipment modifications which are currently in progress.

---

* This work was supported in part under funds supplied by the C.B.S. Laboratories and the Fannie E. Rippel Foundation.

ULTRASOUND IN ORTHOPEDIC DIAGNOSIS

V. Mayer

Hospital for Special Surgery, affiliated with
New York Hospital-Cornell University Medical
College New York, N.Y. 10021

The results of an in-progress feasibility study to
determine the value of ultrasound in orthopedic diagnosis
will be shown. In reviewing the literature on its application to orthopedics the author found remarkably few
reports showing orthopedic studies. Further investigations
revealed that there was a prevailing opinion that the use
in orthopedic surgery was restricted because of the bony
structures which were involved and their poor display by
ultrasound. However, an analysis of orthopedic problems
reveals that the interest in soft tissue structures about
the bones and joints as well as the anatomic relationship
of one bone to another plays an equally important role
in orthopedic investigation and treatment. With this
premise, the author began a survey of various joints and
structures in the body to determine what technique and
which joints would lend themselves to a meaningful investigation. The initial examination was done with the B-mode
and then the Gray scale whenever it was available. Examinations of the shoulder wrist, hand, vertebral column, hips
and knees were done. The cross sectional anatomy of each
of these areas and x-ray examinations were then correlated
with the ultrasound scans and consistent and repeatable
images were obtained.

In the shoulder, cross sectional studies done horizontally at different levels showed clear pictures which could
be related to the anatomy. The same process was applied
to the wrist to investigate the carpal tunnel and showed a
clear outline of the tunnel and on some occasions the con-

tents. Further studies were done of the hand demonstrating the bony outlines of metacarpals and the soft tissue structures which were identifiable such as tendons and fascial planes. The vertebral column, pelvis and hip joints and knees were also surveyed. The maximum amount of studies were done in the knees. After a series of normal asymptomatic knees studies were done of rheumatoid knees as well as osteoarthritic knee joints. The basic changes in the soft tissue outline were clearly defined. As yet, specifics for rheumatoid arthritis were not established. Changes in the knee joint following synovectomy were clearly documented.

A secondary study was then begun since outlines of bony structures could be well demonstrated. It became apparent that where the relationship of one bony structure to another played an important role in the pathologic changes, this could be depicted and recorded. This was done in subluxating patellae and the beginning of an analysis of the patellar pathway, during flexion and extension of the knee. Present studies are continuing and the results will be reported at a later date relating to the various anatomical areas using Gray scale imaging and employing specialized transducers.

PATELLAR TRACKING BY ULTRASOUND

V. Mayer; A. Wardell; J. L. Marshall

Sports Medicine Service, The Hospital for Special Surgery affiliated with New York Hospital-Cornell University Medical College, New York, N. Y. 10021

The patella is known to demonstrate a shift both medial and lateral in the course of its excursion past the femoral condyles as the knee flexes and extends. In addition, a tilting is also noted and rotation is suspected. It is difficult to accomplish the study of these motions in the living knee without invasive techniques. Since bony outlines are needed in this study, the possibility of accomplishing this by ultrasound was explored outlining the patella and femoral condyles in various positions of flexion and extension actively. The technique employed was to have the patient sit with the leg extended beyond the table and to do longitudinal and cross sectional, full circumferential studies of the knee at various levels. The medial epicondyle of the knee was set as the zero baseline and 1 cm. cuts above and below were recorded as plus above and minus below. Studies were obtained using a 5 MHz. transducer. Recordings on the print out were then analyzed by drawing the baseline tangential to the posterior margins of the condyles and then erecting a perpendicular line at the extremes of the medial and lateral femoral condyles. The patellar axis was determined by taking the maximum width of the patella as recorded on the transverse reading. Using this axis and relating it to the baseline at the posterior margins of the condyles offered an opportunity to measure the patellar tilt and the direction of the tilt. The shift of the patella was determined by relating the mid point of the patellar axis to the mid point of the width of the femoral condyles as measured by the baseline. The relationship of these points was then recorded in millimeters.

medial and lateral to the midline of the baseline. The measurements were then plotted for each of the cuts at full extension of the knee, 0°, 20° and 45° of flexion of the knee. Preliminary measurements on the initial cases indicated that thepatellar tilt in the course of flexion of the knee remained facing medially in the normal knee. The shift of the patella was seen to follow a consistent pattern and the mid point of the patella tended to remain in a lateral position in relation to the mid point of the femoral condyles. The study is continuing to establish the range of tilt and shift of the patella in the normal asymptomatic knee. This will be used as a baseline to evaluate the pathologic knee and an effort made to establish reliable patterns for future diagnosis.

Doppler

CALIBRATION OF A DOPPLER BLOOD FLOWMETER FOR MEASUREMENTS

INDEPENDENT OF FLOW ANGLE, VELOCITY PROFILE, AND LUMEN SHAPE

C. Hottinger, L. Gerzberg, J. D. Meindl

Department of Electrical Engineering

Stanford University, Stanford, California 94305

An ultrasonic pulsed Doppler system for unambiguous measurement of blood volume flow is currently under development (1). As shown in Figure 1, a two-element transducer array is used to insonify an arbitrary sample plane cutting across the vessel lumen. The sample volume of the smaller transducer (element 2) lies totally within the vessel lumen, while the sample volume of the combined array is designed to approximate uniform insonification over a plane totally encompassing the lumen projection.

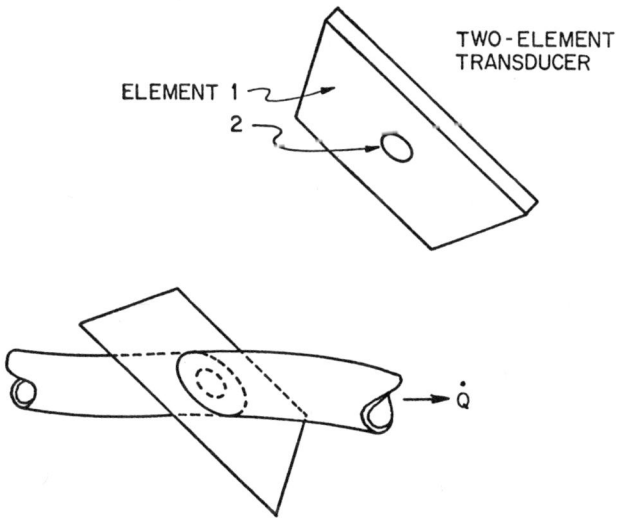

Figure 1. Two-Element Transducer Configuration for Measurement of $\dot{Q}$.

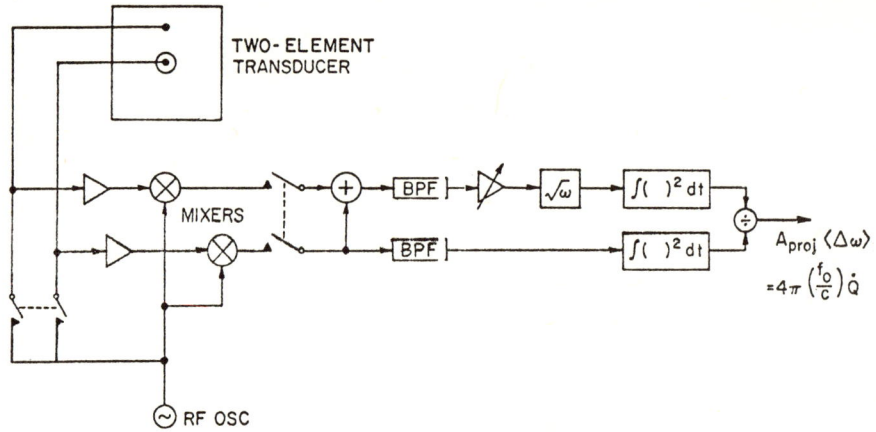

Figure 2. System for Measurement of $\dot{Q}$ Using Two-Element Transducer.

A non-directional demodulator outlined in Figure 2 is now in use. Since the Doppler power spectrum detected by element 2 is $S_2(\Delta\omega)$, with that of 1 and 2 being $S_{1+2}(\Delta\omega)$, the volume flow $\dot{Q}$ is measured by the system following the formula

$$\dot{Q} = (c/f_0)(4\pi)^{-1} \frac{\int (\Delta\omega) S_{1+2}(\Delta\omega) d(\Delta\omega)}{\int S_2(\Delta\omega) d(\Delta\omega)} \frac{|G_2(\vec{r})|^2 d^2\vec{r}}{|G_{1+2}(0)|^2} \quad (1)$$

where $|G_i(r)|^2$ is the antenna beam factor of the respective transducer and (c/f_0) is the ultrasonic wavelength. Under conditions of first-order Rayleigh scattering by particles with constant average density within the lumen (2), Eq. (1) provides an estimate of volume flow independent of flow angle, velocity profile, lumen shape, or size.

Test results are discussed for a 5.7 MHz system with transducer elements having dimensions 24 mm square, and 4.4 mm diameter respectively. The demodulator includes a $\sqrt{\omega}$ discriminator tapered for optimum response, as well as noise cancellation circuitry. Results of in vitro tests demonstrate output invariance with changes in vessel size, orientation, and flow Reynold's number. Errors arising from the transducer beam patterns and demodulator non-linearities are considered and alternate schemes are outlined for minimizing these errors.

The unique versatility of this approach to flow measurement is illustrated by the two extreme examples of transcutaneous aortic flow measurement, and acute measurement of coronary artery flow. The large upper bound on the beam spread permitted of the small transducer (element 2) will allow lower operating frequencies than previously possible (3), while the invariance of the flow estimate will allow measurement without prior knowledge of the lumen geometry and flow distribution (4).

References

(1) C. F. Hottinger and J. D. Meindl. "An Ultrasonic Technique for Unambiguous Measurement of Blood Volume Flow," *Proc. IEEE Ultrasonics Symposium*, Milwaukee, Wisconsin, 1974.

(2) W. R. Brody and J. D. Meindl. "Theoretical Analysis of the CW Doppler Ultrasonic Flowmeter," *IEEE Trans. Biomed. Eng.*, vol. BME-23, pp. 183-192, 1974.

(3) J. E. Jorgensen, D. N. Campau, D. W. Baker. "Physical Characteristics and Mathematical Modelling of the Pulsed Ultrasonic Flowmeter," *Medical and Biological Engineering*, pp. 404-421, July 1973.

(4) D. W. Baker, S. L. Johnson, D. E. Strandness. "Prospects for Quantitation of Transcutaneous Pulsed Doppler Techniques in Cardiology and Pulse Doppler Techniques," in *Cardiovascular Applications of Ultrasound*, ed. R. S. Reneman, North-Holland Publishing, London, pp. 108-124.

Acknowledgement

This investigation was supported by PHS Research Grant No. 1P01 GM17940-05 from the Department of Health, Education, and Welfare.

RESOLUTION PERFORMANCE OF PULSED ULTRASOUND DOPPLER BLOOD FLOWMETERS

J. M. Griffith[*] and W. R. Brody[**]
[*]Biomedical Engineering and Instrumentation Branch, Bldg. 13, Rm. 3W-13, and [**]National Heart and Lung Institute, National Institutes of Health, Bethesda, Maryland 20014

The effectiveness of ultrasound doppler blood flowmeters depends upon both the spatial and velocity resolution afforded. An index is defined here with which the ultimate overall resolution performance of a given instrument in a given application can be estimated. This "resolution product index" can be expressed as:

(1)
$$RPI = \left[(\Delta R)\frac{\Delta V}{V}\right]_{minimum} = \frac{20\,RV}{C}$$

where: V = red cell velocity
R = range
C = acoustic velocity
ΔV = velocity resolution
ΔR = range resolution

The index, applicable to pulsed systems and independent of acoustic beam diameter, establishes a reasonable basis for deciding appropriate compromises between spatial and velocity resolution requirements in design and application. It is derived as follows:

To prevent widening of the doppler sidelobes, a small time-bandwidth product is assumed, i.e.:

(2) $TB \leq 0.1\, C/V$

where: T = coherent signal processing time
B = bandwidth of transmitted signal

and $T \leq T_t$

where: T_t = the transit time. If $T = T_t$ it can be shown that:

(3) $\Delta R \approx 1.25 D$, and

(4) $\dfrac{\Delta V}{V} \approx \dfrac{2C}{D f_o}$

where: D = acoustic beam width to the first null
f_o = signal frequency

Although spatial resolution is assessed in terms of both lateral and range parameters, both depend upon D; and, for the purposes here it is sufficient to consider range effects alone.

Taking the product of (3) and (4) yields:

(5) $(\Delta R) \dfrac{\Delta V}{V} = (1.25 D) \dfrac{2C}{D f_o} = \dfrac{2.5 C}{f_o}$

which demonstrates that range and velocity resolution can be directly traded by changing beam diameter but that the product depends only upon acoustic velocity and signal frequency.

To avoid velocity and range ambiguities the frequency must be less than $C^2/8RV$. Thus the maximum operating frequency is:

(6) $f_{o\,max} = \dfrac{C^2}{8RV}$

Therefore, the minimum RPI, tantamount to best resolution performance, is:

$RPI = \left[(\Delta R) \dfrac{\Delta V}{V} \right]_{min} = \dfrac{20 \, RV}{C}$

For example: given $R = 5$ cm
$V = 200$ cm/sec

$(\Delta R) \dfrac{\Delta V}{V} = 0.13$ cm which could be factored into
$R = 0.65$ cm and $\dfrac{\Delta V}{V} = 0.2$.

Thus the relationship between spatial and velocity resolutions for maximum performance are immediately evident.

In practice the minimum value of the resolution product index may be difficult to achieve; however, it allows the investigator to estimate the highest achievable resolution performance for a given application. In addition, the index allows a simple evaluation of the spatial and velocity resolution trade off which is accomplished by changing beam diameter.

THE DOPPLER ULTRASONIC CEREBROVASCULAR EXAMINATION: IMPROVED

ACCURACY BY REFINEMENT OF TECHNIQUE

H. E. Russell; R. J. Burger; R. W. Barnes

Peripheral Vascular Laboratories, Department of
Surgery, University of Iowa and Veterans Administration
Hospitals, Iowa City, Iowa 52242

INTRODUCTION

Although strokes take the lives of more than 200,000 people annually, 25% of stroke prone patients have occlusive disease amenable to extracranial surgical techniques. Therefore, the diagnosis of extracranial carotid occlusive disease becomes an important priority in health care. One of the simplest, safest and most accurate techniques for evaluating extracranial occlusive vascular disease is the determination of directional flow in the supraorbital artery using the Doppler ultrasonic velocity detector. The 10 megahertz Doppler probe permits detection of flow in the supraorbital artery which is normally out of the orbit and augmented by compression of the ipsilateral temporal artery. In the presence of significant stenosis (>70%) or occlusion of the internal carotid artery, the flow may be reversed and ipsilateral temporal artery compression may diminish or obliterate flow in the supraorbital artery. This technique may detect significant internal carotid disease with 90% accuracy but is associated with both false positive and false negative results. The present study presents the improved results of a modified Doppler cerebrovascular examination of 50 patients who underwent cerebral angiography for suspected arterial occlusive disease.

The frontal artery provided the most prominent arterial signal and was the most reliable indicator of carotid artery patency. Examination of the frontal artery avoided mistaking the supraorbital artery for the palpebral artery which is a branch of the superficial temporal artery. A directionally sensitive Doppler velocity detector was used so that changes in flow direction with compression maneuvers were not misinterpreted as normal velocity augmentation.

The patient was examined in the supine position with the eyes gently closed. A 10 megahertz pencil probe was placed lightly on the skin to locate the frontal artery signal on the superomedial aspect of the orbit. In addition to the classic maneuver of ipsilateral temporal artery compression, the facial arteries were compressed bilaterally. If a decrease in flow resulted the facial arteries were separately compressed to determine which one contributed flow to the frontal artery. Finally transient ipsilateral common carotid compression was performed low in the neck to avoid embolic complications or carotid sinus stimulation. If frontal artery flow augmented with ipsilateral compression, the contralateral common carotid was similarly compressed to determine its contribution to frontal artery flow. The entire sequence was repeated on the opposite side.

Fifty patients underwent both cerebral angiography and Doppler ultrasonic examination. There were 46 males and 4 females ranging in age from 40 to 82 years with a mean of 61 years.

RESULTS

Of the 50 patients, angiography revealed 32 patients to have occlusion or a stenosis greater than 70% of the carotid artery. Utilizing ipsilateral temporal artery compression alone during Doppler examination, 28 of 32 patients (90%) were found to have significant obstruction. Using both temporal and carotid artery compression, the Doppler examination detected all but one patient with significant extracranial vascular disease. This final patient was detected by the use of facial artery compression. Two patients whose carotid obstruction would have been overlooked by temporal artery compression alone had intracranial collaterals supplied by the contralateral carotid system. The third patient had flow via the ipsilateral facial artery which resulted in retrograde flow in the angular artery with subsequent normal directional flow in the frontal artery. The fourth patient whose disease would have been missed demonstrated collateral flow via the contralateral facial artery, detectable by contralateral facial and common carotid artery compression only. Utilizing compression of the ipsilateral temporal, bilateral facial and common carotid arteries all patients with significant cerebrovascular occlusive disease were detected using Doppler examination. The 18 remaining patients with normal or less severely stenotic (<70%) carotid arteries were all correctly identified by Doppler examination.

SUMMARY

The Doppler ultrasonic velocity detector is a reliable, noninvasive method to screen for significant stenosis or occlusion of the internal carotid artery. This study suggests that the application of a methodical Doppler examination directed at assessment of each of the potential extracranial sources of internal carotid artery collateral flow will result in significant improvement in the detection of cerebrovascular disease. We feel that determination of directional flow in the frontal artery coupled with compression of the ipsilateral temporal artery and bilateral facial and carotid arteries will produce maximal accuracy with this instrument.

COMMON CAROTID FLOW DURING GRADED STENOSIS AND OCCLUSION OF THE INTERNAL CAROTID ARTERY

R. R. Gonzalez, Jr. and H. R. Müller

Laboratory of Diagnostic Ultrasound, Neurosurgical Clinic
University of Basel
4004 Basel, Switzerland

Since the introduction of the Doppler ultrasonic transcutaneous flow detector, a host of simplified procedures have been proposed for use in evaluating the resistance, percentage lumen decrease and reduction in flow through the internal carotid artery. These methods generally use information derived from the cervical carotid and/or the ophthalmic branches. One method currently in use employs the relationship between the diastolic and systolic velocities of blood flow in the common carotid artery, as measured with the Doppler flowmeter, to estimate vascular resistance in the carotid system.(3)

An index is computed by dividing the difference in height between the common carotid systolic peak and diastolic trough (that is, the common carotid flow pulse) by the systolic height. This ratio gives a number which is less than one, and varies in normals from 0.55 to 0.75. Indexes greater than this range suggest a high resistance, and indexes lower, abnormally low resistance (e.g. A-V shunts). It is hypothesized that the shape of the flow-pulse is formed by the effective perfusion pressure in the carotid artery. As internal carotid stenosis develops, the diastolic component of the common carotid flow decreases, because the diastolic portion of the perfusion pressure is not high enough to keep blood flowing through diastole. This index is based on repeated measurements of velocity in numerous controls, as well as in patients with cervical carotid vascular occlusive disease. To our knowledge, this index has never been studied under experimental conditions, where the common carotid flow pulse could be observed during various known vascular resistances in the internal carotid artery. We have initiated the following experiments to test this hypothesis.

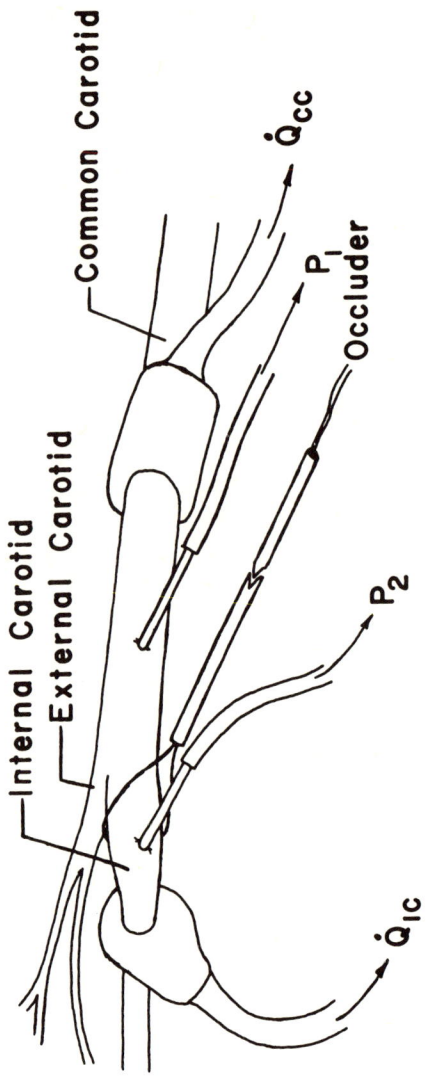

Figure 1. Preparation of the carotid bifurcation with the sensors attached ($\dot{Q}_{ic}$-internal carotid flow, $\dot{Q}_{cc}$-common carotid flow; P_1-common carotid pressure; P_2 internal carotid pressure).

METHODS

Stumptail monkeys were anesthetized with 6 mg/kg ketamine hydrochloride i.m. (Ketalar, Parke Davis), and maintained under anesthesia with a mixture of 2 liters nitrous oxide and one liter oxygen per minute. This ratio could be altered to maintain arterial gas tensions within normal limits. The animals were immobilized with pancuronium bromide (Pavulon, Organon), and artificially respired through an endotracheal tube with a Harvard positive pressure respirator.

Blood flow was monitored from the common and internal carotid arteries. Pressure was taken from the common and internal carotids by needle (0.12 mm by 2.5 cm) tipped catheters (1 mm by 50 cm). A snare ligature was used to make the artificial stenosis and occlusion in the internal carotid artery (Fig. 1).

Blood pressures were measured with Statham P23Db transducers (Fig. 2). These transducers were matched for their hysteresis response to a pulsatile pressure, and their signals were conditioned by a solid state amplifier system, designed and constructed in our laboratory. The amplifier system had a subtraction capability so that instantaneous pressure difference could be obtained (Fig. 3). Blood flow was monitored with the 4 MHz multichannel Delalande Directional Doppler ultrasonic flowmeter (Débitmètre Directionnel Ultrasonique Delalande) in conjunction with periarterial flow sensors which had been calibrated for volumetric flow.

All parameters were registered on an eight channel Elema-Schoenander Mingograph. In addition pressure difference and internal and common carotid blood flows were recorded on a JVC Nivico quadraphonic magnetic tape recorder for later analysis. Pressure and flow signals were frequency modulated prior to tape recording and demodulated before their display. The modulator-demodulator device was designed and constructed by the technical services of the Kantonsspital Basel. Impedance was displayed on the XY coordinates of a Tektronix type 5103N/D11 oscilloscope with the blood flow on the ordinate and the pressure difference on the abscissa. The slope of the loop formed by the pressure/flow relationship represents the vascular resistance to flow.(4,5)

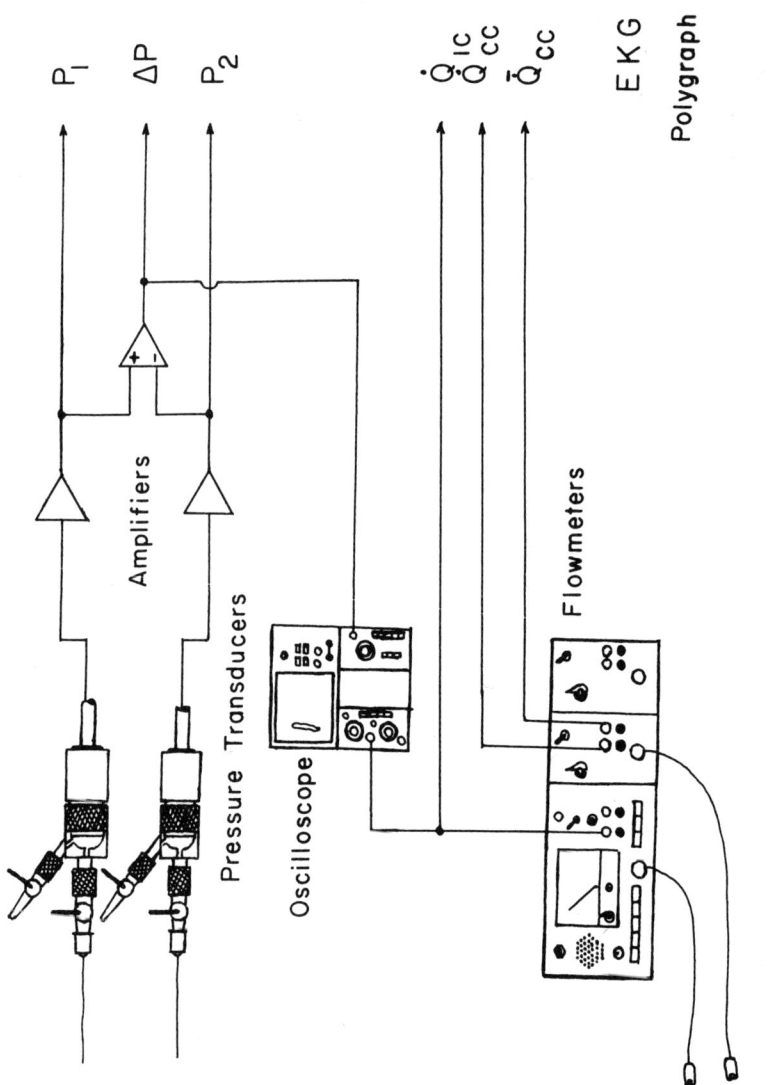

Figure 2. Block diagram of the instrumentation. The parameters measured from top to bottom are: common carotid pressure (P_1), common/internal carotid pressure difference (ΔP), internal carotid pressure (P_2), internal carotid flow ($\dot{Q}_{ic}$), common carotid flow ($\dot{Q}_{cc}$), mean common carotid flow ($\bar{Q}_{cc}$), and electrocardiogram (EKG).

The impedances were expressed in peripheral resistance units (PRU), where 1 PRU is equivalent to 80,000 dynes·sec/cm^5 (absolute units).[1]

RESULTS

Gradual stenosis of the internal carotid artery generally resulted in a decrease of both systolic and diastolic portions of the common carotid flow pulse (Fig. 4). Mean common carotid and internal carotid flows decreased in a linear fashion. Common carotid/internal carotid pressure difference seemed to rise abruptly after a significant internal carotid stenosis had developed (see Fig. 4 phase 4). Even though the internal carotid was eventually totally occluded by the snare ligature, the pressure distal to the snare never dropped below 50 mmHg.

Upon closer inspection (Fig. 5) a small increase in resistance of 0.532 PRU $\pm$ 0.030 S.E. in 24 trials with 10 bifurcations elicited a significant change in the character of the common carotid and internal carotid flow pulses. The total flow pulse of the internal carotid decreased sufficiently to cause a 28% $\pm$ 6 S.E. decrease in internal carotid flow. It appeared that the greatest change in the common carotid flow pulse was a decrease in the systolic component of the pulse with little or no change in the diastolic component. The resistance index had a tendancy to fall rather than rise with small increases in resistance. Common carotid mean flow dropped only 15% $\pm$ 3 S.E. in response to such an increase in internal carotid resistance.

Resistances greater than 1 PRU had to develop before the diastolic trough of the common carotid flow pulse decreased without an accompaniny change in the systolic peak. It was only in these cases of large segmental resistances that the resistance index began to increase into the pathologic range. By this time the internal carotid flow was only 30% $\pm$ 5 S.E. of control and a sizable pressure gradient between the common carotid and internal carotid arteries was evident.

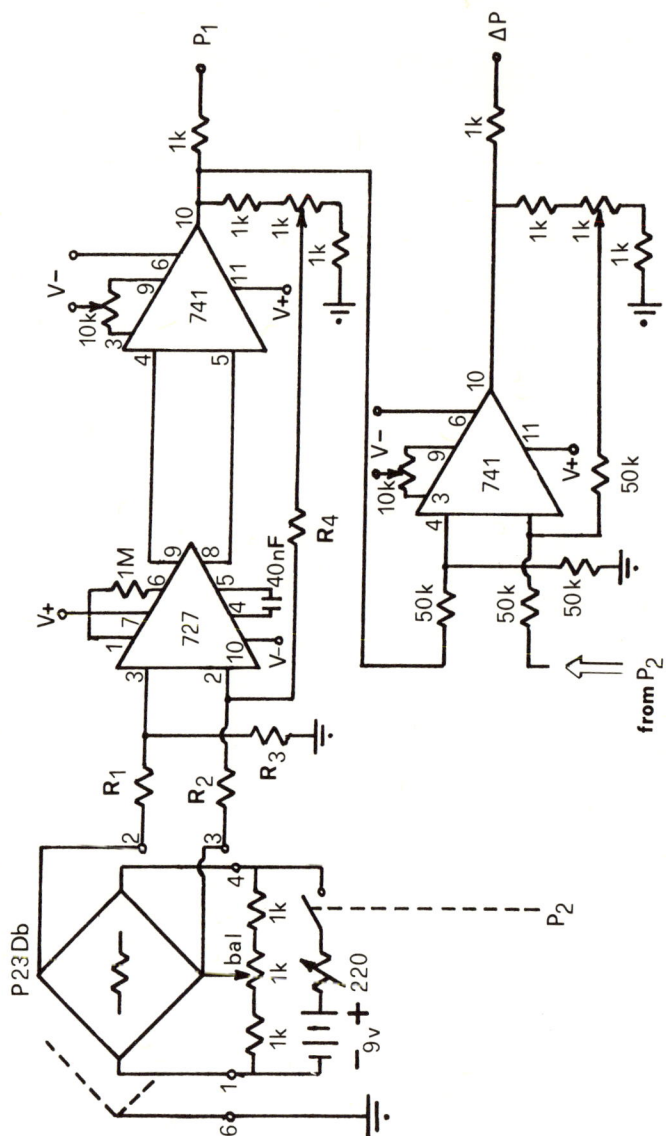

Figure 3. Schematic diagram of the pressure difference amplifier circuit. Only one amplifier and the difference circuits are shown for clarity.

DISCUSSION

The shape of a flow pulse is formed by a variety of kinetic and static elements. Perfusion pressure is only one of these factors, and it is an oversimplification to explain such flow pulse changes as primarily due to alterations in perfusion pressure. As flow pulse configuration is closely related to vascular terminal impedance,[6] an important aspect is the dilatory ability of the terminal vascular bed. In an earlier study[2] with normal subjects we have shown, that by varying the cerebral vascular resistance through one minute of breathholding and hyperventilation, the resistance index can be significantly altered. One can raise the index with hyperventilation, as well as decrease flow velocity in the common carotid. Conversely, breathholding can significantly lower the index and increase flow velocity in the common carotid.

The apparent decrease in resistance index with small degrees of stenosis could be the result of cerebral vasodilation or autoregulation in response to a reduction in perfusion pressure. All organisms studied autoregulated throughout wide variations in perfusion pressure (50-180 mmHg). Therefore it is possible that any impediment in a vascular segment may become critical at different degrees of narrowing or "tightness" depending on the vascular reserve of the terminal vascular bed. Thus the potential exists that one patient with a large vasodilatory capacity and a given degree of stenosis may have an index within the normal range; whereas another individual with the same degree of stenosis, but with a lesser vasodilatory capacity, may exhibit an index within the pathologic range.

Characteristics of the segmental resistance itself, such as its shape or length, can vary the critical impedance necessary to alter flow pulse configuration; however information as to the amount of influence is lacking. It is evident that more needs to be known about the relationship between flowpulse configuration and vascular impedance. It is also apparent that any one simple index or test is not adequate to accurately appraise the status of a vascular segment or vascular bed. Because of the hemodynamic complexity of the cranial vascular bed, and the relative inaccessibility of its collateral circulation, diagnosis must be functional in nature. It is therefore necessary to use a variety of diagnostic methods to evaluate each case.

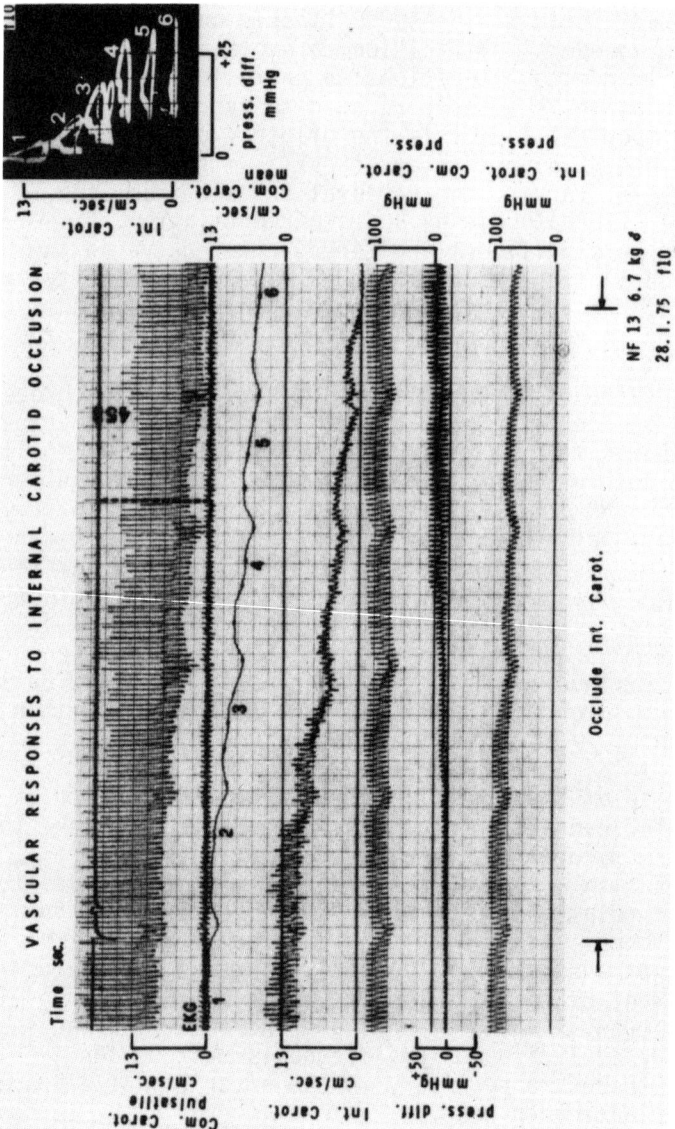

Figure 4. The effect of internal carotid occlusion on the common carotid flow. The upper right polaroid photo is a composite of impedance loops, which represent the instantaneous resistance at the points marked by numerals on the mean common carotid flow channel. (Reproduced by permission from Ultrasound in Medicine, E. Kazner and H. R. Müller (ed.), Exerpta Med., Amsterdam, In press).

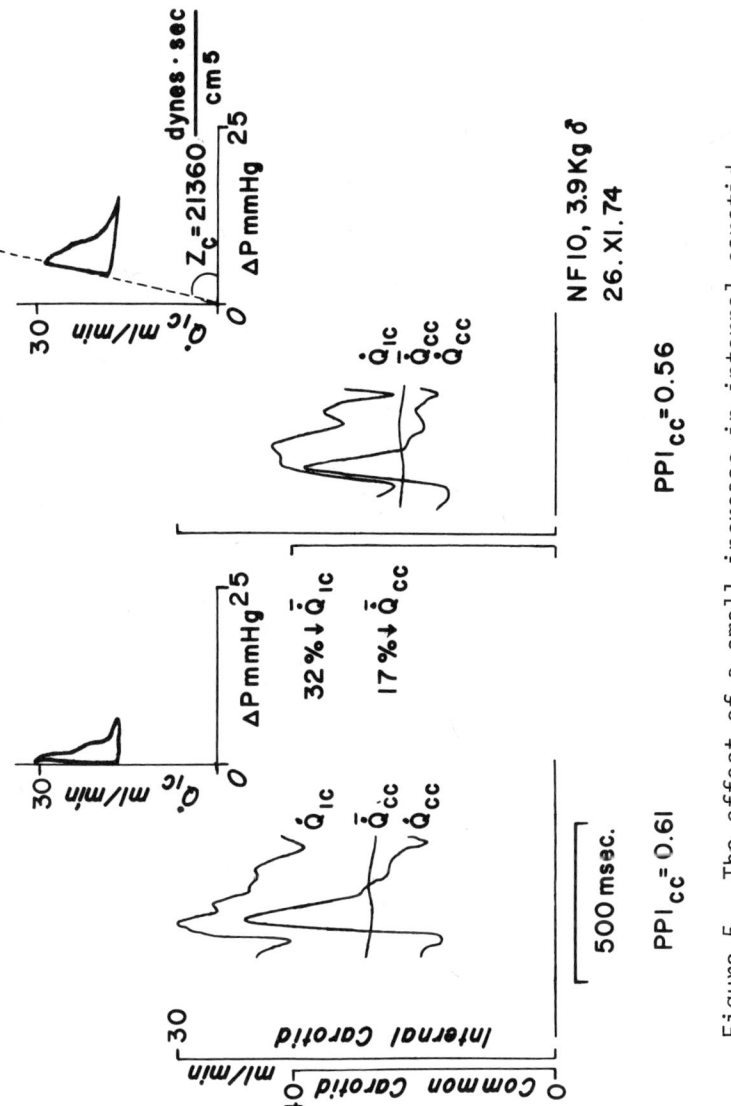

Figure 5. The effect of a small increase in internal carotid resistance on internal carotid pulsatile flow ($\dot{Q}_{ic}$), common carotid mean ($\bar{\dot{Q}}_{cc}$) and pulsatile ($\dot{Q}_{cc}$), flows and resistance index (PPI). The loops on the upper portion of this figure represent instantaneous resistances at control and at 0.267 peripheral resistance units (21360 absolute units).

In summary, in an effort to simplify the evaluation of the status of internal carotid vascular occlusive disease, the use of an index has been proposed. The index is the ratio of the common carotid flow pulse to the common carotid systolic height, and is to represent vascular resistance in the carotid tree distal to the measuring point. We have shown that this index is not reliable in especially low grade stenoses of the internal carotid artery. We have further shown that with small increases in internal carotid vascular resistance the index value can actually decrease, even though mean common carotid flow has fallen slightly and internal carotid flow has lessened by a significant amount. We have concluded that this index can be useful, however, when it is used only as part of the Doppler examination, and in conjunction with other diagnostic procedures.

ACKNOWLEDGEMENTS

The authors thank Miss Marie-Louise Fleissig for technical assistance.

This study was sponsored by grants from the Schweizerische Nationalfonds (3.2020.73) and the Freiwillige Akademische Gesellschaft, Basel.

At the time of this study R. Gonzalez was a postdoctoral research fellow in the Laboratory of Diagnostic Ultrasound of the Neurosurgical Clinic, the University of Basel, Basel, Switzerland, and was supported by the Centre de Recherche Delalande, Rueil-Malmaison, France. His present address is: Department of Physiology, Loma Linda University School of Medicine, Loma Linda, California 92354.

LITERATURE CITED

1. Green, H. D. 1950. Circulatory system: physical principles. In: Medical Physics, Vol. II. O. Glasser (ed.) Year Book Publishers, Inc., Chicago, pp 228-251.

2. Müller, H. R. and R. R. Gonzalez, Jr. 1974. Evaluation of cranial blood flow with ultrasonic Doppler techniques. In: Ultrasonics in Medicine. M. de Vlieger, D. N. White, and V. R. McCready (ed.) Excerpta Medica, Amsterdam, pp 89-96.

3. Planiol, Th. and L. Pourcelot. 1974. Doppler effect study of the carotid circulation. In: Ultrasonics in Medicine. M. de Vlieger, D. N. White, and V. R. McCready (ed.). Excerpta Medica, Amsterdam, pp 104-111.

4. Spencer, M. P., D. L. Johnson, G. H. Lawrence, L. D. Hill, and J. S. Tytus. 1966. Evaluation of cardiovascular lesions by means of an impedance plot at the time of surgical correction. Bulletin Mason Clinic 20:1-12.

5. Spencer, M. P. and L. H. Edmonds, Jr. 1968. Evaluation of operative left ventricular outflow tract lesions with a fluid impedance plot. Circulation 37:912-921.

6. Young, D. F., N. R. Cholvin, and A. C. Roth. 1975. Pressure drop across artificially induced stenoses in the femoral arteries of dogs. Circ. Res. 36:735-743.

AORTIC VELOCITY PATTERNS USING TRANSCUTANEOUS DOPPLER ULTRASOUND

Joan A. Persaud, Derek R. Boughner, M.D.,
Department of Medicine, Cardiac Investigation
Unit, University Hospital and Department of
Biophysics, University of Western Ontario,
London, Ontario, Canada

In 1969, Light demonstrated that descending aortic arch blood velocity could be recorded from the skin surface using Doppler ultrasound (1). The potential value of this technique has not been fully evaluated although its usefulness in the assessment of aortic insufficiency has been suggested (2) and it may have some value in the non-invasive estimation of cardiac output (3). We therefore set out to examine aortic blood velocity patterns in patients with a variety of valvular and myocardial lesions.

METHOD

A 2.2 MHz directional Doppler ultrasound unit (manufactured by Bach Simpson Limited, London, Ontario) was used for this study. The transducer was of the split "D" configuration, focused at 8 cm. A filter was contained in the equipment so that velocities above 100 Hz and below 7 Hz were not recorded. This feature eliminated problems with heart sounds which are of low velocity and high amplitude and could mask the aortic blood velocity recordings.

The unit provided three forms of display for the information: a) The instantaneous peak velocity "away from" and "toward" the transducer was indicated on two calibrated meters on the face of the equipment, b) The Doppler frequency shift produced by the flowing blood was made audible by stereophonic earphones with velocities "away from" and "toward" the transducer on separate channels, c) The output from the unit was

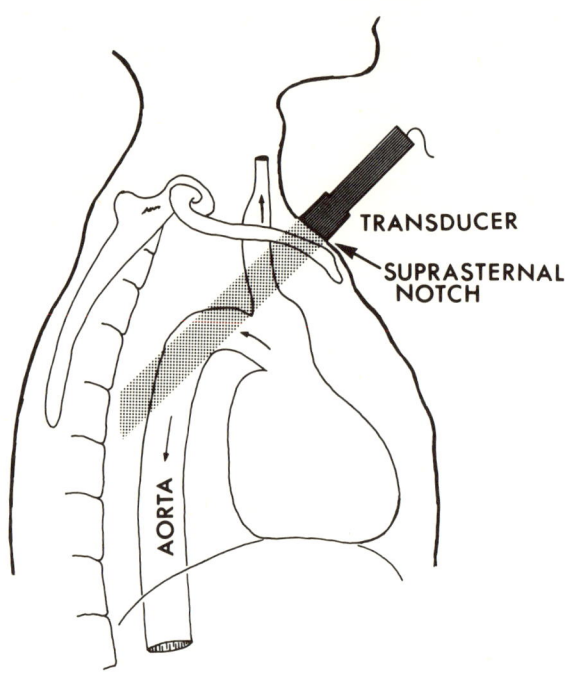

Figure 1
Transducer is positioned in the suprasternal notch and aimed such that the ultrasound beam crosses the aortic arch approximately parallel to flow.

connected directly to a Litton chart recorder with "away" velocity plotted upright and "toward" velocity inverted.

Each examination was performed with the patient supine. The transducer was hand-held against the skin surface in the suprasternal notch and aimed downwards and posteriorly toward the tip of the left scapula, with the beam crossing the descending aortic arch such that the angle of incidence with the blood flow was approximately zero degrees (Figure 1). The transluminal velocity profile in this area of the arch was relatively flat (4) so that the peak velocity reading obtained approximated the mean velocity of the stroke volume. Also since the Doppler shift velocity recording obtained depended upon the cosine of the angle of incidence of the beam with the flowing blood, an angle of $20°$ from parallel produced an error of only $\pm 5\%$ in the instantaneous peak velocity recording.

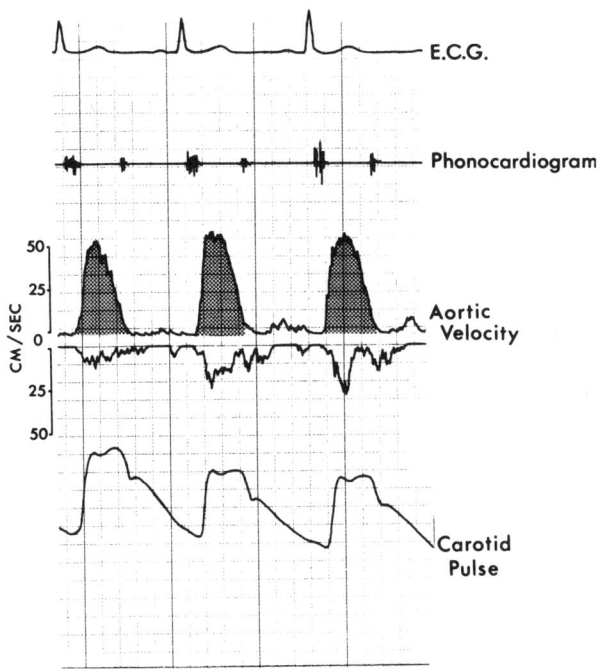

Figure 2
Normal aortic velocity pattern (shaded area) is recorded "away from" transducer in systole and plotted upright. Velocity "towards" transducer, from carotid and other vessels is inverted.

The electrocardiogram, phonocardiogram and carotid pulse tracing were recorded simultaneously with the velocity tracing on the Litton recorder at a paper speed of 50 mm/sec and 250 mm/sec.

The equipment contained an oscillator used for calibration. When activated it produced a signal equivalent to a frequency shift representing 50 cm/sec. In each case the transducer was rotated in the suprasternal notch until a peak velocity "away from" the transducer was obtained. The carotid vessels lay in the path of the ultrasound beam in most patients and therefore simultaneous flow "toward" the transducer was frequently recorded in systole. Ascending aortic arch blood velocity could not be used since it was not possible to differentiate flow in that vessel from flow in the carotid vessels as both were directed towards the transducer. The velocity pattern in vessels other than the aorta has not proven useful since its configuration is altered considerably by reflections from the periphery.

RESULTS

A) Normals

The aortic velocity pattern was recorded in 15 normals with no known cardiac disease ranging in age from 14 - 63 years. All showed an essentially parabolic wave form directed away from the transducer onsetting $\pm$ 20 msec from the beginning of the carotid pulse upstroke and ending at the dicrotic notch of the carotid pulse (Figure 2). Flow in the carotid vessels was usually recorded toward the transducer but separated from the aortic blood velocity by the directional nature of the equipment. In early diastole a small amount of reversed flow was occasionally seen.

By directing the transducer below either clavicle, subclavian artery blood velocity could be recorded. The blood velocity in the superior vena cava could be obtained by aiming the beam almost vertically behind the sternum. Innominate vein flow was occasionally recorded simultaneously with descending aortic arch velocity and was of importance in patients with aortic insufficiency where it obscured the diastolic reversed velocity that was to be expected in that disease. This venous flow was "toward" the transducer beginning in late systole and proceding through much of diastole. Venous flow could be distinguished from arterial flow since it produced a more continuous rushing or rumbling sound, in the earphones, without the rapid rise and fall in amplitude characteristic or arterial flow.

The presence of obstructive airways disease may make it difficult to obtain a definite aortic arch blood velocity signal. In this situation air containing tissue presumably lies between the aortic arch and the transducer. A separate difficulty has been encountered with the extremes of body size since the transducer was focused at 8 cm. In small children this was too deep and in large adults, too shallow.

The velocity tracing recorded on the Litton recorder can provide information in addition to the instantaneous aortic blood velocity (cm/sec). If the area under the velocity curve is measured with a planimeter a value in centimeters is obtained. This represents the distance forward that the stroke volume moves or the length of the aorta filled by the stroke volume.

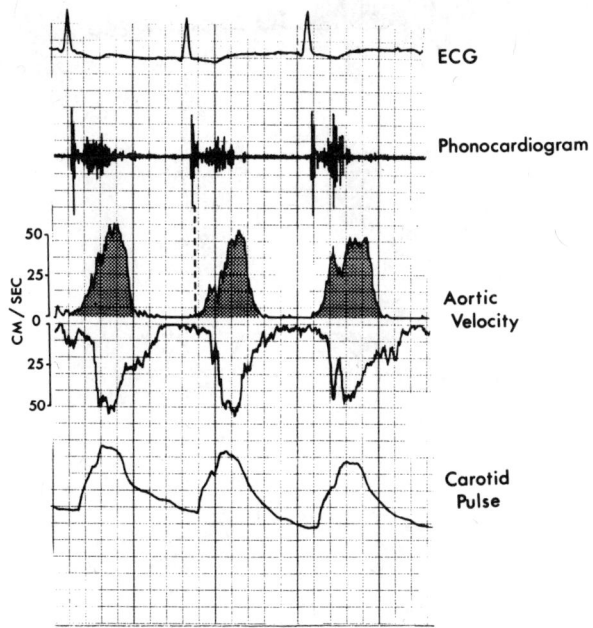

Figure 3
Aortic stenosis produces a variable delay in the rise to peak velocity.

B) Aortic Valve Disease

The aortic blood velocity tracings were obtained in 17 patients with angiographically proven aortic stenosis alone. A variable delay in the rise to peak velocity was seen in 15 of the patients (Figure 3). This delay was as long as 140 msec but was not found to correlate with the valvular gradient. It apparently results from jet formation through the narrowed aortic valve with the formation of large vortices in the ascending aortic arch and thus a delay in the onset of forward movement in the descending arch. With careful aiming of the transducer aortic blood velocity was found to return to the base line coincident with the dicrotic notch on the carotid pulse tracing.

Although the delay did not adequately correlate with the aortic valve gradient to make the findings useful for grading aortic stenosis it did consistently indicate the presence of stenosis.

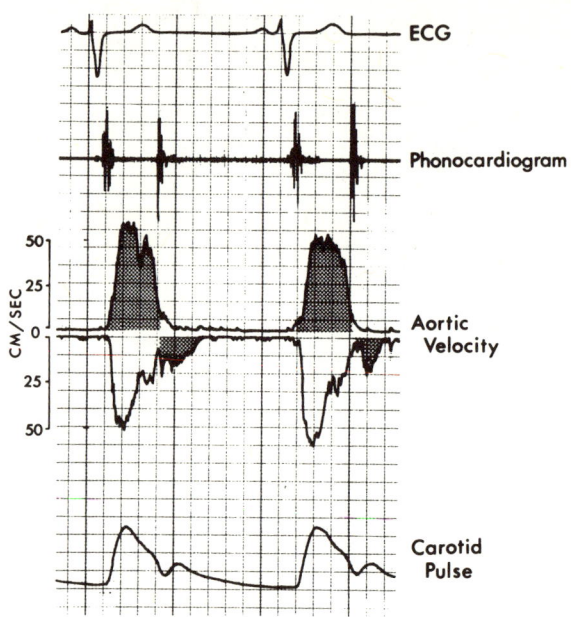

Figure 4
Aortic insufficiency results in abnormal reversed flow "toward" the transducer in early diastole. Measurements and comparison of systolic and diastolic areas provides percent regurgitation.

Aortic insufficiency produced characteristic changes on the velocity tracing. Abnormal diastolic flow "towards" the transducer onsetting in early diastole indicated the presence of regurgitation (Figure 4). In addition, it was possible to estimate the percent regurgitation from the resulting tracing. With a planimeter the area under the systolic and diastolic portions of the velocity tracing was measured. Since the Doppler equipment measures the instantaneous peak aortic velocity in cm/sec, the area under the curve provides a value in centimeters and represents the distance forward that the stroke volumes moves. Thus the ratio of the measured distance forward in systole versus the distance backward in diastole provides an estimate of the percent regurgitation.

This estimate was compared to the results of cardiac catheterization in 14 patients with aortic insufficiency. In each of these patients the percent regurgitation was estimated on the angiograms by comparing

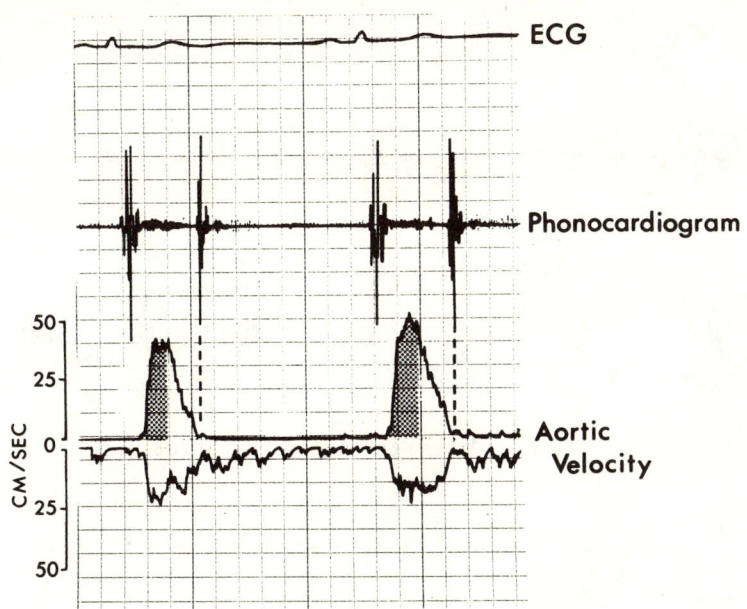

Figure 5

Mild mitral insufficiency. The normally parabolic wave form is skewed leftward with proportionately greater flow in early systole than late systole.

the stroke volume calculated from left ventricular volume measurements with the forward stroke volume calculated by the Fick cardiac output technique. An excellent correlation between the two techniques was obtained (r = 0.91).

C) Mitral Valve Disease

Six patients with pure mitral stenosis showed no abnormalities in their aortic blood velocity tracing.

Mitral insufficiency showed a characteristic change in the velocity pattern previously noted by Elkins et al (5) using cuff flowmeter probes around the ascending aorta at operation. The velocity pattern changed from the normal parabolic shape and became skewed to the left indicating a decrease in the late systolic flow relative to the early systolic flow (Figure 6). As the degree of mitral insufficiency worsened this asymmetry of the curve became more pronounced. By dividing the systolic portion of the velocity tracing in half and estimating,

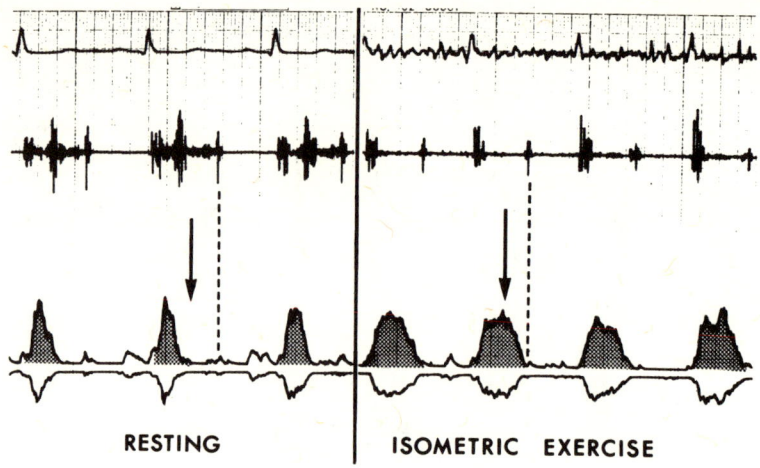

Figure 6
(a) Idiopathic hypertrophic subaortic stenosis, with a high resting subaortic gradient present shows little forward flow beyond mid systole.
(b) After 2½ minutes isometric hand grip exercise the velocity pattern becomes normal with reduction in the subaortic gradient and disappearance of the murmur.

by planimetry, the area in the first and second halves of systole, it was demonstrated that the resulting ratio between the two increased with increasing regurgitation. This was confirmed in 17 patients at cardiac catheterization. All patients catheterized had mitral valve disease alone and the percent regurgitation was again estimated by calculating left ventricular stroke volume from the angiograms and comparing this to the forward stroke output calculated by the Fick cardiac output technique.

On the Doppler tracing the normal ratio of flow in the first and second half of systole was 52:48 ($\pm$ 5 s.d.) and with severe regurgitation the ratio rose in these patients to as much as 78:22. On comparing the percent regurgitation calculated from angiography to the percent flow in the first half of systole a good correlation was obtained (r = 0.80). Since this estimate is indirect it did not appear reasonable to use the technique to accurately predict percent regurgitation but it could clearly grade the regurgitation as simply mild, moderate or severe.

D) Idiopathic Hypertrophic Subaortic Stenosis

The aortic blood velocity pattern was recorded in 14 patients with angiographically and/or echocardiographically proven idiopathic hypertrophic subaortic stenosis (I.H.S.S.). When there was asymmetric septal hypertrophy alone with no evidence of a subaortic gradient at rest, the aortic velocity pattern was normal. In the presence of a significant resting gradient the aortic velocity pattern showed a characteristic rapid rise to a peak then a sharp fall in mid systole with, occasionally, a second late systolic peak or simply a plateau (Figure 6a). If only mild obstruction was present at rest with gradients measured at cardiac catheterization of 10-20 mm Hg the aortic velocity pattern remained normal. However, by administering 7.5 micrograms of isoprenaline intravenously the velocity pattern was altered indicating the development of a significant subaortic obstruction.

Finally the effect of isometric exercise on I.H.S.S. with a significant subaortic gradient can be evaluated and is most helpful in differentiating the velocity pattern seen from that of severe mitral insufficiency. In the patient illustrated with severe outflow tract obstruction little aortic flow could be recorded in late systole (Figure 6a). However, after 2½ minutes of 30% peak maximum hand grip isometric exercise the velocity pattern returned to normal and the murmur was seen to decrease in intensity as the subaortic gradient was removed (Figure 6b).

SUMMARY

This Doppler ultrasound technique adds significant information in the non-invasive assessment of aortic insufficiency, mitral insufficiency and idiopathic hypertrophic subaortic stenosis and is a valuable adjunct to echocardiography.

Although echocardiography can indicate the presence of aortic insufficiency by recording flutter of the anterior mitral valve leaflet it will only grossly estimate the severity (6). Even clinical evaluation and angiographic assessment are of limited accuracy unless time consuming volume estimates are done on the latter procedure (7). Thus the non-invasive recording of the aortic velocity pattern offers a considerable advantage both in ease of operation and accuracy and provides a simple method of assessing and following patients with this lesion

For mitral insufficiency echocardiography is of limited value although various measurements of mitral

valve motion have been recommended (8). By observing
the change in the Doppler aortic velocity pattern in
systole we have been able to easily categorize the degree
of regurgitation. This may be of particular value in
patients with prosthetic mitral valves who have developed
dehiscence of the prosthesis. In such individuals the
regurgitant murmur may be insignificant or absent and in
one such patient we have found the Doppler technique to
be quite accurate in making the diagnosis. In that
patient the aortic velocity pattern returned to normal
after the leaking prosthetic valve was replaced.

Echocardiography is a proven and efficient means
for diagnosing IHSS but here again the Doppler technique
can add useful information. A normal aortic velocity
pattern will agree with suggested minimal subaortic
obstruction while a pronounced decrease in late systolic
flow will indicate the presence of significant obstruction.

As would be expected mitral stenosis produces no
changes in the aortic velocity pattern but aortic stenosis does produce a delay in the upstroke. Although
this latter delay usually indicates the presence of
aortic obstruction it is occasionally seen with aortic
insufficiency and the length of the delay in this study
did not correspond with the aortic valve gradient.

REFERENCES

(1) Light, L.H.: Non-injurious ultrasonic technique for observing flow in the human aorta. Nature 224: 1119, 1969.

(2) Thompson, P.D., Mennel, R.G., MacVaugh, J., Joyner, C.R.: Evaluation of aortic insufficiency in humans with a transcutaneous Doppler velocity probe (abstr). Ann Intern Med, 72: 781, 1970.

(3) Cross, G., Light, L.H.: Non-invasive intra-thoracic blood velocity measurement in the assessment of cardiovascular function. Biomedical Engineering, 9: 464, 1974.

(4) Schultz, D.: Pressure and flow in large arteries: In Cardiovascular Fluid Dynamics, Vol. 1, edited by Bergel, D.H. New York, Academic Press, 1972, p. 287.

(5) Elkins, R.C., Morrow, A.G., Vasko, J.S., Braunwald, E.: The effects of mitral regurgitation on the pattern of instantaneous aortic blood flow. Circulation 36: 45, 1967.

(6) Gray, K.E., Barrett, D.W.: Echocardiographic assessment of severity of aortic regurgitation. Brit. Heart J. 37: 691, 1975.
(7) Hunt, D., Baxley, W.A., Kennedy, J.W., Judge, T.P., Williams, J.E., Dodge, H.T.: Quantitative evaluation of cineaortography in the assessment of aortic regurgitation. Am J Cardiol 31: 696, 1973.
(8) Burgess, J., Clark, R., Kamigaki, M., Cohn, K.: Echocardiographic findings in different types of mitral regurgitation. Circulation 48: 97, 1973.

This study was supported by a grant from the Ontario Heart Foundation. Dr. Boughner is a Senior Research Fellow of the Ontario Heart Foundation.

THE USE OF PULSED DOPPLER ULTRASOUND TO IDENTIFY ARTERIAL FLOW ABNORMALITIES

W. R. Felix, Jr.; Bernard Sigel; Robert Gibson;
James Williams; Annette Edelstein; Jeffrey Justin
Harvard University School of Medicine, West Roxbury VA
Hospital, Boston, Mass. and Abraham Lincoln School of
Medicine, Chicago, Ill.

The Pulsed Doppler Ultrasound Instrument (1) has a feature which distinguishes it from other Doppler Ultrasound blood velocity detectors. It can range across a blood vessel and record the flow velocities in a small sample of blood at a defined position in the cross-sectional diameter of the vessel. This feature makes determinations of the flow condition independent of incident angle since a small sample size is used (approx. 2 mm). Sound spectrograms of Pulsed Doppler signals obtained from a flow model and from the center of the flow stream of human arteries are identical in pattern over a wide range of incident angles (30° to 80°).

Our hypothesis is that blood flow is normally near the threshold of turbulence (2) and that mural abnormalities such as plaques or stenosis produce local flow disturbances which are detected by sound spectral analysis of pulsed Doppler ultrasound signals. We have analyzed ultrasound signals obtained from the center of the flow stream in arteries under laminar and turbulent flow states and developed a method to distinguish laminar (normal) from turbulent (disturbed) flow. The method is based on sound spectral analysis of the Doppler output signal. Under normal (laminar) flow conditions in a flow model the sound spectrograms of pulsed Doppler signals obtained from small samples (2 mm windows) are devoid of low frequency components. The energy is concentrated in a narrow band around the frequency representative of the average velocity at that point in the flow stream. This pattern is seen best in the central portion of the chamber. Under turbulent conditions a wide range of frequencies is seen in all samples taken across the flow stream. This reflects the variety of velocities and vectors of flow which occur during turbulent flow (Figure 1).

Further experiments in the dog (Figure 2) and in axillo-femoral bypass grafts in man (Figure 3) confirm that the same patterns are seen in pulsatile flow as seen in the in vitro model. Center stream samples at 60° gave the best "normal patterns".

Abnormal patterns produced by partial occlusion were seen up to 15 cm (20 diameters) down streatm in an 8 mm graft (Figure 4). Experiments in the aorta of dogs confirmed that turbulence in the vessels produced the same patterns identified with turbulence in vitro. Figure 5 presents the patterns seen in an arteriogram normal femoral artery and in a femoral artery 10 cm distal to an iliac artery arteriotomy site for repair of a complete occlusion.

In a small clinical study of 65 study sites sonograms were made of center stream samples obtained with a transducer angle of 60°. These sonograms were read as "normal" or "abnormal" by seven observers who had no knowledge of the status of the artery under study. There was excellent agreement among the observers. Five of the seven observers agreed on the interpretation of the sonogram in 95% of the cases. In 30 presumed normal carotid studies the seven observers read 23 studies as normal (80% of the cases). The results of the readings of 35 sites proven as normal or abnormal by arteriogram are presented in Table 1. The pulsed Doppler technique was able to identify "disturbed" or "abnormal" flow in 10 of the 12 arteriogram abnormal arteries studied. The sensitivity of the technique is therefore 83%. Of 23 sonograms from arteriogram normal arteries (less than 50% stenosis), 14 were interpreted as normal. The specificity of the technique is therefore 61%.

Table 1

Results of Sonogram Analysis in 35 Carotid and Femoral Sites
Where Arteriogram Diagnosis is Known

Arteriogram Diagnosis	Pulsed Doppler Diagnosis		
	Normal	Abnormal	Total
Normal	14	9	23
Abnormal*	2	10	12
Total	16	19	35

*An arteriogram is read as abnormal if there was greater than 50% stenosis.

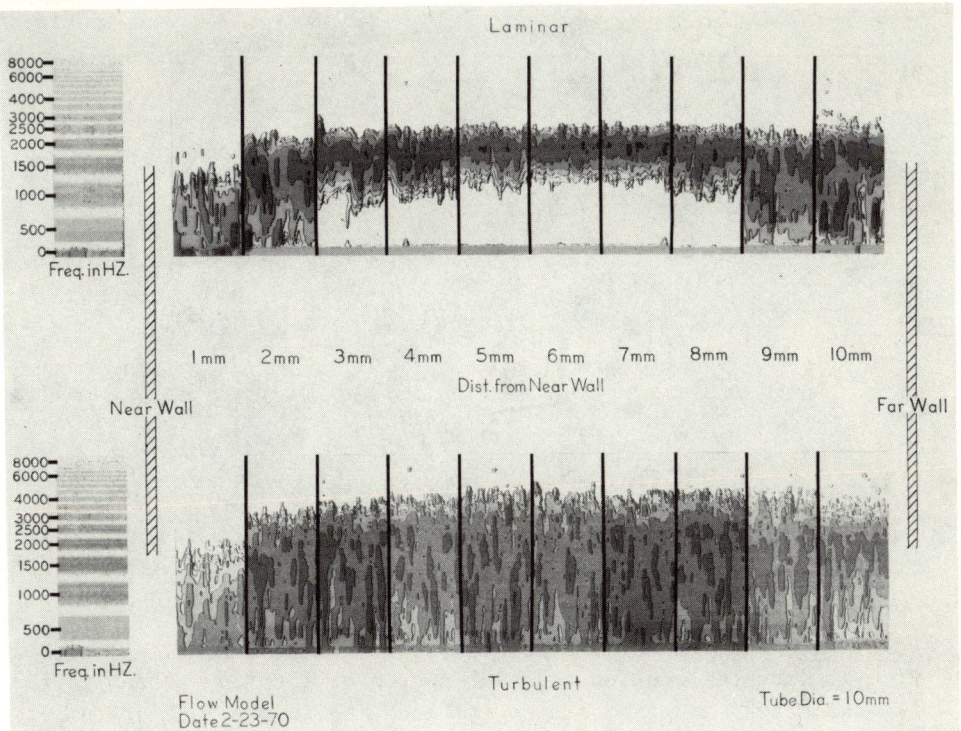

Figure 1 - Sonograms obtained at 1 mm intervals across a 10 mm diameter flow model chamber. Flow velocity is 34 cm/sec. Note the parabolic curve of the profile and the absence of low frequency components in the center stream recordings (3 to 8 mm) when the flow is laminar (upper display). The apparently higher velocities noted near the far wall are probably due to poorer resolution at distance. When the flow is turbulent (lower display) low frequency components are seen at all points across the flow stream; i.e. there is a more uniform distribution of the energy.

This sensitivity implies that in 83% of arterial lesions which reduce the intra-luminal diameter by one-half, this technique will identify a disturbed flow condition. This data does not establish that a disturbed flow condition always exists under these circumstances, but it does imply that the method might be useful in screening and surveillance of patients at risk to develop hemodynamically significant arterial lesions. The low specificity, 61%, might be due to under-reading arteriograms (i.e. not reading the

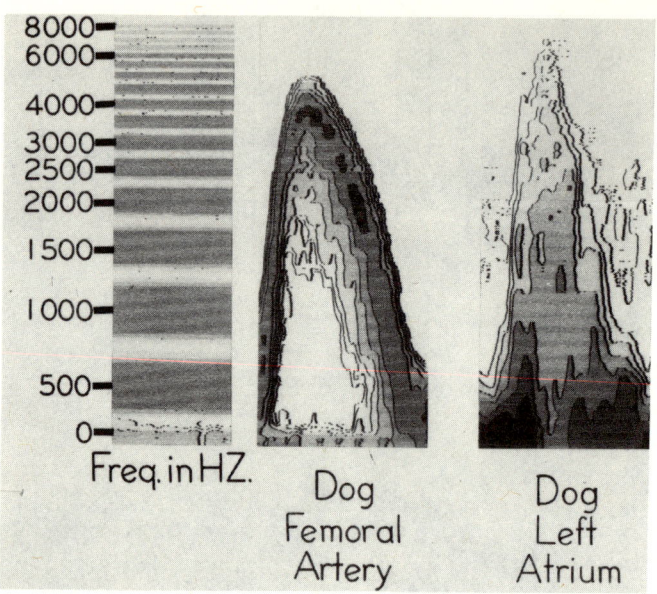

Figure 2 - Sonogram of the pulsed Doppler ultrasound signal obtained from a discrete location near the center of the flow stream in the femoral artery and from a discrete location in the left atrium of a dog. The display depicts the frequency of the ultrasound signal on the ordinate, the time interval (approx. 0.3 sec. per pulse) on the abscissa, and the amplitude (in 6 db increments) by the depth of the shading. Note that in this femoral artery signal, the energy concentrates in a narrow band as the pulse reaches its zenith. There is a marked reduction of the amplitude of low frequency components in the middle period of the pulse (36 db in this case) giving the appearance of a "window" in the pulse contour. In the left atrium, there is a predominence of low frequency components throughout the entire period of the pulse.

arteriogram as abnormal unless a lesion occluded 50% or more of the luminal diameter). Most of the arteriograms used in the study had some degree of abnormality. The "false positive" studies all came from the group of arteriograms which were abnormal but did not have lesions obstructing at least 50% of the lumen. The fact that 80% (23 of 30) studies in presumed normal carotids produced sonograms read as normal is more respectable, and indicates that the technique might have a specificity useful for epidemiologic screening. A more

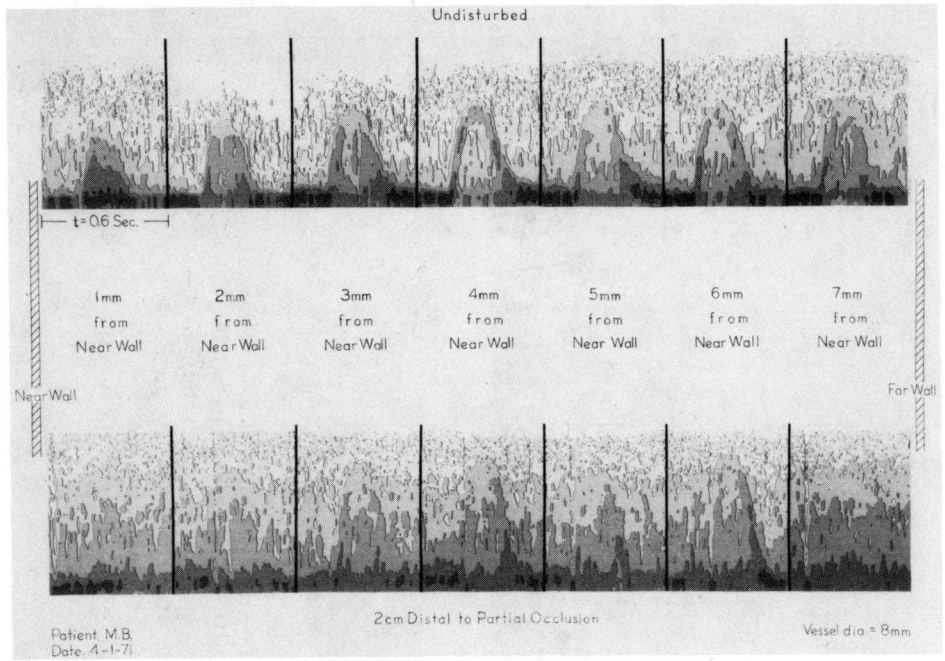

Figure 3 - Sonograms obtained at 1 mm intervals across the distal one-third of an 8 mm x 30 cm axillo-femoral dacron arterial prosthesis under normal conditions and 2 cm downstream from a partial occlusion.

formal validative study in which this Pulsed Doppler technique is compared to arteriograms graded as to severity of disease and to clinical criteria (bruit, pulses, etc.) will better establish the usefulness of this method for early detection of arteriosclerotic vascular disease.

Conclusions:
 1. The Pulsed Doppler Ultrasound blood velocity detector can be used to identify abnormal flow conditions in arteries.
 2. The abnormal patterns persist up to 15 cm (20 diameters) distal to the site of partial occlusion.
 3. The technique can correctly identify disease in 83% of instances of proven arterial lesions, it can accurately identify the normal in 61% of arteriogram proven normal examinations in 80% of presumed normal carotid arteries.
 4. The technique may be feasible as a means of screening for arteriosclerotic lesions in major superficial arteries.

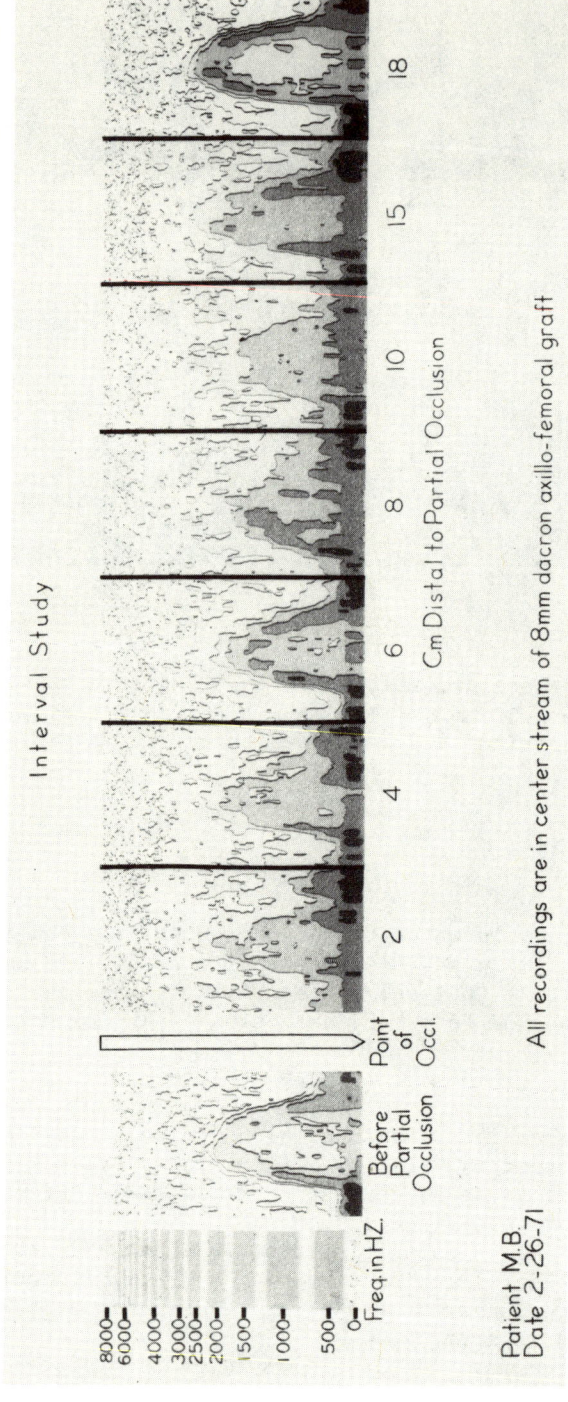

Figure 4 - Sonograms obtained from the center of the flow stream at intervals distal to a partial occlusion of a 8 mm axillo-femoral by-pass graft. The abnormal pattern (i.e. increased amplitude of low frequency components in the mid-portion of the velocity pulse wave) is seen to persist up to 15 cm distal to the occlusion.

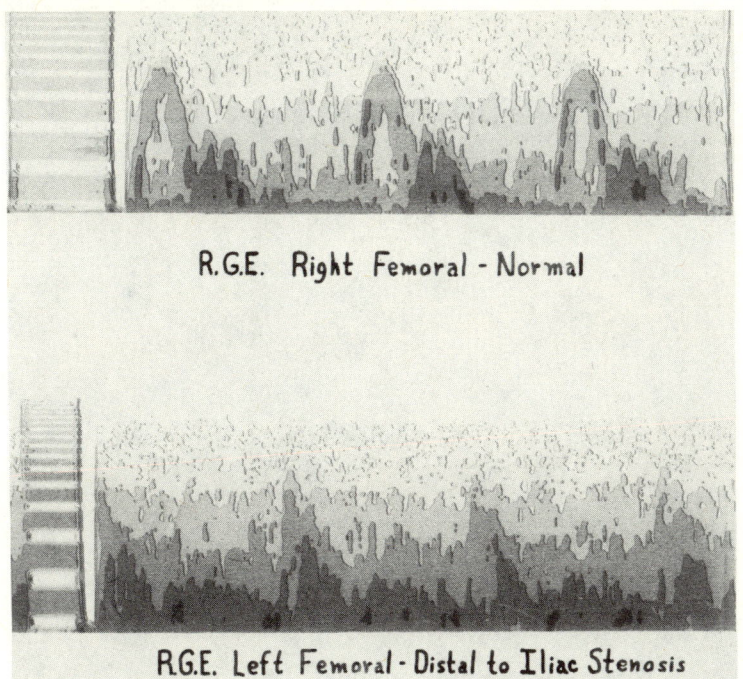

Figure 5 - Sonograms from center stream recordings of femoral arteries. Upper panel is recorded from the arteriogram proven normal right femoral artery. The lower panel is the center stream recording approximately 11 cm distal to an endarterectomy site three days after surgery. This minor alteration in the vessel is apparently sufficient to produce an abnormal sonogram.

References

1. McLeod, Jr., F.D.: Calibration of CW and Pulse Doppler Flowmeters. Proc. 23rd ACEMB 12: 271, 1970.

2. McDonald, D.A.: Blood Flow in Arteries. Arnold Ltd., London, 1960.

CARDIAC BLOOD FLOW DETECTION

Donald W. Baker; Ronald E. Daigle; Vernon Simmons;
Robert Olson
Center for Bioengineering
University of Washington, Seattle, Washington 98195

Real time B-mode sector scanning combined with simultaneous pulse Doppler flow detection provides a method for the more accurate assessment of cardiac performance. The heart is a multichambered, multivalved, variable geometry pump whose comprehensive description requires a multidimensional measurement approach. Each functional defect can be described in terms of a set of interrelated measurements consisting of anatomical as well as flow dynamic components. The relative role of anatomical vs. flow dynamic data will vary with each defect. For example, regurgitant valves may be detected more easily by sensing the resultant flow jet rather than attempting to image the orifice of the regurgitant jet. Similarly small septal defects are detected more easily by flow sensing than by anatomical imaging. The true valve orifice shape and area associated with a stenotic valve might be better evaluated by blood flow rather than following the motion of the valve leaflets.
   The freedom to choose the best measurement approach to a particular diagnostic problem is largely dependent on the availability and effectiveness of the instrumentation.
   The Duplex echo-Doppler concept provides an approach which permits the physician or sonographer this freedom of choice. Real time imaging increases the information rate and makes it possible for the observer to interact with the displays in order to position the Doppler probe at will.
   The cardiac system configuration consists of a real-time sector scanner (54 frames/sec) with a steerable Doppler transducer (3 mhz) mounted adjacent to it. The system displays show the "B" sector scan with an additional Doppler beam trace superimposed in proper orientation over the sector image. An intensified cursor on the Doppler trace indicates the location of the Doppler sample volume.

This cursor moves in or out as the depth select knob on the Doppler is adjusted.

This new duplex approach also has potential application in Pediatric cardiology and abdominal scanning. It has already been proven useful in the evaluation of peripheral vascular circulation.

Blood flow velocity waveforms have been recorded from selected sites and will be presented. A new hardcopy visacorder format is used for flow recording. It consists of Doppler T-M, a real time Doppler spectral analysis, analog flow velocity and ECG signals.

Supported by HL-07293-14

A REAL-TIME HIGH-RESOLUTION ULTRASONIC ARTERIAL IMAGING SYSTEM

J. C. Taenzer; S. D. Ramsey; J. F. Holzemer;
J. R. Suarez; P. S. Green
Stanford Research Institute
333 Ravenswood Avenue
Menlo Park, California 94025

Atherosclerosis is one of the major diseases affecting the health of people throughout the world. Detection of atherosclerotic lesions by invasive techniques presents serious hazards to patients, while current noninvasive techniques often do not yield accurate diagnosis. There is an urgent need for instrumentation that will provide safe, noninvasive, and accurate diagnosis of this disease. Since July 1973, the Mayo Foundation and Stanford Research Institute have been involved in a joint effort to develop high-resolution ultrasonic imaging techniques for clinical application to the diagnosis of human cardiovascular diseases. A first generation, real-time ultrasonic arterial imaging system for the simultaneous visualization of vessel anatomy and blood flow in the carotid and femoral arteries has been developed at SRI for clinical evaluation at the Mayo Foundation. This instrument incorporates both B-scan and Doppler measurement modalities.

A 10-MHz B-scan subsystem displays cross-sectional images of anatomical structure at 15 frames/s. The electronic processor for these images utilizes a special low-noise video preamplifier, an adjustable time-gain-controlled amplifier, and an adjustable compression amplifier to maintain the high dynamic range and wide bandwidth necessary for high resolution gray-scale B-scan images.

Real-time blood flow profiles are produced by a 5-MHz pulsed Doppler subsystem that can measure velocity at 20 individual points along a line segment intersecting the artery. The position and length of this line segment is determined by a joystick servo control, giving the operator complete freedom to make flow measurements anywhere within the field of the B-scan image.

In the clinical instrument a scanning head containing the transducers is supported at the end of a pantograph arm and coupled to the patient's skin by means of a water bag. The B-scan transducer is driven in a linear reciprocating motion while the Doppler transducer position is servo controlled. Both transducers operate in a transmit/receive mode and are focused at the same tissue region by coated ultrasonic lenses.

Initial experiments have shown the importance of the real-time display in both modalities. Simultaneous visualization of tissue detail and flow information promises to greatly enhance the detection and clinical assessment of atherosclerotic disease.

This work was supported by the National Institutes of Health under Contract No. NIH-NHLI-NO1-HT-4-2904.

PRECLINICAL EVALUATION OF THE SRI REAL-TIME ARTERIAL IMAGING SYSTEM

K. W. Marich; P. S. Green; T. C. Evans, Jr.*;
C. E. Harrison*
Stanford Research Institute
333 Ravenswood Avenue
Menlo Park, California 94025
*Mayo Foundation
200 First Street, S.W.
Rochester, Minnesota 55901

Stanford Research Institute (SRI) and the Mayo Foundation have been working together to develop ultrasonic instrumentation for the safe, noninvasive detection of atherosclerotic vascular disease. The advanced concept of this new real-time instrument combines high-resolution B-scans with pulsed Doppler flow profiles to improve diagnosis and provide vital information necessary for better management of this disease.

The preclinical version of the SRI real-time arterial imaging system has been used in laboratory tests to examine arterial anatomy. Preliminary in vivo evaluations of the carotid and femoral arteries were conducted on human volunteers. Subjects were examined while supine, and mineral oil was used to couple the scanning head water bag to the skin. The region of most interest for atherosclerotic pathology lies within 3 cm above and below the carotid bifurcation. Positioning the scanning head in this area to obtain the most useful views of the vessels of interest was greatly facilitated by the real-time image presentation.

Cross-sectional high-resolution gray-scale B-scan images, both transverse and longitudinal, were made of the major vessels in the neck and upper leg. Anatomical structures such as the skin, subcutaneous fat, muscle, nerve bundles, blood vessels, and the thyroid gland were easily visualized. Typical B-scan images of structures in the neck in the region of the carotid bifurcation are presented in Figures 1 and 2.

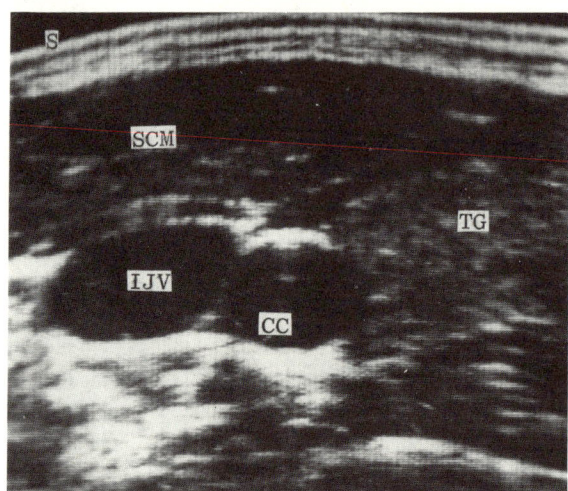

Figure 1. Cross-sectional transverse image of the left side of the neck in the area of the thyroid cartilage. Note the skin (S), sternocleidomastoid muscle (SCM), internal jugular vein (IJV), common carotid artery (CC), and thyroid gland (TG).

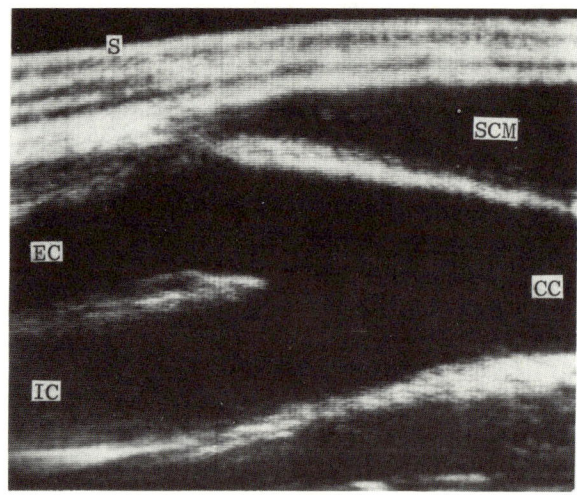

Figure 2. Cross-sectional longitudinal image of the right common carotid artery (CC) in the area of the carotid bifurcation. Note the skin (S), sternocleidomastoid muscle (SCM), external and internal carotid arteries (EC) (IC), respectively.

Pulsatile movements of the carotid arteries were clearly discernible, and in adults a pronounced antiphasic pulsation was seen in the internal jugular vein due to right atrial contraction. Specific identification of this vein was accomplished through the use of the Valsalva (increased intrathoracic pressure) and Müller (decreased intrathoracic pressure) maneuvers to cause the vein to distend or contract. The images obtained allowed measurement of arterial and venous luminal diameters, as well as the determination of the depths and orientations of the vessels.

Blood-flow-velocity profiles were obtained in real-time by use of the 5-MHz pulsed Doppler system. A typical flow velocity profile is presented in Figure 3 (the Doppler presentation was not superimposed on the B-scan in these tests).

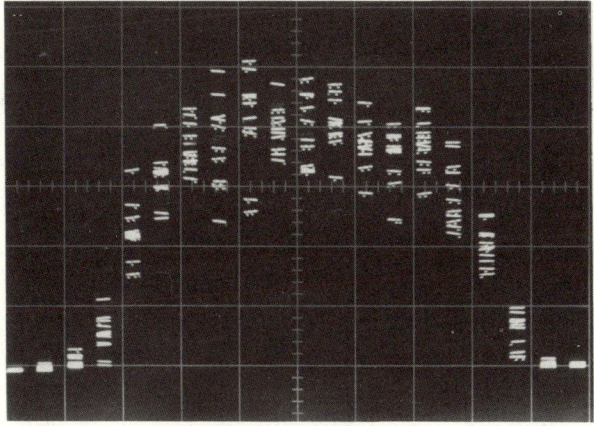

Figure 3. Twenty-point Doppler flow profile showing flow measured transcutaneously in a human artery.

Venous and arterial flow patterns were clearly differentiable in the Doppler profiles by observing the direction and magnitude of the flow in the vessels under examination.

This combination of B-scanning to display tissues and Doppler to display blood-flow profiles provides a complementary presentation of information that will greatly facilitate the clinical assessment and diagnosis of atherosclerotic vascular disease.

This work was supported by the National Institute of Health under Contract No. NIH-NHLI-NO1-HT-4-2904.

NONINVASIVE DETECTION OF THE ATHEROSCLEROTIC PLAQUE: The Carotid Bifurcation

Merrill P. Spencer, M.D.; John W. Li, M.D.;
Edwin C. Brockenbrough, M.D.; John M. Reid, Ph.D.
Institute of Applied Physiology & The Providence Hospital
Seattle, Washington 98122

A new Doppler ultrasonic imaging technique for mapping the course of arterial channels has been applied to the carotid bifurcation in over 800 patients. The technique has proven its ability to detect stroke producing wall disease including calcified plaques and flow disturbances. (Stroke 5:145, 1974) Comparisons with x-ray angiography demonstrates agreement in 89% of hemodynamically significant lesions. When including wall plaques without obstruction, agreement dropped to 79%. The ultrasonic method is more sensitive to elements of the atherosclerotic plaque, including calcium deposits, than is x-ray. Abnormal doppler flow signals associated with the presence of an atherosclerotic plaque beneath the sound beam include low amplitude, coarse quality, and low frequency sounds, as well as weak, biphasic, and inverted velocity flow tracings. Calcium deposits may be responsible for most of these abberations and when present in large quantities, produces silent nonvisualizing segments in the arterial image. The association of these blank segments with symptoms and signs suggestive of embolization leads to the possibility of ulcerated plaque and treatment with antithrombotic agents or endarterectomy.

Narrowing of the channel at the point of the lesion, as evidenced by high frequency and fluttering quality to the doppler sounds, and signs of stenosis or complete absence of the internal carotid image is often associated with abnormally directed flow around the homolateral eye. Obstructive plaques are also diagnosed in the subclavian and vertebral arteries. Long term follow-up by repeating the doppler imaging is useful in following the course of atherosclerotic lesions in both pre- and post-operative patients.

VELOCITY MAPS IN THE CANINE AORTA

C. W. Miller; F. D. McLeod; R. C. Nealeigh

Department of Physiology and Biophysics and the
Collaborative Radiological Health Laboratory
Colorado State University, Fort Collins, CO   80523

Velocity distributions (maps) have been recorded at six locations along the aorta in awake and anesthetized beagle dogs using implanted flow cuffs and a pulsed Doppler. The recordings of the velocity maps have been made in 60° intervals around the circumference of the aorta in order to document the influence of individual arterial outflow tracts and curvatures upon the local velocity characteristics.

The pulsed Doppler employed for this study has considerably improved resolution over earlier versions and the depth resolution is about ½ mm. A continuous scan system has been implemented which permits rapidly recording the velocity maps from each of the 6 piezoelectric crystals encased in the cuff. In addition, a display scheme has been used which provides a rapid velocity distribution display at 16 times in the cardiac cycle. These velocity maps have been recorded at three locations in the thoracic aorta and at three locations in the abdominal aorta. A typical recording session consists of making 36 velocity maps.

From these data considerable information concerning development of the velocity distribution patterns along the irregularly curved and branched aorta has been obtained in both awake and anesthetized dogs. Coupled with a power scan across the vessel which permits localization of the vessel walls, the profiles can be used to estimate the shear force on the vessel wall.

In the awake dog, the peak velocities frequently exceed 1m/sec and the profiles are blunt. A variety of reverse flow patterns exist which may be related to the location of the outflow tract and the degree of peripheral vascular constriction. These data point out the influence of curvature and branchpoints upon local velocity characteristics in both awake and anesthetized dogs and demonstrate the variations that normally exist.

MEASUREMENT OF HEMODYNAMIC PROPERTIES IN THE ABDOMINAL AORTA AND ILIAC ARTERY VIA AN INTRAVENOUS CATHETER-TIP PROBE

R. C. Nealeigh; C. W. Miller; F. D. McLeod

Collaborative Radiological Health Laboratory and the
Department of Physiology and Biophysics
Colorado State University, Fort Collins, CO   80523

Comparisons of local blood velocity, flow, vessel wall motion and diameters using standard implanted pulse Doppler ultrasonic flow cuffs and an intravenous catheter-tip probe were made on the abdominal aorta and iliac arteries of 5 Beagle dogs.

The catheter-tip device is a relatively nontraumatic intravenous approach and eliminates several problems encountered using other methods. Since the catheter is not in the artery problems of flow stream disturbances and vessel trauma are minimized. The close proximity of the vein and artery allows easy access to the artery and eliminates the problem of penetrating several layers of tissue which may jeopardize transcutaneous measurements. The problems encountered when placing a monitoring device directly on the artery, although permissible in some studies, are eliminated.

To accurately measure blood velocity using ultrasound the angle between the sound beam and the flow axis must be accurately determined. This angle is calculated using a ratio of the flow stream velocities measured by two opposing crystals. A third crystal centered between the two opposing crystals is set at 90° to the probe axis to allow recording vessel wall motion and diameter using an echo track instrument.

Vessel wall motion and instantaneous diameter measurements are easily obtainable along 4-6 cm of the abdominal aorta and 2-3 cm of the iliac artery. Calculations of pressure-strain elastic modulus are therefore obtainable when blood pressures are recorded. Segmental pulse wave velocities can also be calculated providing data related to arterial wall elasticity.

Divergence of the vena cava and abdominal aorta along with flow stream disturbances from large vessel branches such as the renal arteries are an example of some of the difficulties encountered using the venous probe, these are minimal however, and present no real problems when recording distal to the renal arteries.

We have found this method for measuring arterial hemodynamic properties in the abdominal aorta and iliac artery reliable, relatively nontraumatic and easy to perform. This technique may be valuable in assessing the severity of atherosclerotic disease, normal aging changes, normal arterial behavior, and could be used as a monitoring device during surgical or physiological procedures.

TRANSCUTANEOUS ASSESSMENT OF FOREARM REACTIVE HYPEREMIA BY DOPPLER ULTRASONOGRAPHY: CORRELATION WITH VENOUS OCCLUSION PLETHYSMOGRAPHY

R. W. Barnes; P. G. Miller; E. V. Miller

Peripheral Vascular Laboratories, Division of Thoracic and Cardiovascular Surgery, Department of Surgery, University of Iowa and Veterans Administration Hospitals, Iowa City, Iowa 52242

The magnitude and duration of increased limb blood flow (reactive hyperemia) following temporary tourniquet ischemia are useful clinical indices of the peripheral arterial circulation. Recently Fronek and colleagues[1] utilized Doppler ultrasonography to noninvasively assess leg reactive hyperemia but the method has not been compared with an established technique of measuring limb blood flow. This investigation compared transcutaneous Doppler ultrasonography with venous occlusion plethysmography in the assessment of reactive hyperemic blood flow in the forearm of normal adults.

METHODS

Seven normal adult volunteers were studied in an air-conditioned laboratory with a temperature of 23-25° C. With the individual positioned supine and the forearm elevated above the level of the heart, pneumatic cuffs were placed on the upper arm and the wrist. A pencil probe of a 9.4 megahertz continuous-wave directional Doppler velocity detector was coupled to the skin of the antecubital fossa over the brachial artery. The probe was immobilized in an adjustable clamp at a 45° angle with the skin surface. A mercury-in-silastic strain gauge was placed around the mid-forearm and was connected to an automatic plethysmograph which permitted electrical calibration of the gauge. The outputs of the Doppler detector and the plethysmograph were connected to a multi-channel recorder. A low frequency filter with a time constant of 0.3 seconds permitted continuous recording of mean brachial artery flow velocity.

After exclusion of hand blood flow by the wrist cuff, the arm cuff was repeatedly inflated to 50 mm Hg to permit determination of resting forearm blood flow from the initial upslopes of the recorded forearm circumference. Resting mean brachial artery flow velocity was simultaneously recorded by Doppler ultrasonography. The arm cuff was then inflated to 250 mm Hg to temporarily induce arm ischemia. After one minute, the cuff was rapidly deflated and then repetitively reinflated to 50 mm Hg to determine forearm blood flow while brachial artery flow velocity was simultaneously assessed during the ensuing reactive hyperemia. The procedure was successively repeated after periods of arm ischemia of 2, 3, and 4 minutes with intervening rest periods of 5 minutes each. Each determination of reactive hyperemia was analyzed by the percent increase in peak blood flow ($\%\Delta Q$) or flow velocity ($\%\Delta V$) relative to resting values and for the recovery half-time ($T_{\frac{1}{2}}$) for these measurements to return to 50% of the peak values.

RESULTS

The mean values ($\pm$ 1 S.D.) for the $\%\Delta Q$ (plethysmography) and $\%\Delta V$ (Doppler) of reactive hyperemia after 1, 2, 3, and 4 minutes arm ischemia were: 653 $\pm$ 182 and 1176 $\pm$ 330, 922 $\pm$ 222 and 1575 $\pm$ 215, 1261 $\pm$ 269 and 2192 $\pm$ 326, and 1174 $\pm$ 193 and 1933 $\pm$ 356, respectively. Linear regression analysis of the results of these two techniques of measuring peak reactive hyperemia revealed a correlation coefficient of 0.95 ($p < 0.001$) and an equation of $\%\Delta V = 1.46\ (\%\Delta Q) + 260$. The mean values of $T_{\frac{1}{2}}$ for the plethysmographic and Doppler assessments of reactive hyperemia after 1, 2, 3, and 4 minutes ischemia were 10.0 $\pm$ 2.1 and 9.8 $\pm$ 1.8, 13.1 $\pm$ 1.0 and 12.5 $\pm$ 1.1, 15.2 $\pm$ 2.6 and 13.6 $\pm$ 2.0, and 19.9 $\pm$ 7.2 and 19.2 $\pm$ 7.0 seconds, respectively. The correlation coefficient of these values was 0.97 ($p < 0.001$) and the linear equation was $T_{\frac{1}{2}}$ (Doppler) = 0.97 $T_{\frac{1}{2}}$ (plethysmography) - 0.56.

DISCUSSION

This study indicates that there is excellent correlation between transcutaneous Doppler ultrasonography and venous occlusion plethysmography in the assessment of reactive hyperemic blood flow of the forearm. The systematically greater values of percent change in velocity at peak blood flow by Doppler ultrasonography may in part be explained by a relatively low mean resting velocity as a result of marked diastolic flow reversal in response to the inflated wrist cuff. The systematically shorter $T_{\frac{1}{2}}$ for the Doppler technique may reflect the earlier detection of flow alterations in the brachial artery compared to venous occlusion plethysmography. Inasmuch as the latter technique has been a diagnostic standard for noninvasive assessment of limb blood flow, we would conclude that transcutaneous Doppler ultrasonography is a reliable and simple technique for continuous determination of limb reactive hyperemia in man.

[1] Fronek, A., Johansen, K., Dilley, R. B., and Bernstein, E. F.: Ultrasonographically monitored post-occlusive reactive hyperemia in the diagnosis of peripheral arterial occlusive disease. Circulation 48:149, 1973.

New Techniques

OCTOSON - A NEW RAPID GENERAL PURPOSE ECHOSCOPE

        G. Kossoff;   D.A. Carpenter;   D.E. Robinson;
        G. Radovanovich
          Ultrasonics Institute
          5 Hickson Rd., Millers Point, Sydney, and
W.J. Garrett
          Department of Diagnostic Ultrasound
          Royal Hospital for Women, Paddington
          Sydney, Australia

A new multi-purpose ultrasound scanner has been designed from experience, both technical and clinical, gained from over 12 years usage of various scanners. These have covered the areas of obstetrics, gynecology, breast, thyroid, abdominal organs and the brain in children[1-5]. The unit was designed around the following objectives in order to improve on presently used skin contact scanners and water coupling echoscopes.

1. To achieve a high quality compound scan[6] in the shortest possible time. The scan time is limited by the resolution required and the travel time of the ultrasound to the order of 2 seconds.

2. To give the highest resolution and sensitivity to achieve maximum information display in the echogram.

3. The unit to be capable of scanning a wide range of organs and be flexible in providing a wide range of movement of the plane of scan and capable of measuring other parameters such as velocity, attenuation and echo scattering cross section.

4. To allow simple operation with small dependance on operator skill and ease of coupling to the various organs. The unit to be capable of examining the sickest patients.

Principle

If we consider a typical high quality 10cm x 10cm display unit screen used for the display of echograms the spot size will of the order of 0.3mm. For a sector scan displayed on this screen the angle between lines which is just discernible is of the order of $0.1°$. Hence a $50°$ sector will contain 500 lines. A full compound scan from many different directions requires the superposition of eight such sectors and hence contains 4000 lines. In a water coupling echoscope for general purpose scanning we need to examine a depth of tissue of over 20cm and the transducer must stand back from the patient a distance slightly greater than this to avoid multiple reflection artifacts. The average velocity of ultrasound in water and tissue is 1530 m/sec which gives a travel time of 13 μsec/cm on a there and return basis. This gives typical timings of 300 μs travel in water, 300 μs travel in tissue and 100 μs recovery time between lines for equipment to recover and echoes to die away. Hence the practical minimum time for a 4000 line scan is 2.8 seconds and the theoretical minimum (tissue travel time and recovery) is 1.6 seconds. These times can be further reduced if a simpler scan is acceptable as a single $30°$ sector requires less than 0.3 seconds.

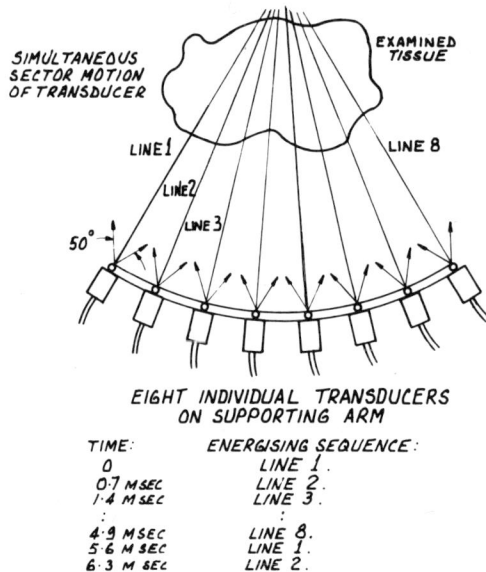

Figure 1. The principle of operation

A single transducer cannot produce 8 sector scans from different directions in such short times due to mechanical inertia limitations and turbulence generated in the water. In the Octoson 8 transducers are used and switched in sequence, and simple mechanically sectored about their origin points. Fig. 1 shows how a compound scanned echogram is obtained by simultaneously sectoring all the transducers which are mechanically linked and mounted on a common arm. The transducers are sequentially energised and the received echo displayed, the sequential rate of energising being such that each transducer is energised when the trace representing its line of sight has moved to its next discernible position. Hence the compound scan is easily obtained in one sector of the transducers[7], which can easily be achieved in the order of 2 seconds.

The Octoson

The complete echoscope is shown in Fig. 2. A water bed approach is adopted in which the scanner is immersed in the tank and the patient lying on the couch is examined through a polythene membrane.

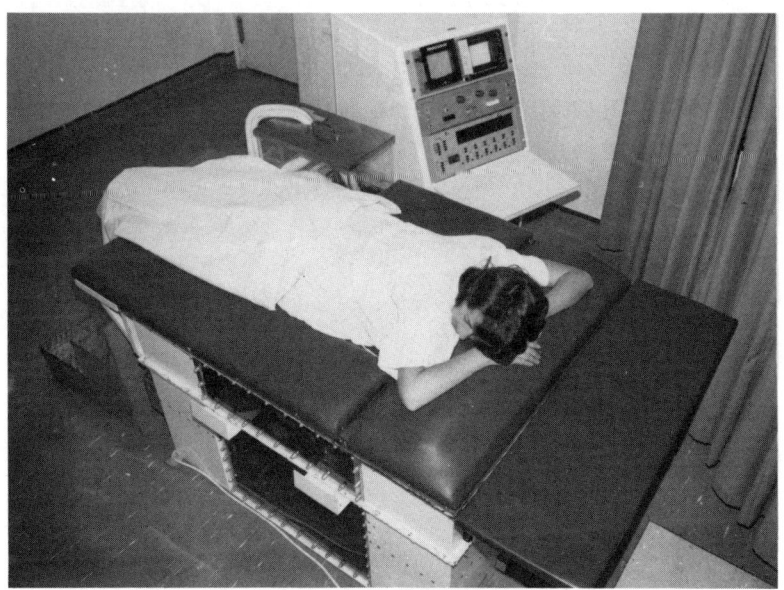

Figure 2. The Octoson

The water coupling method was used so that high resolution can be obtained from the use of large diameter transducers. Also a greater sensitivity against artifacts in tissue is obtained with water couplings. The transducers can be fixed focus or dynamically variable focus annular array types. Large aperture focused transducer are less dependant on the inclination of interfaces. The water coupling method also allows the scanner to be fully motor driven so an even scan rate is achieved and the quality of the echogram is less dependant on operator skill.

The ease of coupling allows the sick patient to be examined. Optimum coupling to various organs is assured by a number of different shaped membranes which have a quick change mechanism. Also the water level in the tank can be raised or lowered to make the membrane wrap around the area of the patient being scanned.

The mechanism of the scanner is shown in Fig.3. The scan plane is normal to the face of the eight transducers mounted on the supporting arm. The transducers can sector through an angle of $50°$ to produce a compound scan and the scan plane has five degrees of movement. The scan arm holding the transducers can be translated along the X and Y axis in increments from 1 mm to 2 cm to give automatic acquisition of a set of parallel echo-

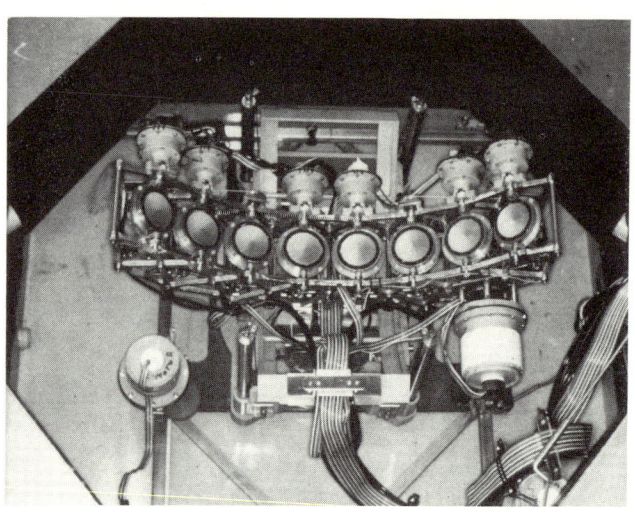

Figure 3. The scanning arm of Octoson

grams at a selected uniform spacing. A set of 15 such echograms can be acquired in order of 1 minute. The arm can also be moved up and down in the Z axis to correctly position the focus of the transducers in relation to the organ being scanned. The arm may be rotated by $180°$ to give transverse, longitudinal or oblique scans and it can be tilted through an angle of $+ 30°$ to give inclined sections. This tilting is designed to centre about the patient's skin line so that no translational movement of the scan plane is involved. Stepper motor drives are used to give even scan rates and because they are amenable to automated drive systems.

Excellent correlation is possible between sections at various positions and angles as there is no need to alter the patient position due to the water coupling employed. The high acquisition rate of echograms minimises the blurring of detail due to respiration, fetal activity and other movement of tissue. The formation of a picture in around 2 seconds offers quasi-real time viewing and this time can be reduced further by using a simpler scan with less transducers and sectoring them through a smaller angle. Also a given volume of tissue can be scanned from a number of different angles in rapid succession. As well as reducing the total examination time the total irradiation to the patient is significantly reduced as any area within a scan receives no more than eight ultrasound pulses. This is further assisted by the fact that the attenuator controls the size of the transmit pulse and not the receiver gain. At present the echoscope has been in use for seven months, and full details of results obtained are given in a joint paper.

Extended Modes of Operation

The availability of eight transducers and the many degrees of movement of the Octoson extends its use to a variety of modes of operation. If the scanner arm undergoes a translational movement along its length as the transducers are scanning this will allow the transducers to 'look' around some overlying structure such as the ribs. In another mode of operation all the transducers can be made to function as a single large transducer with extremely high resolution in one plane. The scanner is then translated normal to this plane to give a high resolution linear scan.

The eight transducers can be used to provide a single transmitter, multiple receiver mode of operation akin to that used in seismology. Correlation of inputs from many receivers can be used to reduce multiple reflection artifacts and to measure local values of velocity throughout the organ.

Echo scattering cross section is a recently discovered property of tissue^9 in which the echo level from a given volume of tissue varies depending on the direction from which the tissue volume is viewed. The two angular motions give rotation and tilting, thereby give two methods of measuring this property. By using the tilting action with a transducer facing vertically upwards the tissue at the centre of the tilting movement is examined. This gives the echo scattering cross section as a function of angle in a fixed plane. Alternatively by pointing the transducers so that their lines of sight cross at the centre of curvature of the arm, the echo scattering cross section of tissue at this point is obtained by rotating the arm. This gives the value when viewed at a fixed angle from variable planes. If all eight transducers are used in either method a reasonably co rse estimation of echo scattering cross section is obtained in two dimensions.

Conclusion

The Octoson represents an advance into a new class of echoscope by giving high quality compound scan echograms in the shortest period limited by the travel time of the ultrasound in tissue. Every transmitted pulse is effectively utilised to form the echogram and this has the advantage that the tissues are scanned with the minimum number of pulses. The dependance on operator skill is minimised by a fully motor driven scanner and the simplicity of the coupling makes it a general purpose instrument capable of examining the sickest patient.

References

1. G. Kossoff, W.J. Garrett and G. Radovanovich. Grey Scale Echography in Obstetrics and Gynaecology. Australasian Radiology, 58, 63-111, 1974.

2. W.J. Garrett, G. Kossoff and D.E. Carpenter. Grey Scale Compound Scan Echography of the Normal Upper Abdomen. J. Clin Ultrasound (in press).

3. W.J. Garrett, G. Kossoff and R.F.C. Jones. Ultrasonic Cross Sectional Visualisation of Hydrocephalus in Infants. Neuroradiology, 8, 279-288, 1975.

4. J. Jellins, G. Kossoff, T.S. Reeve and H. Barraclough. Ultrasonic Grey Scale Visualisation of Breast Disease. Ultrasound in Medicine and Biology 1, 393-404, 1975.

5. J. Jellins, G. Kossoff, J. Wiseman, T. Reeve and I. Hales. Ultrasonic Grey Scale Visualisation of the Thyroid Gland. Ultrasound in Medicine and Biology 1, 405-410, 1975.

6. G. Kossoff. Technical Procedures and Imaging - Diagnostic Ultrasound 75. Present and future of Diagnostic Ultrasound Ed. S. Levi, Proc. of 3rd International Symposium of the FRESERH, Brussels, May 1975.

7. G. Kossoff, G. Radovanovich, W.J. Garrett and D.E. Robinson. Annular Phased Arrays in Ultrasonic Obstetrical Examinations. Ultrasonic Diagnostics, Milan, June 1974, Plenum Press (in press).

8. Garrett, W., Kossoff, G., Carpenter, D.A., Radovanovich, G. The OCTOSON in Use. Ultrasound in Medicine 2. Edited by D.N. White and R.W. Barnes. Plenum Press, New York pp. 341-349   1976.

9. C.R. Hill. Interactions of Ultrasound with Tissues. Ultrasonics in Medicine. Ed. M. deVlieger, D.N. White and V.R. McCready, Excerpta Medica, Amsterdam   pp. 14-20   1974

THE OCTOSON IN USE

>W.J. Garrett
> Department of Diagnostic Ultrasound
> Royal Hospital for Women, Sydney 2021, and
>G. Kossoff; D.A. Carpenter; G. Radovanovich
> Ultrasonics Institute
> 5 Hickson Road, Millers Point
> Sydney 2000, Australia

The Octoson, a rapid acting two dimensional echoscope designed and built at the Ultrasonics Institute in Sydney[1], was installed in the Department of Diagnostic Ultrasound at the Royal Hospital for Women in February, 1975. Now, seven months later, we report our experience of its use in a service environment and compare it with the Ultrasonics Institute's manual contact and earlier water delay echoscopes both of which we still have in the Department.

First, from our experience it may be said that Octoson combines the good points of the manual contact and earlier water delay machines while avoiding the disadvantages of both of those systems. Secondly, we find that Octoson has advantages peculiar to itself. Its rapid action produces an echogram in two to three seconds so movement from respiration or by a wriggling fetus is minimised. With automatic level incrementing a series of ten echograms is obtained in less than one minute, so for small children deep sedation with ketamine is largely avoided. Octoson's rapid action means that the patient through-put is four times that of a standard contact machine. Cost per examination is therefore on a different basis and where an examination room is built to house an Octoson, at least three patients dressing cubicles must be allowed. Octoson's smooth mechanical scanning action is excellent for simple sector scans as the motion is absolutely even. This eliminates the operator skill content of simple scans which is an integral part of the manual contact method. Being a water delay machine, the focused wide aperture transducers in Octoson provide good resolution without the artifacts in skin and superficial tissues associated with contact echoscopes. This is significant in studies of the breast and of small subjects such as abdominal examinations of the newborn. Octoson is truly a general purpose machine and we have been able to examine subjects as diverse as the brain of a three and a half pound premature baby and the full term pregnant uterus of a 230 lb woman. We have also found Octoson suited to the examination of a very sick or weak patients as the patient is recumbent during the examination. Our earlier water delay abdominal echoscope is not so successful in this respect as the patient has to stand up. Finally, we find Octoson an impersonal machine. This is an advantage in that operator skill is not demanding and its operation can be left completely in the hands of a suitably trained technician.

For the examination, the patient lies on the padded top of the Octoson with the part to be examined in direct contact with the polythene membrane of the water bed section. An oil or jelly coupling medium is used. Young babies are given a feeding bottle to avoid movement. Active two or three year old children may require light sedation if they regard the water bed as a trampoline. Older children are easily persuaded to lie still for the two or three periods 60 to 90 seconds during which echograms are taken. Adults find the whole procedure quite acceptable. A few examples will illustrate the work.

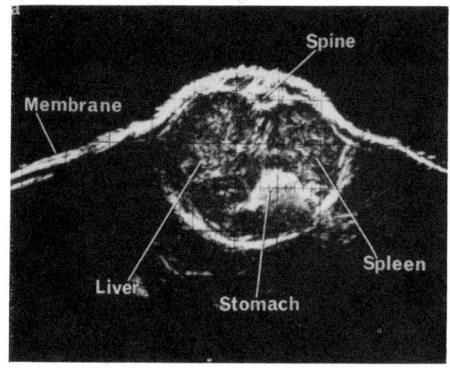
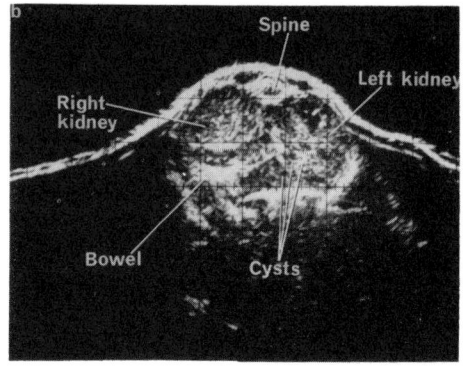

Figure 1. Transverse section echograms of a five day old baby, a. liver and spleen, b. polycystic kidneys

Figure 1 shows bilateral polycystic kidneys in a five day old baby weighing 3050 gms. Figure 1a is a transverse section through the liver and spleen. The line on each side of the abdomen is the polythene membrane of the water bed. This picture has been published with the back uppermost to keep it in line with standard contact echograms but it will be appreciated that the picture was in fact obtained the other way around with the back down as the child was lying on the polythene membrane. Figure 1b is a transverse section echogram 16mm below 1a. It shows the enlarged neonatal kidneys almost filling the abdomen at this level. On close inspection of the renal parenchyma minute black echo free areas are seen. These are the little cysts which characterise polycystic disease.

Figure 2 is from a child aged 3 months with marked hydrocephalus. For this examination the hair on one side of the head is filled with coupling medium and the head is placed against the polythene membrane. There is no need to reposition the head when coronal sections are taken as scanning arm of Octoson simply rotates to the desired plane before starting another automated series of cross sections. In figures 2a,b,c,d transverse sections of the brain are seen. Figure 2a shows the dilated anterior horns, bodies and atria of the lateral ventricles. The cortical thickness of the compressed cerebrum is less than 5mm in the parietal region. Figure 2b is 32 mm below 2a. It shows the choroid plexuses which stand out clearly in cases of hydrocephalus. Figure 2c, 24 mm below b is at the level of the third ventricle whose transverse diameter is 15 mm. The septum pellucidum and foramina of Monro are seen. Figure 2d, 32 mm below c, shows the brain stem with the characteristic black appearance[2]. This section clearly shows the inferior horns of the lateral ventricles which are not usually seen with contact echograms of babies' heads as the ear gets in the way[3]. With Octoson this is not a problem and the inferior horn is regularly outlined.

Figures 2e,f,g are coronal sections from the same patient. Figure 2e shows the foramen of Monro opening to the third ventricle. Figure 2f, 8 mm behind e shows the thalamus on each side of the third ventricle standing out like two great ganglia. On the left, the choroid plexus is particularly obvious in cross section on the floor of the body of the lateral ventricle and on the roof of the inferior horn. The brain stem stands out in the mid line. Figure 2g, 64 mm behind f, shows the dilated atria of the lateral ventricles and the compressed cerebral cortex. Cerebral scanning with Octoson is easier and far quicker than with a contact machine. Sedation requirements are minimal and results are of the same quality as in our earlier publications with the UI contact echoscope or, as in this case, better than before in that the lower part of the brain is seen clearly.

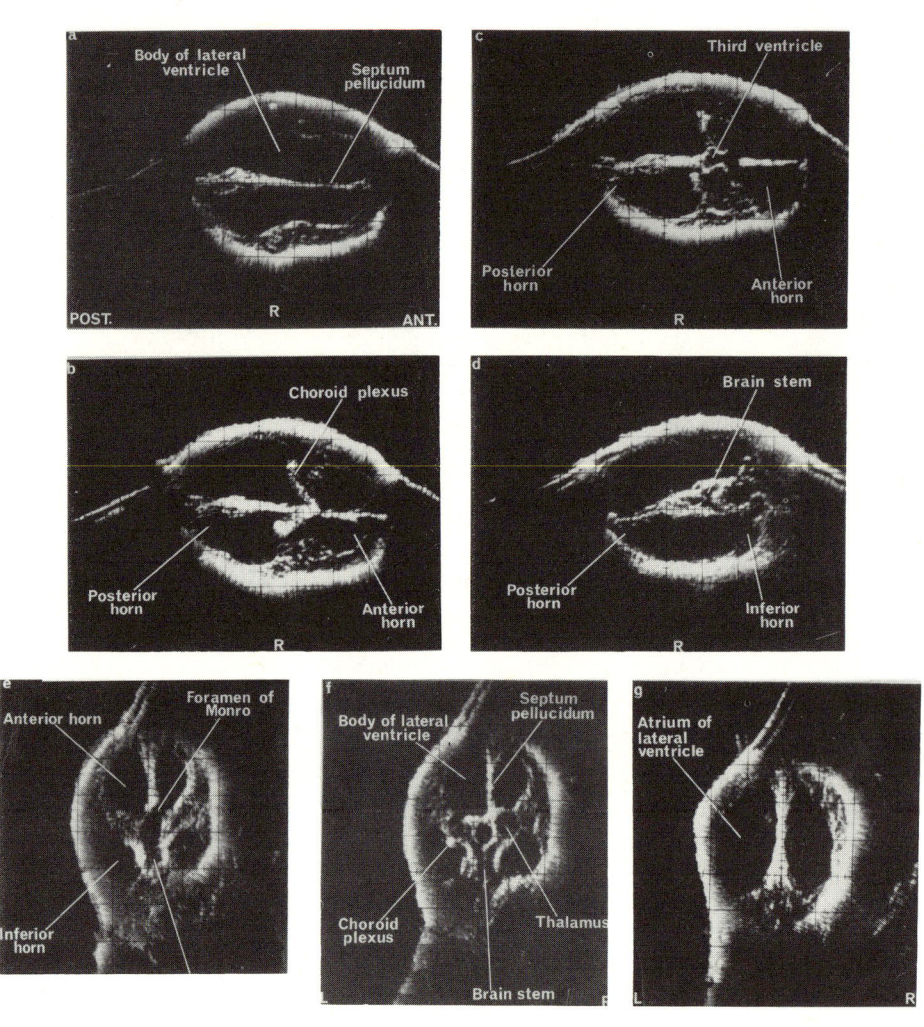

Figure 2. Hydrocephalus in a child aged three months, a,b,c,d transverse section echograms, e,f,g coronal section echograms. Examinations such as these obviate the use of X-ray air studies in many cases.

THE OCTOSON IN USE

For breast examinations, the polythene membrane is lowered by pumping some of the water from the main tank of Octoson to a reserve tank. This produces a basin like concavity in the membrane into which water is poured. The breasts are then placed into this water. Alternatively, the polythene membrane is removed and the breasts are placed directly in the main tank. Figure 3 shows both breasts from one patient. The echograms of each breast were taken separately and assembled for this illustration but it is possible to examine both breasts simultaneously. In the left breast a benign cyst with its echo free content is seen. This is compared with a solid malignant lesion in the right breast.

Large abdominal cysts are equally well defined by Octoson as with any other echoscope. Figure 4 shows a monolocular benign ovarian cyst in transverse section compared with a similar section from a malignant ovarian cyst. The malignant cyst shows plaques of solid tissue distributed irregularly among the cystic areas.

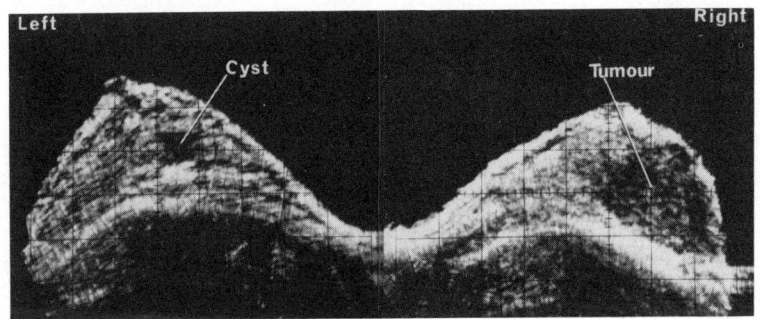

Figure 3. Transverse section echograms of breasts

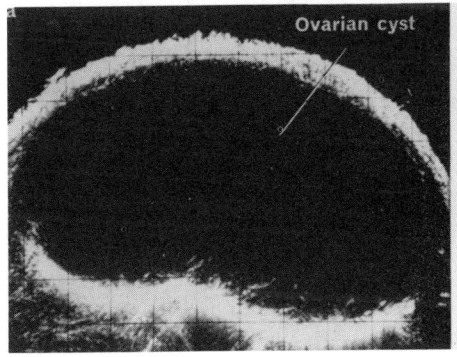
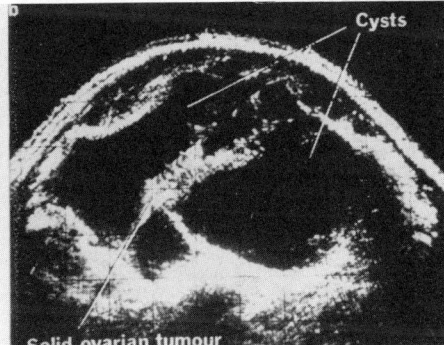

Figure 4. Ovarian cysts <u>a</u>. benign <u>b</u>. malignant

Renal abscesses, cysts and tumours are well defined by Octoson. Figure 5a is a longitudinal section simple scan using a transducer. Note the even quality of this mechanically produced scan. It is very difficult to achieve this quality of simple scan with a hand held transducer. The section shows the expanded upper pole of the right kidney with an abscess cavity. The adrenal which is of normal shape and size is displaced upwards. The liver is normal. Figures 5 b,c,d are compound scan transverse sections through the liver, the abscess and the normal lower pole of the kidney respectively.

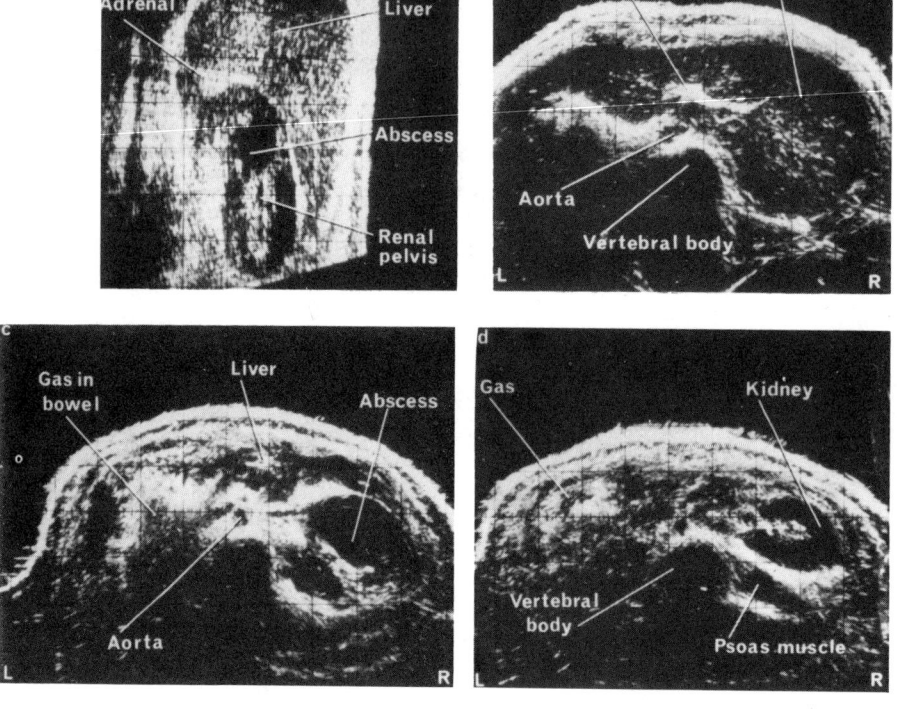

Figure 5. Renal abscess a. longitudinal simple sector scan b,c,d. transverse section compound scan

Liver scans with Octoson are similar to those[4] obtained by our earlier water delay machine but the new machine seems to have solved the problem of seeing the dome of the liver more clearly. The water bed section of Octoson wraps itself around the patient giving good contact over the ribs. Figure 6a is a true transverse section over the lower ribs and not a tilted plane. In this particular patient the anatomy is slightly unusual in that the dome of the liver is at the level of the heart. The heart would have contracted twice while this echogram was being taken but could have been in diastole for most of the time during which the heart was being written. Figure 6 b shows a section 10cm below a.

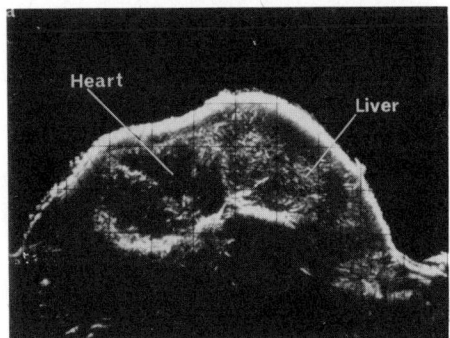 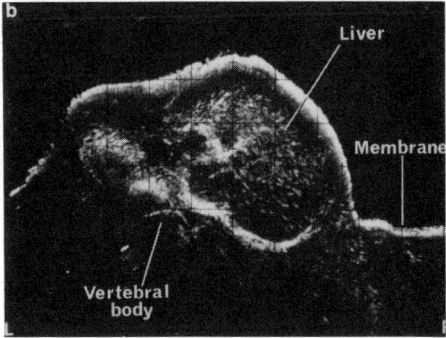

Figure 6. Transverse section echograms of the liver 10cm apart.

Octoson is quick and easy to use for obstetric examinations. Fetal movement is reduced and this is particularly helpful with small fetuses. Figure 7 is one section from a series taken to diagnose twin pregnancy in a patient with a history of 20 weeks amenorrohea. The fetal membrane separating the two sacs is outlined. With the earlier UI water delay echoscope in which the patient stands up, some difficulty is experienced in longitudinal sections in clear definition of the lower part of the field. This difficulty is solved by Octoson where the lower pole of the uterus, the bladder and the vagina are regularly seen with clear detail as in Figure 8.

In late pregnancy the resolution which has characterised echograms obtained in the past with UI echoscopes[5,6] is obtained with Octoson. Figure 9 shows a transverse section of a fetal trunk at the level of

the kidneys. The placenta containing odd flecks of
calcification is on the anterior uterine wall and loops
of umbical cord are seen floating freely in the amniotic
fluid. Figure 10 is from a different patient. The echogram is a transverse section through the fetal chest
showing the heart and lungs. Note the grayness of the
long tissue compared with the black echofree areas of
the chambers of the heart.

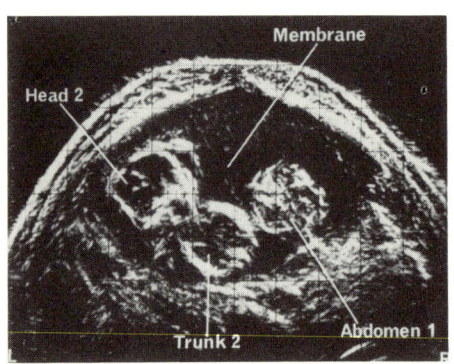

Figure 7. Twins, showing membrane between sacs.

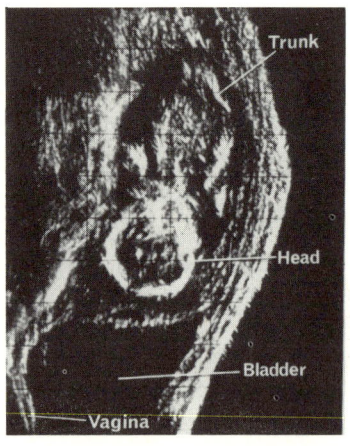

Figure 8. Longitudinal section showing lower segment and vagina.

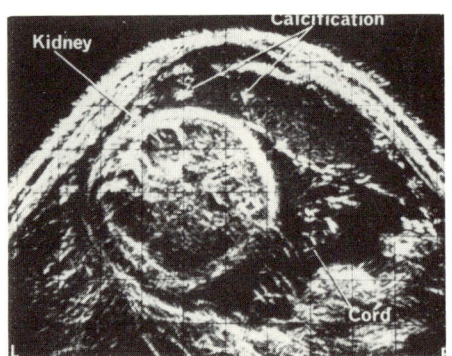

Figure 9. Fetal kidneys, cord and placenta.

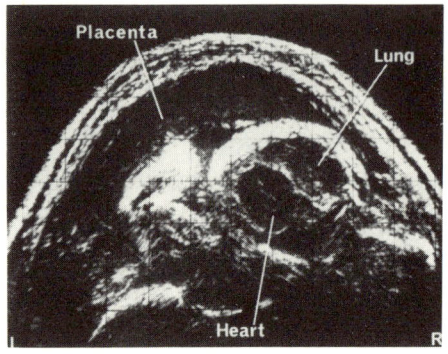

Figure 10. Fetal heart and lungs.

Summary and Conclusion

From seven months experience of its use we find Octoson a general purpose echoscope which, in many ways is ideal in the service environment. It is quick and easy to operate. It can be used for very sick or weak patients. It is equally suited to small and large subjects and its picture quality equals that of our previously published work. Fine quality compound and simple sector scans are a regular feature with Octoson and no special dexterity on the part of the operator is necessary to obtain them.

References

1. Kossoff, G., Carpenter, D.A., Robinson, D.E., Radovanovich, G., Garrett, W.J., Octoson - A new rapid general purpose echoscope, *Ultrasound in Medicine 2. Edited by D.N. White and R.W. Barnes, Plenum Press, New York. pp. 333-339, 1976.*

2. Kossoff, G., Garrett, W.J., Radovanovich, G., Ultrasonic atlas of normal brain of infant, Ultrasound in Med. & Biol., 1, 259-266, 1974.

3. Garrett, W.J., Kossoff, G., Jones, R.F.C., Ultrasonic cross-sectional visualization of hydrocephalus in infants, Neuroradiology, 8, 279-288, 1975.

4. Garrett, W.J., Kossoff, G., Carpenter, D.A., Gray scale compound scan echography of the normal upper abdomen, J. Clin. *Ultrasound 3, 199-204, 1975.*

5. Kossoff, G., Garrett, W.J., Radovanovich, G., Gray scale echography in obstetrics and gynaecology, Australasian Radiology, 18, 62-111, 1974.

6. Garrett, W.J., Kossoff, G., Lawrence, R., Gray scale echography on the diagnosis of hydrops due to fetal lung tumor, J. Clin. Ultrasound, 3, 45. - 50, 1975.

AN ANALOG ECHOCARDIOGRAM FOR ESTIMATING VENTRICULAR STROKE VOLUME

M.L. Petrovick, G.S. Malindzak, Jr., and E.D. Haak, Jr.

Environmental Protection Agency

Chapel Hill, North Carolina 27514

ABSTRACT

A multiple range-gated echocardiographic signal processor has been developed for the purpose of converting the complex ultrasonic image of the left ventricular anterior and posterior wall boundaries to equivalent analog signals as a means of estimating stroke volume and computing cardiac output.

Two conventional time-analog range-gated modules have been redesigned and synchronized with the initial transmit pulse of 1000 hz, for the purpose of simultaneously gating echocardiographic images of the anterior and posterior left ventricular walls. Each echocardiographic image boundary is selectively gated in the A-Mode and adjusted to a width exceeding the maximum wall motion. The gated echocardiographic boundary of each time-analog channel is processed by a fast-attack envelope detector and a low-pass filter network to produce a D.C. analog signal corresponding to the motion of the left ventricular anterior and posterior wall. These analog signals serve as the basis for the estimation of ventricular stroke volume and the computation of cardiac output.

Pilot studies were conducted in six healthy male subjects to evaluate the feasibility of producing the analog signals equivalent to the echo image boundaries of the anterior and posterior left ventricular walls on a beat-by-beat basis. The results of these studies have shown a favorable comparison between the conventional echographic analysis and estimation of stroke volume and cardiac output based on the analog method described here. These findings are encouraging and serve as a basis for continuing developments and studies to provide for automatic tracking of wall boundary echos and computational procedures through microprocessor techniques.

INTRODUCTION

Studies of dynamic ventricular geometry have yielded important information relative to the understanding of cardiac function and its performance. The non-invasive determination of ventricular volume, ejection fraction and myocardial contractility have served as a valuable resource in caring for cardiac patients(1) and as the basis for the development of sensitive health indicators resulting from air pollution exposure(2).

In the last decade imaging the heart and quantitation of ventricular stroke volume and cardiac output have been based on visual identification of cardiac structural boundaries through a variety of complex biomedical instrumentation systems including such techniques as: cineangiography(3), video-densitometry(4) and radioisotometry (5). While these systems provide a means for "visualizing" dynamic and pulsatile cardiac performance, they require procedures that are invasive and utilize material that present some hazard to the subject.

The development of echocardiography has, in the last five years, provided an alternative procedure for determining ventricular stroke volume and cardiac output non-invasively. The practical problems associated with the processing of non-invasive clinical echocardiographic boundary signals in the determination of changing cardiac geometry has been difficult. Usually interpretation and analysis of the displayed ultrasonic signals have been accomplished manually by outlining the boundaries of echo patterns from cardiac structures with a line drawing superimposed on the oscillographic tracing of the echo pattern in the M-Mode(6). This process is always time consuming and usually requires some arbitrary decision on the part of the analyst.

Methods and procedures for converting echocardiographic image boundaries to an analog signal with a sonic or light pen have been useful but complex(7). One desirable requirement for effective echocardiovascular research is to have available the capability for producing instantaneous analog signals from echo profiles of cardiac structures on a continuous beat-by-beat basis.

It is the major purpose of this paper to present a working design of a signal processor for a single plane time-motion echocardiographic system as a means of converting echo patterns of two ventricular boundaries simultaneously to analog signals for the purpose of estimating stroke volume and determining cardiac output. The substance of this presentation will be to describe: a) the specific modifications made to existing conventional echocardiographic equipment, b) the interface design required for synchronous operation, and c) the pilot studies upon which the system operation was evaluated.

SYSTEM DESIGN

A signal processor has been designed as a means for converting video echocardiographic images of cardiac structures into equivalent analog signals for ease of analysis and processing. It was the purpose of this design to utilize the echocardiographic image-to-analog conversion processor to provide for the capability of identifying and converting two cardiac images (near and far) simultaneously; specifically for estimating stroke volume and computing cardiac output from the image-to-analog converted anterior and posterior ventricular wall echo boundaries.

The system design is based on a modified Smith Kline Instruments SKI-20 Echocardiograph which operates at a frequency of 2.25 Mhz with an output power of 10 milliwatts, utilizing focused and unfocused transducers (Aerotech) with a single time-analog module. Specific modifications of the original time-analog module involve the peak envelope detector and range-gate synchronization. The purpose for these modifications was to improve the analog signal quality of the envelope detector output by significantly reducing the internally generated artifact inherent in the original time analog system.

The original peak envelope detector was replaced with a Paynter envelope detector coupled to a low-pass filter network. The Paynter envelope detector operates with a time constant of 5 milliseconds, permitting nearly instantaneous tracking of the near and far (video) targets. The frequency response of the envelope detector was flat from D.C. to 3 megahertz (3 db) with a 12 db per octave roll off. The low-pass filter was a 3-pole Butterworth design with a frequency response flat from D.C. to 100 hertz (3 db) with a 12 db octave roll off.

These specific modifications were performed on two off-the-shelf time-analog modules. The two modified time-analog modules were combined in a way to permit selective and synchronous range-gating of near and far echocardiographic video targets (Figure 1).

Functionally, the transmit pulse A (Figure 2), triggers a monostable Q-1 (Figure 1), resulting in pulse B, the length of which may be adjusted to coincide with the maximum duration of the transducer artifact. The output of Q-1, pulse B, is then differentiated to produce pulse C, and diode clipped and inverted to produce pulse D; a trailing edge of which enables the near-depth range-gate. The near-depth range-gate is then positioned in range and adjusted in width (depth) to coincide with the maximum motion of the near target. The output of the near-depth range-gate, pulse E. The inter-channel inverter functions to provide a trigger between the near and far range-gates which synchronizes the near and far time-analog modules. The trailing edge of pulse G, provides a new trigger for the second

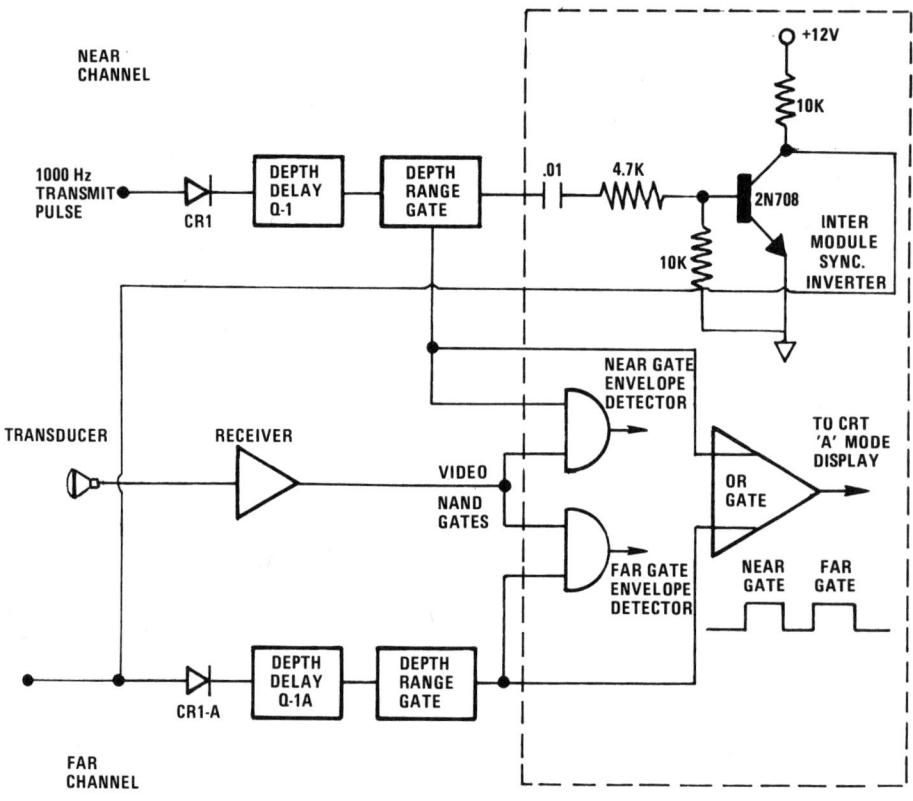

Figure 1. Functional block diagram of the dual time analog echocardiographic signal processing system. The modifications of the basic time analog modules are outlined by the dashed lines.

time-analog module and enables Q-1A, the delay monostable of the far-depth range-gate, producing pulse H. The output delay monostable Q-1A (pulse H) is adjusted in range so that the trailing edge is within the far range target area. This pulse is differentiated to produce pulse I, diode clipped and inverted to produce pulse J, providing a trigger which in turn enables the far-depth range-gate and produces pulse K. The timing logic of A through E and H through J (Figure 2) is basic to the functional characteristic of each time-analog module. In addition, modification of the basic time-analog module was necessary to provide a differentiated output of the near-depth range-gate E, and the trailing edge G, as part of the inverter inter-channel synchronization process. This procedure is essential for the generation of the near and far range-gates simultaneously.

ANALOG ECHOCARDIOGRAM

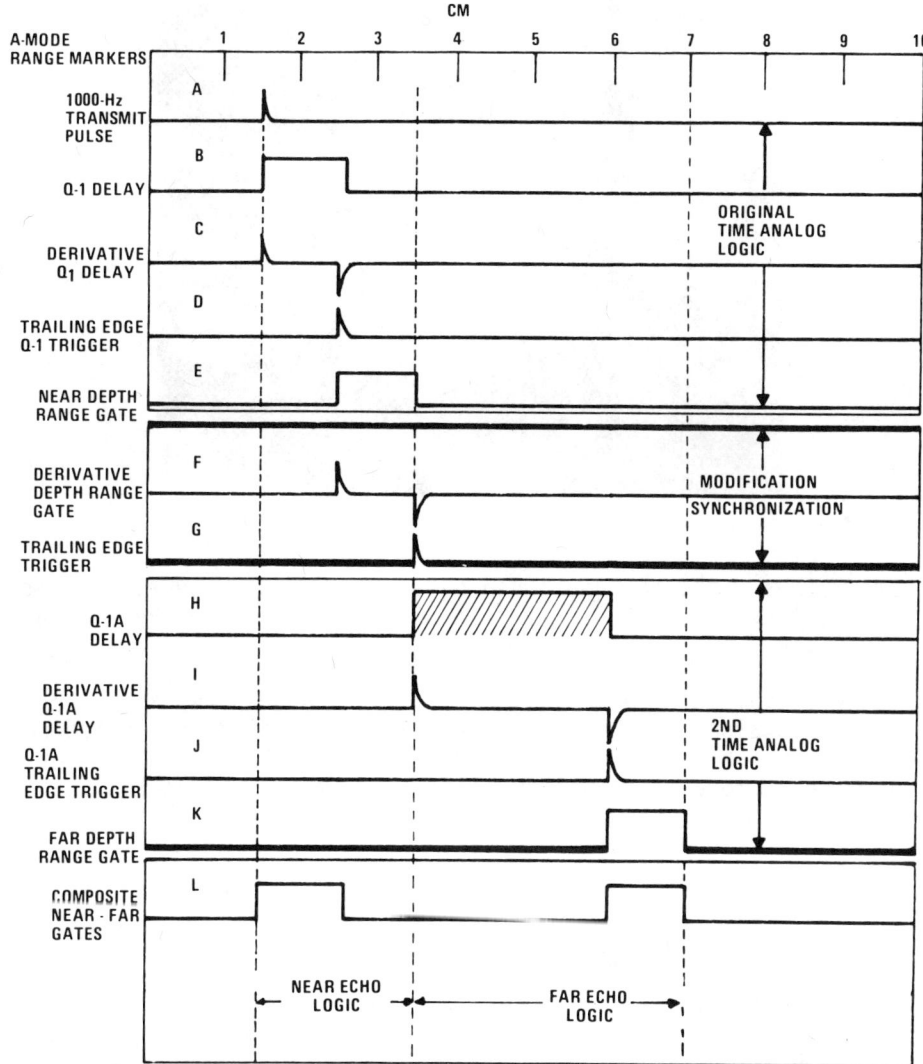

Figure 2. Timing logic for the dual channel analog echocardiographic processing system.

The output of each near- and far-depth range-gates serve as the inputs to an "OR" gate (Figure 1), the output of which is displayed on the cathode ray tube in the A-Mode. This results in a composite signal display on the cathode ray tube consisting of near- and far-depth range-gate outputs superimposed on the existing conventional A-Mode video echos (Figure 3).

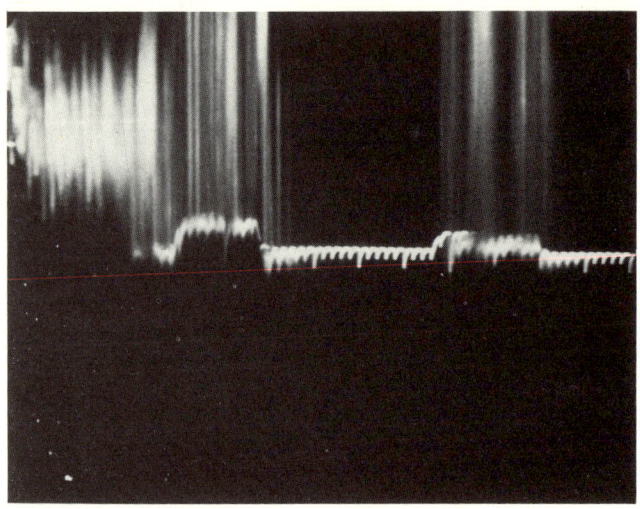

Figure 3. Near and far depth range gates positioned over the left ventricular anterior and posterior walls in the A-Mode.

The outputs of the near- and far-depth range-gates also serve as input signals to the video "NAND" gates providing only gated echo boundary signals to the envelope detector and low-pass filter for final signal processing and conversion into two near and far analog boundary signals (Figures 1 and 4).

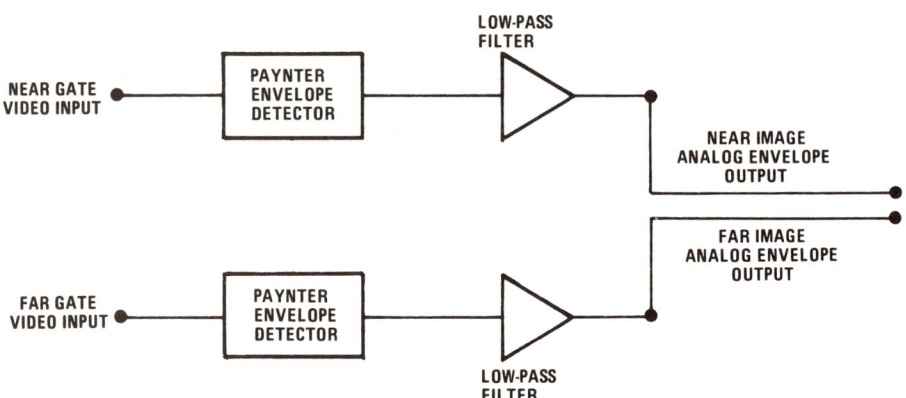

Figure 4. The envelope detector and low pass filter.

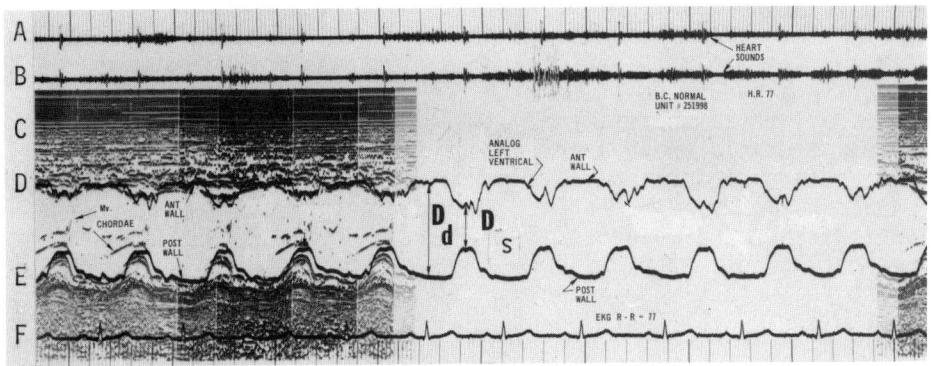

Figure 5. (A) and (B) heart sounds, (C) conventional echo display (D) and (E) analog profile of anterior/posterior walls of left ventricle (F) ECG.

In actual practice, the near and far echos are viewed in the A-Mode. The transducer damping and gain controls are adjusted to enhance the near and the far echo to be range-gated. The near-depth range-gate is manually positioned and superimposed over the near echo and the width (depth) adjusted to encompass the range of motion. Once the near-depth range-gate is adjusted, the far-depth range-gate is manually positioned and superimposed over the far echo and the width (depth) adjusted to encompass the range of motion. At this point, the CRT displays (in the A-Mode) the output of each range-gate (near and far), superimposed on the echocardiographic image which includes echos from the selected near and far targets (Figure 3). Each selected target falls within the width of its respective range-gate. The system control is then switched to the M-Mode display (on the graphic recorder). Then the position and gain controls for the analog boundary signals are manually adjusted so that they are superimposed over the boundary of the M-Mode video images, corresponding to the near and far targets. In this particular application, the product of this effort is two analog signals which correspond to the motion of the left ventricular anterior and posterior wall boundaries (Figure 5). The graphic analysis of this analog output is then performed for the estimation of ventricular stroke volume and computation of cardiac output.

APPLICATION

A pilot study was conducted based on six healthy male subjects (age range from 22 to 31) who were examined for the purpose of determining the feasibility of estimating left ventricular stroke volume and computing cardiac output based on two echocardiographic techniques; one based on the analysis of the conventional video image in the M-Mode, and the other based on the analog technique described in this presentation. The study was conducted with the subject in a supine position with the head and shoulders elevated to the horizontal approximately 15 degrees. A standard electrocardiogram was taken on each subject for the purpose of providing a time reference for identifying the diastolic and systolic events of the cardiac cycle. The modified echocardiographic instrumentation* (with output power of 10 milliwatts) and 2.25 Mhz transducer** (0.5" diameter unfocused) was calibrated with a standard plastic test block supplied by the manufacturer for the purpose of establishing calibrated depth in the A-Mode.

The transducer was placed in the left parasternal position between the third and fourth intercostal space. A standard arc scan view with the transducer was performed until the anterior and posterior wall of the left ventricle was clearly identified. All measurements, calculations and comparisons were made with the transducer fixed in the left ventricular view position. A conventional echocardiographic record was then taken on each subject in the M-Mode. The near and far range-gates were positioned to correspond to the anterior and posterior ventricular wall echos and adjusted in width to encompass the range of motion of each boundary for further processing and conversion into respective analog signals. The analog output of the echocardiographic processor was positioned (in the M-Mode) to superimpose each analog boundary signal over its corresponding video image. The display of each analog boundary signal alone and in combination with the echocardiographic video image is shown in Figure 5. This display option is accomplished by reducing the video threshold level in the graphic recorder to eliminate the video image from the M-Mode display, while retaining it for the depth range-gate processor.

An M-Mode oscillographic tracing of the combination echocardiographic video image and analog envelope was obtained for analysis. Each oscillographic record on each subject was analyzed for stroke volume and cardiac output based on the following equations(6):

$$SV = D_d^3 - D_s^3, \quad (1)$$

where, SV = stroke volume (ml), D_d = diastolic dimension (cm), and D_s = systolic dimension (cm), and,

$$CO = SV \times HR, \quad (2)$$

where, CO = cardiac output (liters/min), and HR (beats/min) = heart rate (determined from the R-to-R interval).

* Smith Kline Instruments/SKI-20
**Aerotech

For the purpose of comparing the systolic and diastolic dimensions extracted from oscillographic tracings corresponding to the conventional video echo and the analog boundary signals, an estimation of stroke volume and cardiac output from each subject was computed using equations 1 and 2 and tabulated (Table 1).

Table 1. Echocardiographic Estimates of Left Ventricular Stroke Volume and Cardiac Output

Subject #	CONVENTIONAL ECHO STROKE VOLUME (ml)	ANALOG PROCESSED ECHO STROKE VOLUME (ml)
1	55	55
2	52	51
3	56	55
4	62	60
5	125	134
6	85	77

Subject #	CARDIAC OUTPUT (liters/min)	CARDIAC OUTPUT (liters/min)
1	4.2	4.2
2	3.9	3.8
3	4.3	3.9
4	4.9	4.8
5	9.1	9.7
6	5.9	5.4

DISCUSSION

The analog echocardiogram processor described in this presentation has demonstrated the feasibility of range-gating two simultaneous ventricular echos separated in depth, and converting their respective complex videos to analog signals (in the M-Mode) corresponding to the motion of the anterior and posterior ventricular wall boundaries. The design presented here and its implementation provides an alternate means of performing analyses of echocardiographic signals on a beat-by-beat basis, including digital computer processing. Provision for automatic digital computer processing is not included in the current design; however the analog signals produced from the present system are easily digitized for this purpose. Implementation of a more complete data processing system is being undertaken in combination with a microprocessor and will be the subject of a future report.

The position and depth adjustments of each range-gate is performed manually. This adjustment procedure is tedious and cumbersome. In addition, the ability for the analog to track the video image with excellent fidelity is not possible. A noticeable phase shift or tracking error may be detected when the echo image and analog envelope signal are superimposed (Figure 5). Provisions are being made to correct for some of these inconveniences by providing for an automatic range-gate tracking feature utilizing the same microprocessor currently scheduled to perform the automatic data processing function. At the present time, the manual method is simple and reliable, but frustratingly slow. In addition, part of the phase shift error is being corrected by using logrithmic amplifiers and digital filtering techniques.

The application of the analog echocardiogram processor is not limited to ventricular measurements alone. Depending on the echos to be analyzed, it is possible to range-gate other structures such as the anterior and posterior walls of the aorta(8), aortic valves, mitral valves and convert the gated motion of these structures to analog boundary signals for further analysis of cardiac performance.

At the present time the authors have undertaken a further study which involves the use of a microprocessor to perform computations, coordinate the timing logic and provide for the automatic range-gate tracking function. The substance of this study will be reported at a future date.

CONCLUSIONS

This study has demonstrated the practicality of redesigning a conventional echocardiograph to provide for more than one time analog signal from a single transducer. Specifically, this redesigned system provides two simultaneous analog signals corresponding to the near and far boundary echos of a complex echocardiographic ventricular image from which stroke volume and cardiac output was estimated. The analog echocardiographic method compares favorably with the conventional echo image method for this determination. This system of echocardiographic processing and signal analysis for evaluating dynamic cardiac changes without the loss of conventional echocardiographic information enhances the ease of signal analysis.

ACKNOWLEDGEMENTS

The authors wish to express their appreciation to Mrs. Sally Moos of the Division of Cardiology, University of North Carolina School of Medicine and the North Carolina Memorial Hospital, Chapel Hill, N.C. for her assistance in echocardiographic techniques.

This work was conducted at Clinical Studies Division, Health Effects Research Laboratory, U.S. Environmental Protection Agency, University of North Carolina School of Medicine, Chapel Hill, North Carolina 27514.

REFERENCES

1. Fortuin, N.J., Hood, W.P., Sherman, M.E. and Craige, E.: Determination of left ventricular volumes by ultrasound. Circulation 54: 575-584, 1971.

2. Shy, C.M. and Finklea, J.F.: Air pollution affects community health. Environmental Science and Technology 7: 204-208, 1973.

3. Marcus, M.L., Schuette, W.H., Whitehouse, W.C., Bailey, J.J., and Glancy, D.L.: An annotated method for the measurement of ventricular volume. Circulation 55: 65-76, 1972.

4. Bursch, J.H., Heintzen, P.H. and Simon, R.: Videodensitometric studies by a new method of quantitating the amount of contrast medium. Europ. J. Cardiol. 1: 437-446, 1974.

5. Johnson, S.A., Robbi, R.A., Greenleaf, J.F., Ritman, E.L., Lee, S.L., Herman, G.T., Sturm, R.E. and Wood, E.H.: The problem of accurate measurement of left ventricular shape and dimensions from multiplane roentgenographic data. Europ. J. Cardiol. 1: 241-258, 1974.

6. Feigenbaum, H.: *Echocardiography*, Philadelphia, Lea and Febiger, 1972.

7. Van Wijk van Brievingh, R.P., Richtering Blenken, A., Van Poelgeest, R., Sneek, J.H.J., Zimmerman, A.N.E. and Meijler, F.L.: A measurement system for left ventricular volume determination. Europ. J. Cardiol. 1: 259-277, 1974.

8. Petrovick, M.L., Malindzak, G.S., Jr., and Knelson, J.H.: A non-invasive cardiac output processor for clinical echocardiography. 27th Annual Conf. on Eng. in Med. and Biol. 267, 1974.

A NEW THREE-DIMENSIONAL RANDOM SCANNER FOR ULTRASONIC/COMPUTER GRAPHIC IMAGING OF THE HEART

Donald Latham King, M. D.
Sami J. Al-Banna, EngSc.D. David R. Larach, A.B.
Division of Ultrasound, Department of Radiology,
Columbia University College of Physicians and
Surgeons and the School of Engineering and Applied
Science, Columbia University, New York, N. Y.

Echocardiography is a valuable technique for cardiac diagnosis. It is now routinely used in many clinical situations to evaluate the aortic and mitral valves and to diagnose pericardial effusion. Although useful for many applications it does not meet urgent clinical needs for easier and faster diagnosis of structural abnormalities and for accurate, non-invasive evaluation of cardiac function. The use of echocardiography to establish the nature of a congenital cardiac malformation requires an unusually high degree of technical skill and knowledge of congenital heart disease. Such examinations are so difficult and time consuming that they are beyond the capability of all but the most dedicated and expert echocardiographer. In addition, while many studies have attempted to establish the usefulness of echocardiography for evaluation of cardiac function (1-5) the results have been disappointing. Recently an awareness of the limited usefulness of echocardiography for this purpose has developed (6,7). Echocardiography cannot provide precise estimations of ventricular volume although calculation of ejection fraction from the chordal echo diameter may be clinically useful (6). Furthermore, echocardiography, by its nature, can only detect abnormal ventricular wall movement. It cannot accurately

Supported in part by the Judith Harris Selig Memorial Foundation and the Picker Foundation.

localize or quantify the size of abnormally contracting segments. These limitations have led us to an assessment of the technical aspects of echocardiography and to the development of a new, alternative type of instrumentation that will overcome its limitations and fulfill the clinical needs referred to above. The objective of this effort has been to develop a non-invasive technique using diagnostic ultrasound that would compete with or surpass quantitative angiocardiography in clinical usefulness. In so doing it would provide a means for rapid, easy and reliable diagnosis of congenital and acquired morphologic abnormalities of the heart. It would also yield accurate quantitative determinations of ventricular volume and it would be a means for qualitative and quantitative assessment of regional abnormalities of left ventricular wall motion. The purpose of this report is to present the rationale for the development of the new instrumentation, the concept of its operation and the general features of its design.

Echocardiography is a one dimensional technique. Each echo is a measure of the range or distance of its source from the transducer. At any given instant the echoes are related to one another only in terms of depth along the sound beam. They are not related spatially to any external reference point and hence are not related to one another as the sound beam is moved. The ultrasound beam lacks spatial orientation. There is no means for registering the position of the transducer in space , nor for recording its direction or angulation. As a consequence the relationship of spatially separate structures in the heart cannot be determined by echocardiography. Areas or volumes cannot be measured directly and images of structures cannot be created. In echocardiography the echoes are displayed in a time-motion format that does not resemble the appearance of the heart. The technique of an M-mode sweep across the left ventricle from aortic root to apex has been developed to compensate for this as far as possible by producing a pseudo-image. Because of its lack of spatial orientation and its time-motion display format echocardiography utilizes diagnostically only a small portion of the available echo data. That data, varying in time and space must, to be interpreted, be mentally integrated by the observer using his proprioceptive position sense. This is a difficult skill requiring extensive knowledge and experience in order to achieve morphologic diagnoses and estimates of ventricular size and function. The lack of spatial orientation and integration of the data by echocardiography will be overcome by the new instrumentation described herein.

A variety of techniques for planar, two-dimensional, cross-sectional imaging of the heart have been developed(8-12) in an attempt to overcome some of the limitations of echocardiography. Integration of echo data into an image has aided visualization of some morphologic anomalies but has been less helpful for evaluation of cardiac function. Although an improvement, planar imaging techniques nevertheless have inherent limitations. The echo data in a planar image is characterized in only two dimensions. The position of the plane in space is not defined. That is, two-dimensional scanners do not relate the orientation of successive planar images to each other. This fact, as in echocardiography, requires the observer to assume the difficult task of mental integration of the time and space-varying images. An additional limitation of the real-time planar imaging techniques is their limited field of view. Except in the case of infants and children the sector or linear scanner will depict only a small portion of a planar cross section of the heart. While planar images represent a step toward our objectives they do not provide a complete image of the heart that will allow direct measurement of ventricular volume or easier quantification of wall motion.

A general problem faced by ultrasonic scanners is the specular nature of ultrasound reflections from tissue structures. Larger surfaces and structures in the body such as the heart valves and walls, tend to act as mirror-like reflectors in which the angle of reflection equals the angle of incidence. For echo-ranging instruments in which the reflected sound wave must return to the transmitting transducer the angle of incidence of the wave must be nearly perpendicular to the reflecting structure. In the heart, as in the body generally, the geometry and orientation of reflecting surfaces is highly variable and complex. Therefore to optimize echo return from any given surface an ultrasound scanner should be capable of scanning freely in any direction, that is, it should be able to compound scan in three dimensions. Only by means of a freely moving compound scanner may the position of the transducer and direction of the sound beam be optimized by the operator to collect all available data.

To overcome the limitations of one and two-dimensional techniques and the problems posed by the specular nature of echo reflections a new type of instrumentation is essential. An ideal new instrument will compound scan freely in three dimensions and will collect, store and integrate all echo data available from the heart into a complete three dimensional ultrasonic image of the heart, an image volume of a tissue volume. Achievement of this requires an unconstrained scanner capable of compound scanning freely in three dimensions while continuously registering the position of the ultrasound beam in space and of characterizing each echo source by a complete set of X,Y and Z coordinates. An instrument which will accomplish this is a three-dimensional random scanner. In addition, achievement of a three-dimensional ultrasonic image requires integration and storage of the image echo data in a suitable three-dimensional memory, such as provided by a digital computer. Display of the image in computer memory may be carried out by advanced computer graphic techniques for simulating a three dimensional display. A complete instrument system will therefore be a three-dimensional ultrasonic/computer graphic random scanner.

A three-dimensional scanning system requires a means other than an oscilloscope or television storage tube for image integration and storage. Conventional ultrasonic scanners developed as two-dimensional systems because image integration and image display were combined into a single two-dimensional device, the screen/film combination. The screen/film combination is only capable of integrating and displaying two-dimensional data. The third dimension perpendicular to the plane of the screen cannot be depicted. Therefore the registration of echoes was confined to two dimensions. Correspondingly the movement of the transducer was confined to a two dimensional plane. The two-dimensional memory-image format dictated the use of a two-dimensional scanning format. The plane of the oscilloscope screen (the image plane) had to have a direct correspondence to the tissue plane under examination. Therefore, scanners were built as two-dimensional planar scanners. Analog systems such as these had no capability for storing or integrating into the planar image echoes recorded outside the tissue plane giving rise to the echoes and corresponding to the image plane. There was no means for dissociating the direct correspondence of the scanning plane and the image integration and display plane. Achievement of this dissociation and three-dimensional scanning requires separation of the image integration and image display functions. The image integration function has to be performed by a device capable of three dimensional memory, that is, a digital computer. A three-dimensional memory system in conjunction with a three-dimensional scanning system solves the problem of specular echo collection and creates an image volume of a tissue volume. It registers the spatial relationship of sequentially obtained echo data, whether acquired by parallel, orthogonal or non-parallel planar scans, or by other scanning formats such as spiral scanning.

In the past Fry (13) has proposed a system for "omnidirectional" scanning. This apparatus however required rotation of the subjects (dog) head and time-gating to achieve a single planar image scanning from many angles. Brown (14) has discussed the limitations and development of two and three dimensional scanning. Recently Dekker (15) has described a mechanical system for three dimensional scanning. This apparatus utilizes a mechanical arm linkage with five potentiometers to register the position of the ultrasound transducer. It also utilizes a digital computer for three-dimensional image integration. The ultrasound transducer in this system is a conventional single element transducer. The new random scanner ultrasonic/computer graphic system described herein consists of four major components:

1) a real-time cardiac scanner,
2) A three-dimensional sonic locater,
3) a digital mini computer, and
4) a scheduler/controller.

The real-time cardiac scanner may be of any suitable type, such as a linear array, phased array, or mechanical sector scanner. It appears probable that one type will be more suitable than another in specific clinical situations and age groups. The real-time scanner provides a maximal rate of data acquisition for spatially varying lines of echo data. The same signals that are used to coordinate the real-time image display with scanner transducer operation are utilized as system synchronizing signals and are transmitted from the real-time scanner to the scheduler/controller. In addition the R-wave signal of the patients electrocardiogram is transmitted to the scheduler/controller and is utilized as a primary sequencing signal. The processed video signal carrying the echocardiographic data is transmitted to a 0.77 megaHerz 3-bit analog-to-digital converter and subsequently to computer memory. The real-time scanner transducer is attached by a fixed, mechanical apparatus to the transmitter apparatus of the three-dimensional sonic locater.

The sonic locater consists of three major components, a transmitter apparatus, a sensor apparatus, and electronic circuits to operate them. The transmitter apparatus consists of three spark gaps in a triangular arrangement. The sensor apparatus consists of three orthogonal 24 inch linear electret microphones. The microphone array is positioned over the scanning area, that is, above the patient, in such a way that the volume it defines encompasses all movements of the transmitter apparatus. The spark gaps, when fired electrically, produce a hypersonic wave front which travels outward through the air in all directions at a known velocity. When the wave front arrives at each microphone the transit time to each is measured and, using the known velocity, the distances from the spark gap to each microphone are calculated. Subsequently, the X,Y and Z coordinates of each point are calculated, digitized and transmitted to the computer. The accuracy of localization is to the nearest 0.1 millimeter. Because three spark gaps are utilized a plane is defined and therefore the position and orientation of the real-time scanner transducer in space can be continuously tracked.

The R-wave of the patients electrocardiogram triggers a 50 millisecond clock in the scheduler/controller that defines a 50 millisecond segment of the cardiac cycle. This segment is divided into thirds. During the first third a frame of echo data is transmitted to computer memory. During the second third the three spark gaps are sequentially fired defining the spatial coordinates of the frame of echo data. The last third of the segment is used for computer processing. The 50 millisecond segments are repeated until the next R-wave. Depending upon the heart rate 10 to 20 segments will be recorded during each R-R interval. Each R-R interval is measured. Provisions are made to interrupt any segment due to the occurrence of an R-wave and begin the cycle over again.

The fundamental assumption of stop-action imaging of the heart (9) is that the mechanical events of systole and diastole occur in a regular, predictable sequence after the R-wave when the patient has normal sinus rhythm and a constant heart rate. Variation in mechanical events are slight with sinus arrhythmia and occur at the end of diastole. Consequently echo data recorded at the same interval after the R-wave of successive heart beats from different portions of the heart may be integrated into an image that will depict the same mechanical events of the cardiac cycle.

During an examination the transducer is held over the

heart and the sound beam directed into it. The position is
adjusted for optimal echo collection using the real-time
display. Slowly, as the examination progresses, the position
of the transducer is moved slightly so that new data is
recorded with each heart beat. Data collection in this
manner may be carried out for five or ten minutes, or a
total of 400 to 500 heart cycles, until the entire heart
has been scanned. Using the R-wave as a timing signal echo
data recorded during sequential but corresponding segments
of the heart cycle is then integrated into single, static
three-dimensional images. That is, all echo data recorded
from the first segment immediately after the R-wave is
integrated to produce a three-dimensional image of the heart
at end-diastole. Similarly a 3-D image may be constructed
for the end-systole segment as well as for all other segments.
Currently the images are not corrected for the blurring effects
of respiratory motion. Previous experience has indicated that
in most patients this is not a serious problem. Additional
gating of the data for respiratory motion may be added at
a later date.

Data processing is done by computer programs. The computer software is divided into five logical parts:

1. data collection and storage,
2. data display,
3. data transformation to a body image matrix,
4. body image matrix display,
5. interactive calculation of physiologic parameters.

The data collected is stored in data blocks which include
a sequence number, the R-R interval, a frame of echo data and
the spatial coordinates of the three spark gaps corresponding
to that frame. The unprocessed data may be displayed for
verification and then transformed into the body image matrix
coordinate system, a digital image in which each memory location corresponds directly to a cubic millimeter tissue volume
within the patient. Display of the body image matrix is
carried out using advanced three-dimensional computer graphic
techniques. Initially the data, that is, any of the three-
dimensional images of the heart, may be leafed through from
front to back. During this process the end points of the
long axis of the left ventricle are identified. The data may
then be leafed through in the direction of the long axis
sequentially viewing the short axis cross-sections of the left
ventricle. The ventricle may be bisected and the medial and
lateral walls viewed en face. At any given view or cross-
section the image may be animated by displaying in rapid

sequence all corresponding views or cross-sections from subsequent 50 millisecond segments. By using these images and by interactively defining the borders of the chambers the ventricular volume may be directly determined. Similarly, using interactive techniques and animation of the wall images throughout the cardiac cycle areas of abnormally contracting segments may be measured along with their amplitude and velocity of motion.

Three-dimensional random scanning and three-dimensional image integration and display of the heart promise to overcome many limitations of current one and two-dimensional ultrasonic techniques. The three-dimensional approach will increase the quantity of echo data incorporated into an ultrasonic image by several orders of magnitude. The quality of the data will also be markedly improved by the addition of a third dimension, by random scanning for specular echo collection and by three-dimensional integration of echo data. The new system allows dissociation of image integration and image display functions and therefore permits incorporation into a image display echo data recorded outside of the corresponding tissue plane, that is, out-of-plane echo collection. These improvements make possible a global approach to cardiac imaging and to image analysis. It is believed that such an approach will revolutionize left ventricular function evaluation and will produce data far superior to that now available with invasive radiological techniques. The volume of the ventricle will be measured directly and repetitively without use of mathematical assumptions every 50 milliseconds. These measurements will allow calculation of peak velocity and acceleration of left ventricular ejection and relaxation. Similarly, having defined the ventricular walls throughout the heart cycle visual display of their movement will permit evaluation for abnormally contracting segments and interactive definition and quantification of their size and movement. Lastly, because the technique is non-invasive and carries no greater potential risk than echocardiography it may be repeated for serial evaluation of patients in a manner impractical with angiocardiography. It will be possible to study the evolution of cardiac disease and its response to therapy as well as the effects of various types of diagnostic interventions.

REFERENCES

1. Feigenbaum H, Zaky A, Nasser WK: Use of Ultrasound to Measure Left Ventricular Stroke Volume. Circulation 35: 1092, 1967.

2. Pombo JF, Troy BL, Russell RO: Left Ventricular Volumes and Ejection Fraction by Echocardiography. Circulation 43: 480,1971.

3. Fortuin NF, Hood WP, Sherman ME: Determination of Left Ventricular Volume by Ultrasound. Circulation 44:575,1971

4. Belenkie I, Nutter DO, Clark DW: Assessment of Left Ventricular Dimension and Function by Echocardiography. Am J Cardiol 31:755, 1973.

5. Cooper RH, O'Rourke RA, Karliner JS et al: Comparison of Ultrasound and Cineangiographic Measurements of the Mean Rate of Circumferential Fiber Shortening in Man. Circulation 46:914, 1972.

6. Linhart JW, Mintz GS, Segal BL et al: Left Ventricular Volume Measurement by Echocardiography: fact or fiction? Am J Cardiol 36:114, 1975.

7. King DL: Stop-action Imaging. In: Cardiac Ultrasound. Ed: Gramiak R, Waag R. C. V. Mosby Co., St.Louis, 1975.

8. Kikuchi Y, Tanaka M; Some Improvements in Ultrasonotomograph for the Heart and Great Vessels. Part II Tomography synchronized with any Cardiac Phase. IEEE Symposium on Ultrasonics, J-3, Cleveland, Ohio. Oct,1966.

9. King DL: Cardiac Ultrasonography. A Stop-action Technique for Imaging Intra-cardiac Anatomy. Radiology 103:387-392, 1972.

10. Bom N, Lancee LT, van Zwieten G et al: Multiscan Echocardiography. I. Technical Description. Circulation 48:1066, 1973

11. Griffith JM, Henry WL: A Sector Scanner for Real-time Two-dimensional Echocardiography. Circulation 49:1147, 1974.

12. Thurstone FL, von Ramm OT: A New Ultrasound Imaging Technique Employing Two-dimensional Electronic Beam Steering. In: Acoustical Holography, Volume 5. Ed: Green PS. Plenum Press. New York, 1974. pp. 249-259

13. Fry WJ, Leichner GH, Okuyama D et al: Ultrasonic Visualization System Employing New Scanning and Presentation Methods. J. Acous Soc Amer 44:1324, 1968.

14. Brown TG: Visualization of Soft Tissues in Two and Three Dimensions - Limitation and Development. Ultrasonics 5:118, 1967.

15. Dekker DL et al: A System for Ultrasonically Imaging the Human Heart in Three Dimensions. Computers and Biomedical Research 7:544-553, 1974.

REAL TIME B-MODE ECHO-ENCEPHALOGRAPHY

S.W. Smith[1]; D.J. Phillips[2]; O.T. von Ramm[3];
F.L. Thurstone[3]
1. Food and Drug Administration, Rockville, Maryland 20852
2. Center for Biomedical Engineering University of Washington, Seattle, Washington
3. Department of Biomedical Engineering Duke University, Durham, N.C. 27706

Since the initial development of B-mode ultrasonography, there have been many attempts (Fry et al, 1974; Brinker & Taveras, 1966) to produce high quality cross-sectional images of the brain through the intact adult skull. Real time B-mode echo-encephalography was initially demonstrated by Somer in 1968 using phased array techniques. Despite these efforts, however, B-mode echo-encephalography is not used clinically in the United States because of the poor quality of the images obtained with current techniques. The intervening presence of the skull results in poor signal to noise ratio, large reverberation artifacts, limited dynamic range and reduced lateral resolution.

Three characteristics of skull bone are responsible for poor quality brain images. These include: (1) high attenuation of diagnostic ultrasound by the skull bone; (2) rapid variation of that attenuation with the frequency of ultrasound; (3) the variation in thickness of the inner table of the skull. Therefore, in order to optimize B-mode ultrasound images of the brain, the imaging system must be desensitized to these effects of the skull bone. By a proper choice of transducer frequency, aperture size, and image format, significant improvement can be made in ultrasound tomograms of the brain.

A propagating ultrasonic pulse is severely attenuated after two passages through the skull by such phenomena as diffractive

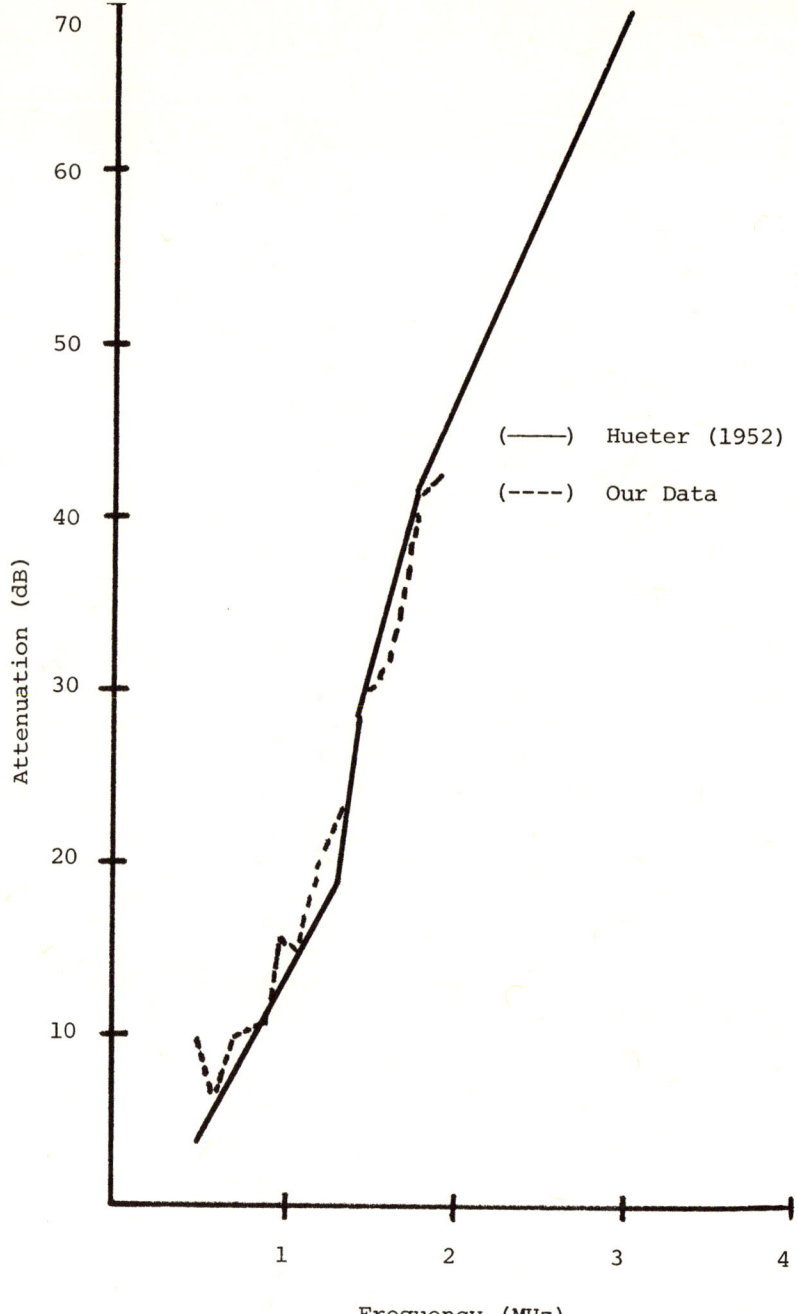

Figure 1. Variation of Attenuation Versus Frequency for a 1 cm Section of skull bone.

scattering, mode conversion, absorption and the impedance mismatch at the skull-brain interface (White, 1970).

In Figure 1 the solid curve shows skull attenuation data from Hueter (1952) normalized to a 1 cm thickness. The dashed line shows similar data which we obtained from a preserved segment of an adult skull. The data indicate that a 2 MHz signal is attenuated approximately 50 db per cm of travel through skull bone. The attenuation at 1 MHz is approximately 12 db per cm. Much of the energy lost from the interrogating pulse returns to the imaging system as unwanted acoustic noise. Such a high background reduces the signal to noise ratio obscuring low level echo information and restricting the useful dynamic range of the imaging system. The result is usually a high contrast B-mode image of the brain in which only the strong specular echoes are displayed. From the figure it can be seen that using a 1 MHz transducer substantially reduces the problem of high attenuation due to the skull.

The rapid variation of attenuation also degrades the lateral resolution of a B-mode imaging system. For a typical broadband diagnostic transducer, the ultrasonic pulse contains significant amounts of energy at higher and lower frequencies. After two passes through an adult skull the high frequency content of the pulse has been significantly reduced relative to the low frequency components. The center frequency of the ultrasound is effectively shifted to a lower frequency. For a fixed transducer aperture, such a frequency shift will result in degraded lateral resolution. Our own experience with linear array transducers and broadband piston transducers has indicated that an interrogating 2 MHz pulse will show a center frequency of approximately .8 MHz after two passes through the temporal region of an adult skull. This results in more than a twofold loss in lateral resolution capability. A 1 MHz ultrasonic pulse is also shifted to approximately .8 MHz but the resultant loss of resolution is not as significant since the original transducer aperture will normally be larger at 1 MHz. One can conclude, then, that the high attenuation of the skull at ultrasound frequencies above 1 MHz is an important factor to consider when choosing an optimum transducer size and center frequency.

Of perhaps equal importance is a consideration of the effects of the thickness variation of the skull bone. In the temporal and parietal areas of the skull where most neurological ultrasound examinations are made, the inner table of the skull bone undergoes rapid variations on the order of 1-2 mm. Phase variations are introduced across the transducer aperture when acoustic energy propagates through a section of skull varying in thickness. Figure 2 shows two elements of a transducer array simultaneously transmitting an acoustic pulse through a section of skull. Due to the factor of two difference in velocity between bone and soft tissue,

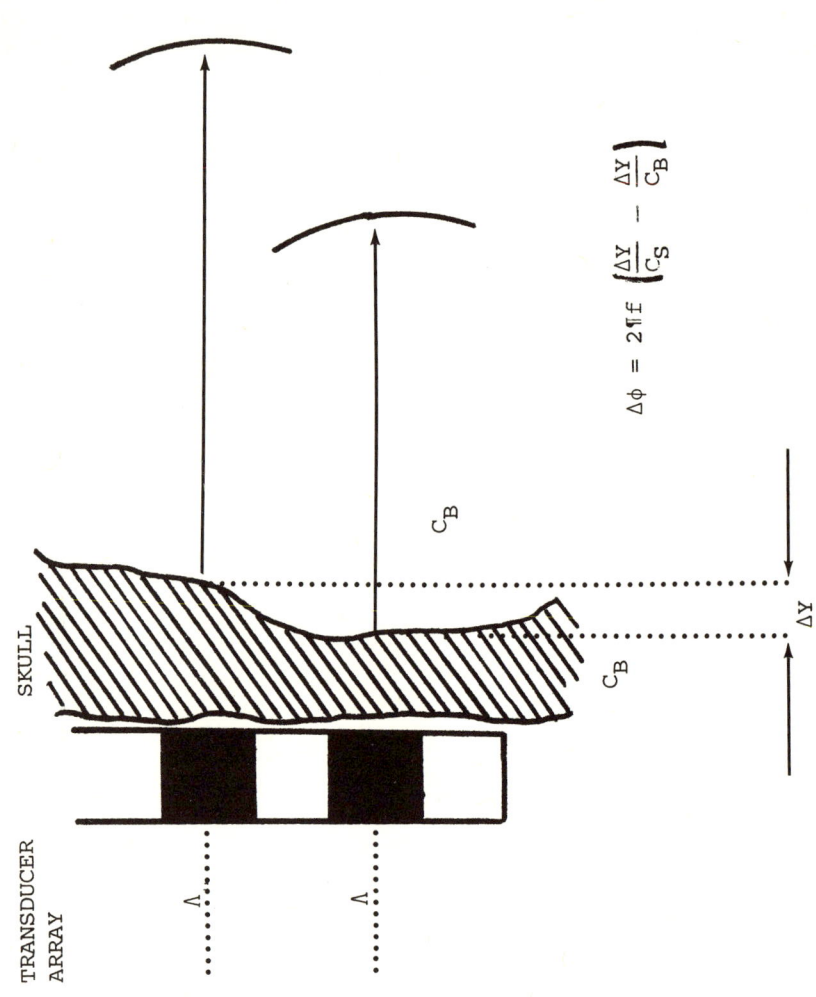

Figure 2. Phase Aberrations Introduced by the Presence of Skull

variations in skull thickness will produce relative changes in the phases of the acoustic wavelets emerging from the inner table of the skull. The phase variation, $\Delta\phi$, is described by

$$\Delta\phi = 2\pi f \left(\frac{\Delta y}{C_S} - \frac{\Delta y}{C_B}\right) \quad (1)$$

where Δy is the thickness variation of the skull bone; C_S is the velocity of sound in skull and C_B is the velocity of sound in brain. Such a phase variation degrades the resolution capability and useful dynamic range of the ultrasonic imaging system. The resolution capability is given by

$$\text{Resolution} = \frac{R\lambda}{D_{eff}} \quad (2)$$

for a one dimensional focussed aperture, where R is the focal distance and D_{eff} is the effective aperture of the transducer. It has been shown for optical imaging (Fried, 1965, 1966) that if a random phase variation is introduced across an aperture, the effective aperture, D_{eff} is reduced. This has been further described by Goodman, 1966 as

$$D_{eff} = \frac{R}{R - \rho} \Delta \quad (3)$$

where Δ is the coherence length, i.e., the linear dimension on the transducer over which the phase variation is less than, say, 1 radian; R is the focal distance and ρ is the distance from the transducer to the skull.

For a contact B-scanner ($\rho \approx 0$), the effective aperture is approximately equal to Δ, the coherence length. Therefore to optimize the resolution capability of a contact B-scanner, steps should be taken to maintain the effective aperture as large as possible. From measurements taken at 160 points on two preserved skull samples, the relation between rms phase variation and transducer aperture has been determined.

In Figure 3 the upper curve shows the relation between the rms phase deviation from the mean phase versus the aperture size in one dimension. On the average, the data predict that for a 1.8 MHz transducer used for contact linear B-scans, the rms phase deviation reaches 1 radian at an aperture size of 6 mm. Thus the maximum effective aperture size at 1.8 MHz is 6 mm for a 1-D aperture; and according to the Rayleigh criterion, the imaging system focussed at 7 cm would be able to resolve point targets spread 1 cm apart. A contact electronic sector scanner such as described by Somer (1968) and by Thurstone and von Ramm (1974) is unaffected by linear phase variations. In Figure 3, the lower line shows the relation between the rms deviation from the mean phase slope versus transducer aperture size at 1 MHz. Extrapolating from the data the rms phase deviation appears to reach 1 radian at approximately

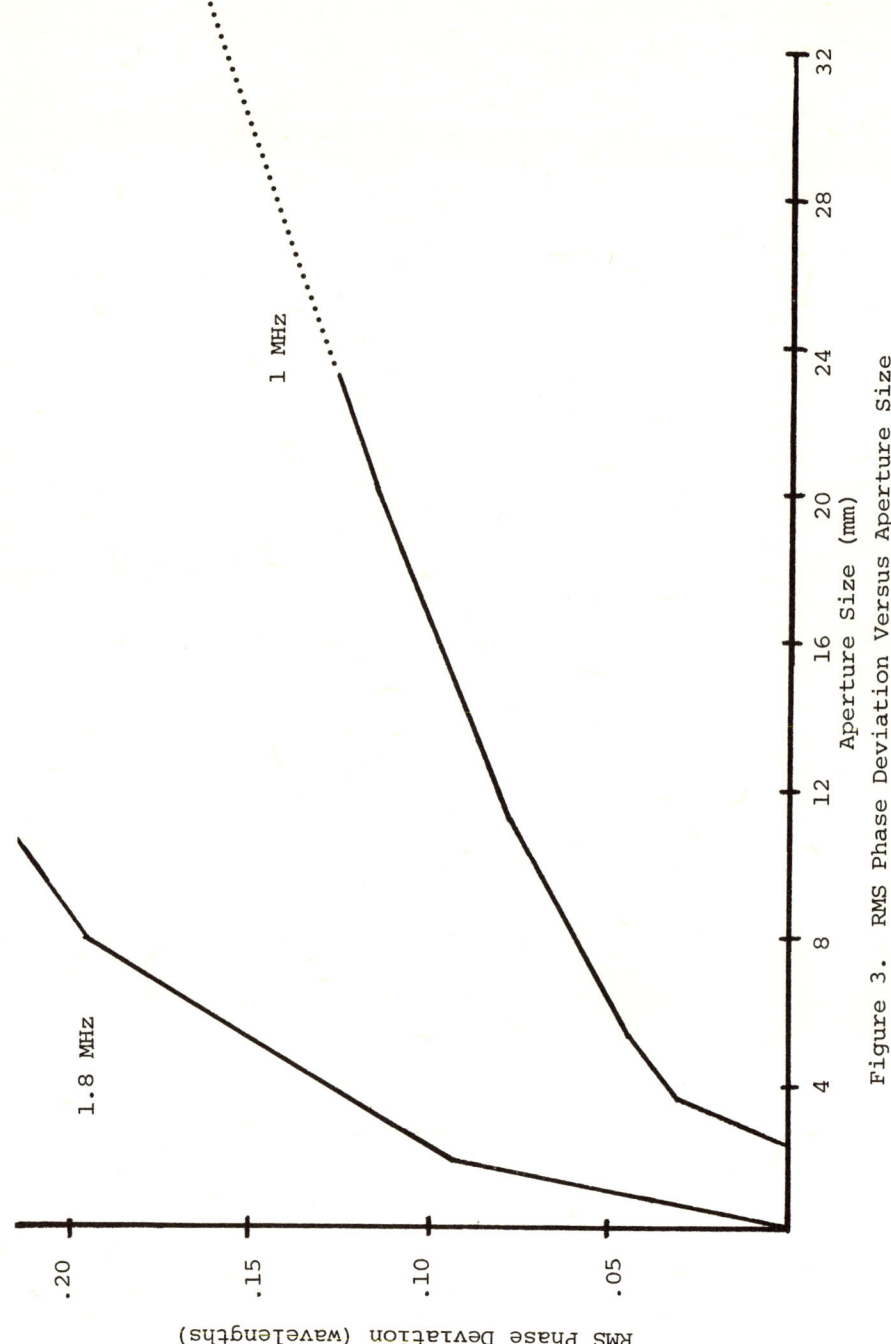

Figure 3. RMS Phase Deviation Versus Aperture Size

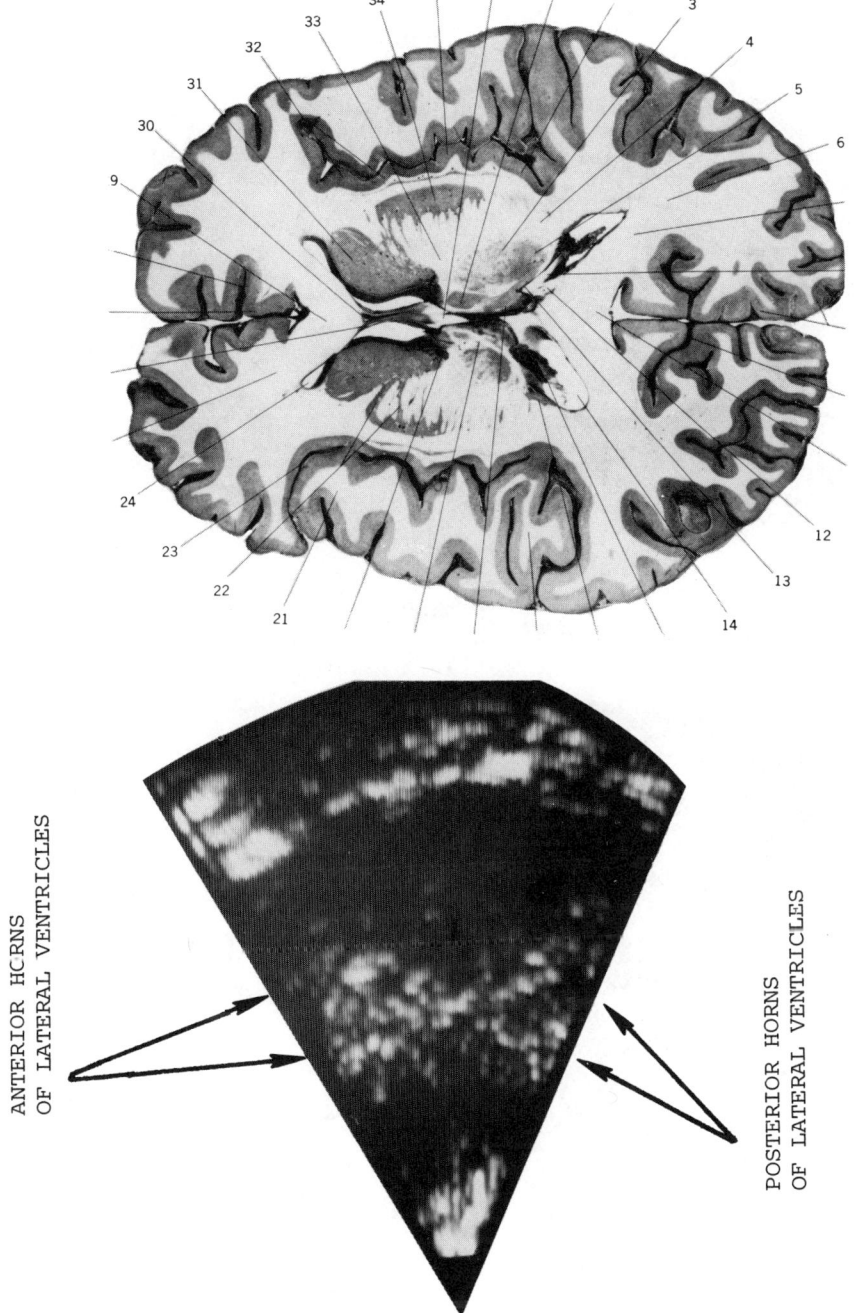

Figure 4 - Comparison of Ultrasound Tomogram with Anatomical Cross Section of Human Brain

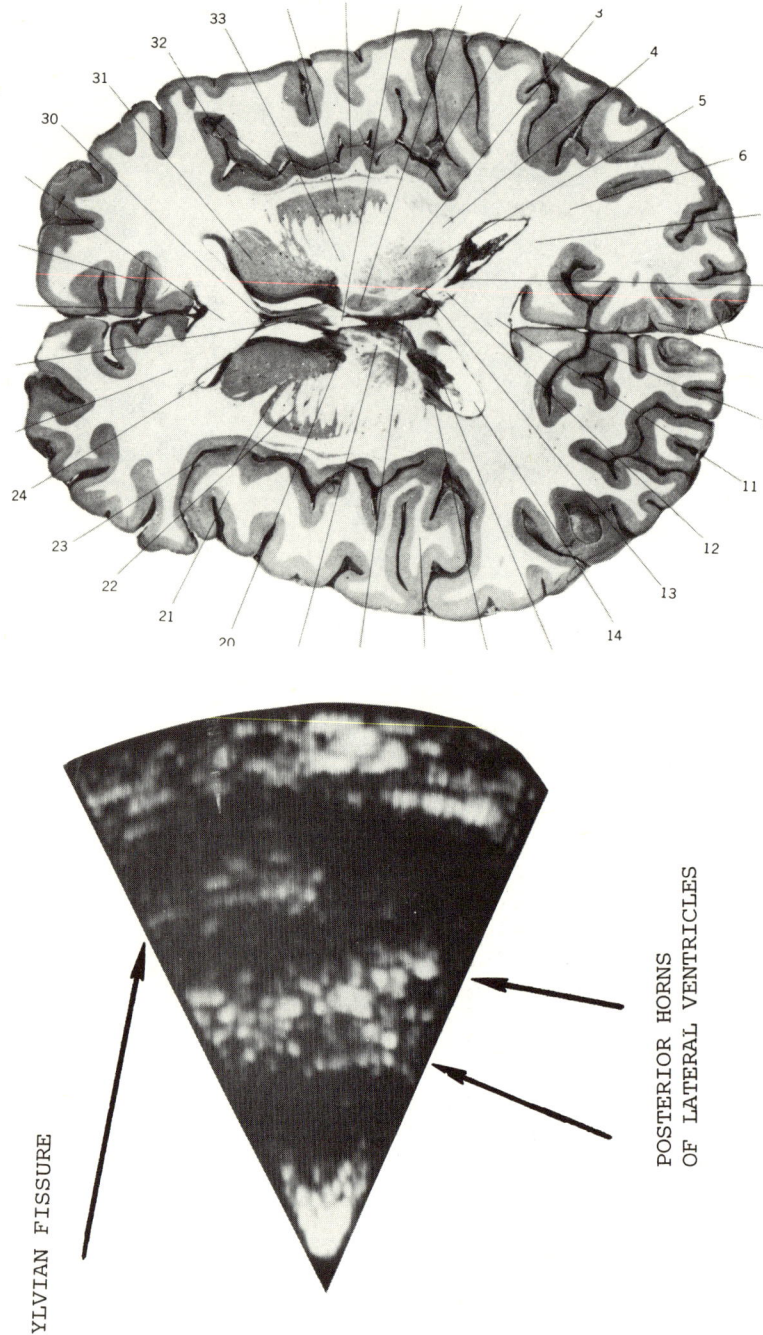

Figure 5 - Comparison of Ultrasound Tomogram with Anatomical Cross Section of Human Brain

36 mm or 1-1/2 inches. Thus the maximum effective aperture at 1 MHz is 36 mm for an electronic sector scanner. Such a scanner focussed at 7 cm would be able to resolve point targets spaced 4 mm apart. That is a 2-1/2 times improvement over a conventional B-scanner at 1.8 MHz.

Based on the limited data which has been presented here, there seems to be some criteria for selecting an optimum transducer and scan configuration for ultrasonic imaging of the brain through the skull. A real time, swept focus, electronic sector scanner operating at 1 MHz with a 1-1/2" transducer aperture would seem to offer distinct advantages over conventional B-scanners operating at 2 MHz.

Representative images using the Thaumascan system under evaluation at Duke University are shown in the next two figures. Using a 1-1/2 inch 1 MHz linear array transducer, horizontal scans were made at the level just above the ear.

Figure 4 compares a horizontal ultrasound scan in a 21 year old female with an anatomical cross section of the brain (Roberts and Hanaway, 1970). The echoes at the point of the sector and on the far right of the image originate from the skull bone. The echoes in the center of the scan compare favorably with the anterior and posterior horns of the lateral ventricles in the anatomical cross-section. One can note the several shades of gray in the image indicating a reasonable dynamic range. Figure 5 shows a similar scan for a 32 year old female. In this image one can see portions of the anterior horns, the midline and posterior horns. In addition there are definite indications of echoes from the Sylvian fissure at the far side. Such images in real time show several discrete pulsations both in the area of the lateral ventricles and in the area of the Sylvian fissure.

These images are the results of preliminary work to improve B-mode echo-encephalography by using optimized transducer parameters and scan format. It is our belief that further improvements in the resolution and dynamic range can be made using signal processing techniques previously described (Phillips et al., 1975). The ultimate goal is to resolve the pulsating lumens of major cerebral blood vessels. Hopefully real time B-mode echo-encephalography will then become a useful diagnostic tool in clinical neurology.

REFERENCES

1. Brinker, R.A., and Taveras, J.M., "Ultrasound Cross-Sectional Pictures of the Head." Acta. Radiol. Diag., 5:745-753, 1966.

2. Fried, D.L., "Statistics of a Geometric Representation of a Wavefront Distortion." Journal of the Optical Society of America, 55:1427-1435, 1965.

3. Fried, D.L., "Optical Resolution Through a Randomly Inhomogeneous Medium for Very Long and Very Short Exposures." Journal of the Optical Society of America, 56:1372-1379, 1966.

4. Fry, F.J., Eggleton, R.C., and Heimburger, R.F., "Transkull Visualization of Brain Using Ultrasound: An Experimental Study." Ultrasonics in Medicine. M. de Vlieger, D.N. White, and V.R. McCready, Editors. American Elsevier Publishing Company, Inc., New York, pp. 97-103, 1974.

5. Goodman, J.W., Huntley, W.H. Jr., Jackson, D.W., Lehman, M., "Wavefront-Reconstruction Imaging Through Random Media." Applied Physics Lett., 8:311, 1966.

6. Hueter, T.F., "Messung der ultraschallabsorption im menschlichen schädelknochen und ihre abhängigkeit von der frequenz." Naturwissenshaften, 39:21-22, 1952.

7. Phillips, D.J., Smith, S.W., von Ramm, O.T., and Thurstone, F.L., "Sampled Aperture Techniques Applied to B-Mode Echoencephalography." Sixth International Symposium on Acoustical Holography and Imaging, February 4-7, 1975.

8. Roberts, M., and Hanaway, J., Atlas of the Human Brain in Section. Lea and Feiberger, Philadelphia, 1970.

9. Somer, J.C., "Electronic Sector Scanning for Ultrasonic Diagnosis." Ultrasonics, 6:153-159, 1968.

10. Thurstone, F.L., von Ramm, O.T., "A New Ultrasound Imaging Technique Employing Two-Dimensional Electronic Beam Steering." Acoustical Holography, 5. P.S. Green, Editor, Plenum Press, New York, pp. 249-259, 1974.

11. White, D.N. Ultrasonic Echo-encephalography. Medical Ultrasonic Laboratory, Kingston, Ontario, Queen's University, 1970.

Acknowledgements

This work was supported by USPHS grants HL 12715, HL 14228, HS 01613, and by the Food and Drug Administration, Bureau of Radiological Health.

VERSATILE ECHOSCANNER

James B. Williams; Thomas B. Smith

Diagnostic Electronics Corporation
Box 580, Lexington, Massachusetts 02173

Real-time imaging of soft-tissue structures in any part of the body can be achieved for the first time by a new, completely electronic ultrasound system. High scanning speed, small detector size and wide-angle sector allow live visualization of cardiovascular structures such as valves and intracranial arteries.

At great cost, nuclear and x-ray instruments have recently been computerized for soft-tissue analysis. However, the low sensitivity of their high energy interactions limits them to the delayed reconstruction of images of non-moving organs.

By contrast, ultrasound, although relatively unexploited to date, exhibits wave properties which can provide soft-tissue image information beyond that of any other energy form. The following list summarizes some primary characteristics of ultrasound interactions and their consequences:

1. _Reflectivity_ at interfaces and density changes gives _depth/time_ information.

2. _Amplitude_ of signal indicates _size/orientation_ of echo source.

3. _Phase_ of echoes characterizes the _nature_ of tissue.

4. _Speed_ of response permits _real-time imaging_.

5. _High frequency_ allows _resolution_ of the order of 1mm.

6. _Interference_ properties permit directional steering and dynamic _focussing_ of the beam on both _transmission and reception_.

7. <u>Single plane</u> motion of the beam produces true <u>laminographs.</u>

8. <u>Low-energy</u> tissue interactions are <u>non-ionizing.</u>

Although no static-imaging instrument can be optimized for multiple applications, a versatile real-time echoscanner can be designed to balance the above features.

For example, in cardiovascular studies a live moving picture introduces a new dimension. The emphasis is on structure identification and speed of response. However, in organ imaging and obstetrics, picture detail is most important. To image the soft tissues of the brain through the intact skull a relatively low frequency of the order of 1-2 MHz must be used. Because of the consequently longer wave length the resolution is limited to approximately 1mm. Therefore, a balance must be realized between penetration and resolution.

One of the most important features of a live imaging system is that visual surveys of large regions can be made very rapidly. Detailed examinations can then be directed to selected areas. The resulting increase in operational efficiency with which routine procedures can be performed is an important step toward achieving widespread clinical use of ultrasound.

In addition to the many practical features inherent in a good clinical instrument, the following list describes the general specifications of a versatile echoscanner:

1. <u>Real-time imaging</u> with response fast enough to follow the motion of any structure in the body. This should include the capability of stop-action image storage as well as provision for dynamic recording.

2. <u>Hand-held contact probe</u> with a very small transmit/receive aperture for application to any point of the body at any angle.

3. <u>Wide-angle field</u> of view with provisions for magnification and minification in a large screen format.

4. <u>Image quality</u> properties such as resolution and gray scale should permit general clinical use including intracranial procedures.

Such a system has general applicability in the fields of cardiology, neurology and obstetrics, as well as in general organ imaging. The practical embodiment of these features has been achieved.* It is a wide-angle electronic sector scanner based on the original work of

---

* The ECHOSTAT^{Tm}, Diagnostic Electronics Corp., Lexington, Mass.

Somer[1,2] beginning in 1967 and resulting in the clinical neurological use of prototypes in Holland and Germany. The incorporation of state-of-the-art electronic techniques permitted significant improvements over the original design and the later one by von Ramm[3].

The principle of operation is the electronic phasing of a small (½" x ½") array of crystals (Fig. 1). Because the radiating/receiving surface consists of many small elements, it can be electronically controlled not only to generate and steer a beam of ultrasound, but also to focus it. In essence, it can simulate a single large curved crystal with an electronically-variable focal point (Fig. 2).

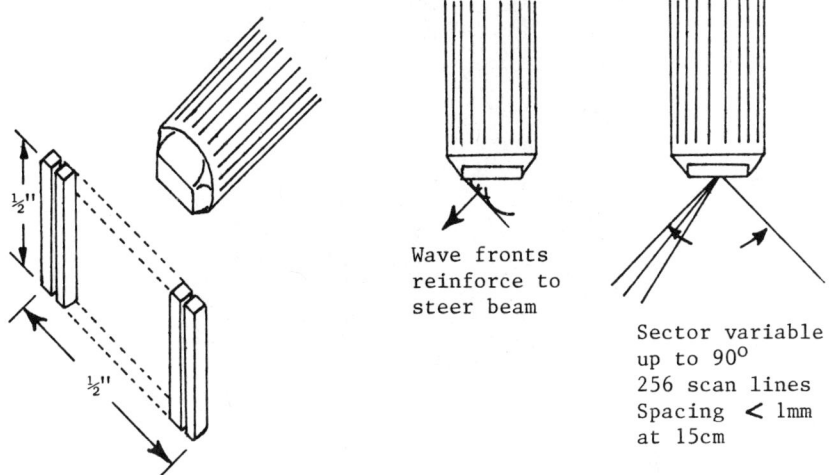

Wave fronts reinforce to steer beam

Sector variable up to 90°
256 scan lines
Spacing < 1mm at 15cm

Figure 1. Principle of Electronic Sector Scanning

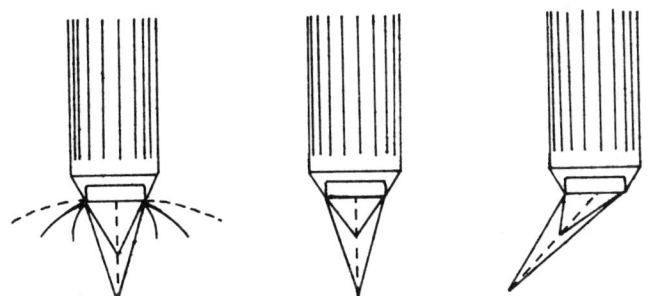

Transmission: Focus on a designated area
Reception: Array continuously focussed on the receding echo point

Figure 2. Dynamic Electronic Focussing of Phased Array

The complete system (Fig. 3) has mobility, a built-in scan converter for image storage, a 19-inch high-performance CRT display, hand-held phased-array probe, and an integrated control panel (Fig. 4).

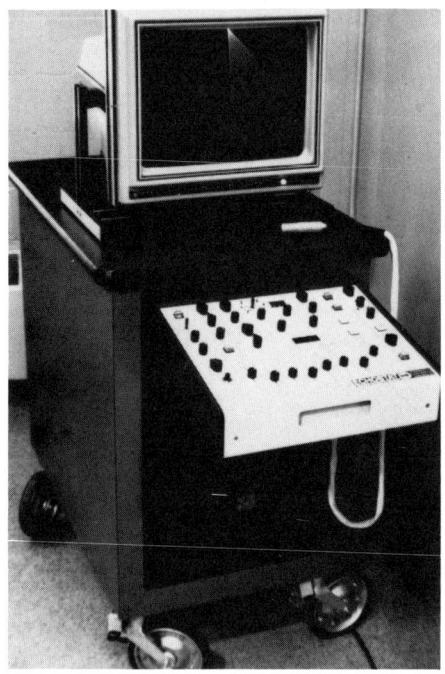

Fig. 3   The ECHOSTAT^{Tm}

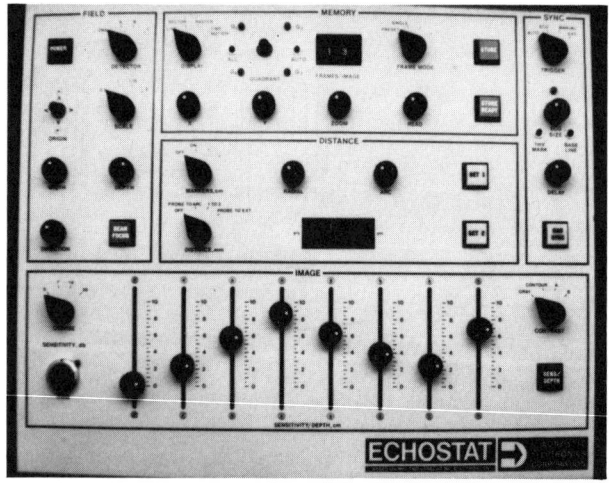

Fig. 4   The ECHOSTAT^{Tm} Control Panel

VERSATILE ECHOSCANNER

The <u>field</u> of examination can be electronically varied in depth, width and direction (Fig. 5). The origin of the display sweep can be oriented to agree with the position of the probe on the patient for a particular clinical measurement. The scale of the display can be 0.5, 1.0, 1.15 or 2.0. The 1.15 scale approximates standard x-ray magnification. The width of the field can be varied from a sector of 0° to 90°; the depth from 3 to 30cm; the direction of the sector to any part of the full 90°.

The <u>image</u> quality (Fig. 6) can be optimized independently by controlling the signal sensitivity for tissues at different depths in the body. Several signal processing modes may be chosen, including gray scale and edge detection. Dynamic focussing may be used during transmission and reception.

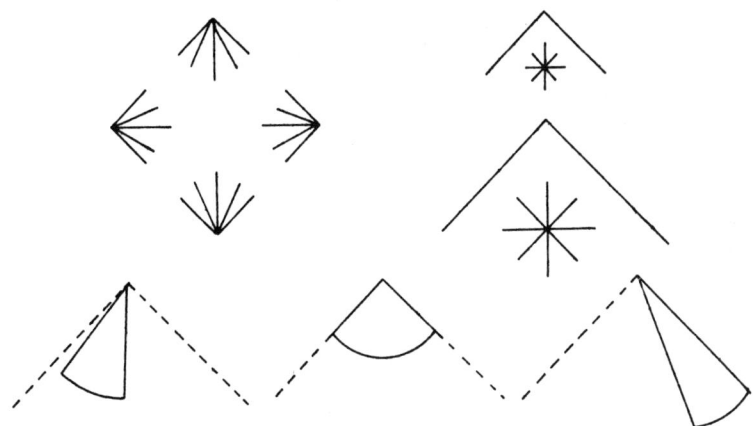

Figure 5.   Orientation, Scale and Field Size

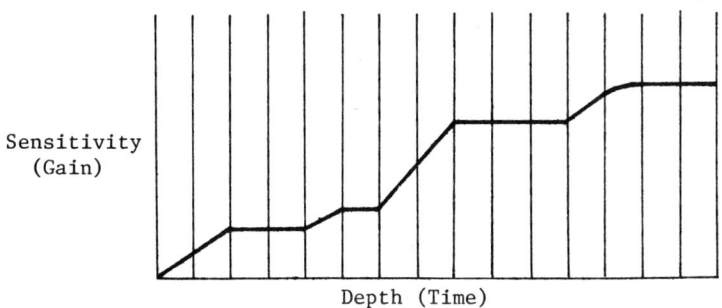

Figure 6.   Image Sensitivity

Interstructure distances (Fig. 7) in mm. can be indicated automatically on the digital panel display by manually setting arc and radial cursors at any points in the field. Centimeter depth markers can be displayed and any one of 256 radial scan lines can be selected for external A-mode display. This radial may be used to produce a simultaneous time/motion recording of moving structures such as valves and arteries.

Cardiac synchronization is provided by a built-in diagnostic grade ECG channel (Fig. 8) to permit triggering single frames from the R-wave or later in the cardiac cycle. Single or multiple frame scans may also be triggered manually or from an external source.

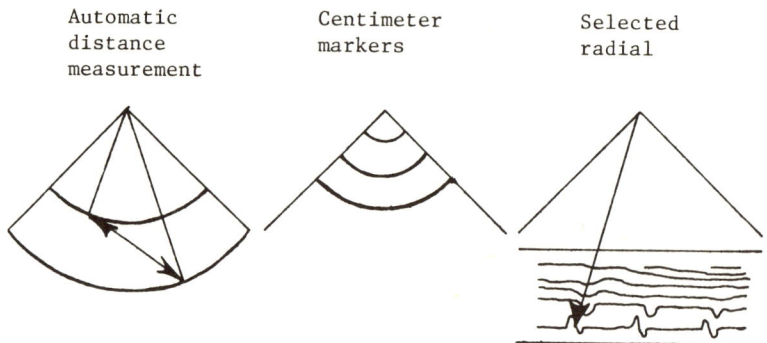

Figure 7.   Electronic Distance Measurements

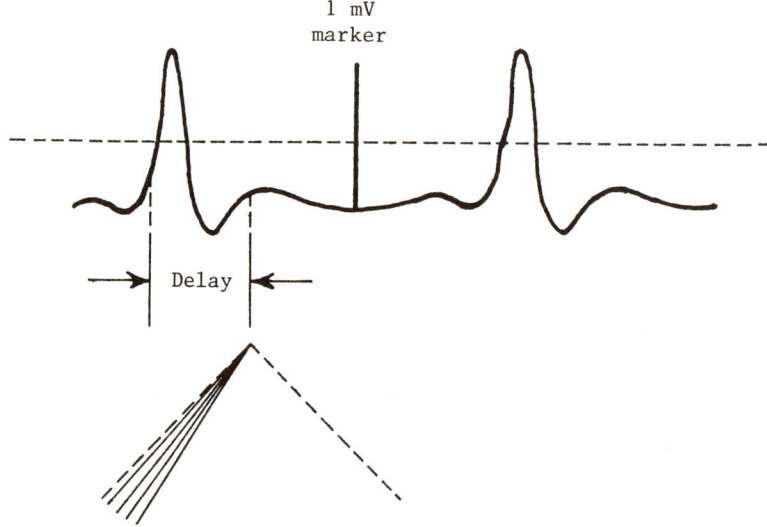

Figure 8.   Synchronization of Image Frames

Finally, any live image can be frozen by storing it in the built-in scan-converter. It can be displayed in either the sector format in which it was recorded or in a TV raster scan mode compatible with monitors and video tape recorders. The unique properties of the scan-converter include storage in quadrants and zoom capabilities.

References

1. Somer, J.C., Instantaneous and continuous pictures obtained by a new two-dimensional scan technique with a stationary transducer. Proceedings in Echo-Encephalography. Edited by Kazner, E., Schiefer, W. and Zulch, K.J. Springer-Verlag, New York pp. 234-238 1968.

2. Freund, H.J., Somer, J.C., Kendel, K.H. and Voigt, K. (1973) Electronic sector scanning in the diagnosis of cerebrovascular disease and space-occupying processes. Neurology 23:1147-1159

3. von Ramm, O.T. and Thurstone, F.L. THAUMASCAN: Improved image quality and clinical usefulness. Ultrasound in Medicine II. Edited by White, D.N. and Barnes, R.W. Plenum Press pp. 463-464 1976.

ULTRASOUND TRANSAXIAL TOMOGRAPHY BY RECONSTRUCTION*

P. L. Carson; T. V. Oughton; W. R. Hendee

Department of Radiology
University of Colorado Medical Center, Denver, CO 80220

ABSTRACT

The diagnostic potential of transmission imaging with ultrasound has stimulated many attempts to utilize the large differences in ultrasound attenuation between various soft tissues. Most such attempts have met with very limited success due to practical difficulties including scattering and phase distortion by bones, air spaces, and fat. Imaging a transverse plane in the body by transmission scanning of that plane from a large number of angles, and subsequent reconstruction of the transmission image by computer may provide the long desired diagnostic information in many areas of the body. Just as with computerized axial tomography now used successfully for enhanced x-ray imaging, ultrasound transaxial tomography by reconstruction (UTTR) displays those objects causing distortions of the ultrasound and allows, in effect, averaging of data from scans at many angles. Others have investigated UTTR for soft tissue imaging. The present results simulate with phantom measurements the image of soft tissues adjacent to bone-equivalent objects.

INTRODUCTION

Previous studies (1,2) of ultrasound transaxial tomography have included imaging of soft tissue samples and resolution test objects

---
*This project was supported in part by General Research Support Grant 5 S01 RR 05357 from the U.S. Public Health Service and Grants 5D12 AH 00346 and 5D12 AH 00041 from the U.S. Department of Health, Education and Welfare.

which did not obstruct transmission of the ultrasound beam as do bones in the body. In the present investigation of Ultrasound Transaxial Tomography by Reconstruction (UTTR) a phantom was employed to simulate imaging of soft tissue in planes containing bones. The phantom consisted of an aluminum rod to simulate bone, and balloons filled with castor oil and silicone fluid, to simulate soft tissue organs. Emphasis was placed on Ultrasound Transaxial Tomography of Attenuation by Reconstruction (UTTAR) although Ultrasound Transaxial Tomography of Velocity by Reconstruction (UTTVR) also was considered.

The convolution method (3-7) of reconstruction was employed primarily in this study, although a comparison also was made with a more rigorous reconstruction method described by Perry, Altschuler and Altschuler (8). Descriptions of the principles of reconstruction of UTTAR and UTTVR images is given in References 1, 2 and 9. In essence, UTTAR image reconstructions are almost identical to reconstruction of x-ray computerized axial tomography images. The transmitted ultrasound pressure wave amplitude is measured with a receiving transducer, and exponential attenuation of a pencil-shaped beam is assumed for homogeneous materials. For UTTVR imaging, relative ultrasound transit time is measured to give a reconstructed velocity image.

In the present tests, pulsed ultrasound was employed for maximum sensitivity with minimum average acoustic intensity and for compatibility with future instruments combining pulse-echo and UTTR imaging. A diagram of the scanning motion and pulse transmission is shown in Figure 1. However, acoustic waveforms other than short pulses may serve just as well if some form of coding is employed to allow rejection of multiple scattered ultrasound.

UTTAR RECONSTRUCTION OF HYPOTHETICAL DATA

To test the feasibility of using available reconstruction algorithms for UTTAR imaging in planes containing bones, transmission functions were calculated for two concentric cylinders viewed in a plane normal to their axis of rotation and positioned in a nonattenuating medium. The inner 5 cm diameter cylinder was assigned an attenuation of 100 dB/cm and the outer 20 cm diameter cylinder was assigned 2 dB/cm attenuation.

An image of the cross-section reconstructed with the convolution method is shown in Figure 2. The image indicates that large oscillations in the reconstructed attenuation coefficients are restricted to a narrow region at the discontinuities in attenuation coefficients. A slight nonuniformity is caused by the graticules on the display oscilloscope.

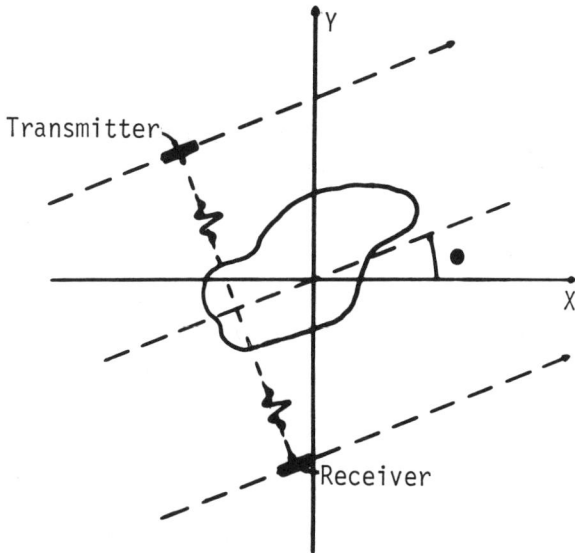

Figure 1. Diagram of transducer motion and pulse transmission through the body to obtain UTTR images.

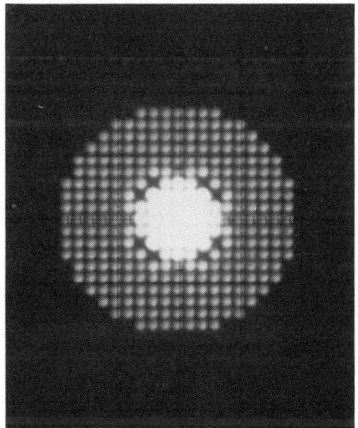

Figure 2. Reconstructed image of hypothetical 20 cm diameter and 5 cm diameter cylinders with 2 dB/cm and 100 dB/cm attenuation coefficients, respectively.

Plotted in Figure 3 are initial and reconstructed attenuation coefficients along one radius of the image. Throughout the soft tissue equivalent outer cylinder, in the region from 4 to 9 cm from the center of the cylinders, a digital printout shows that the standard deviation of the reconstructed attenuation coefficient for the 2 dB/cm tissue is less than 0.1 dB. This corresponds to less than 1.2% and 2.3% imprecision, respectively, in the transmitted amplitude and power per cm. By comparison, the attenuation coefficients for various tissues differ by considerably more than 0.1 dB.

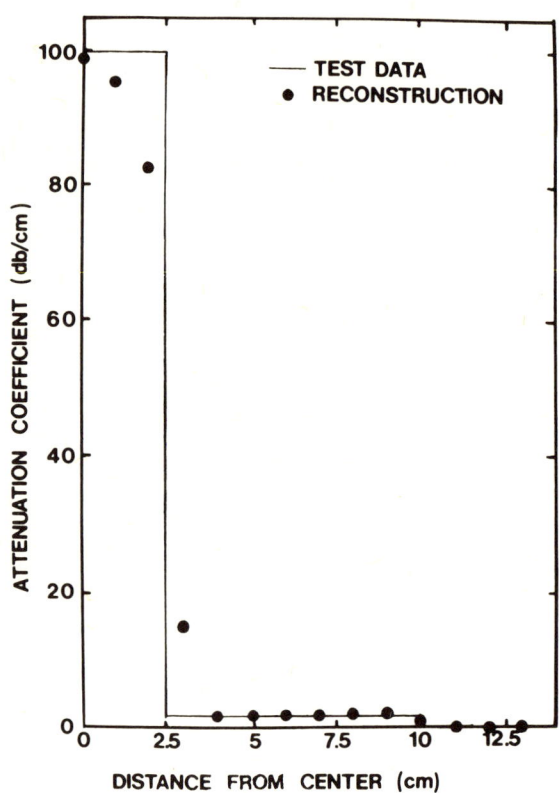

Figure 3. Attenuation coefficients along one radius of the cylinders depicted in Figure 2. Shown are reconstructed attenuation coefficients (dots) and attenuation coefficients on which the calculation was based (solid line).

UTTAR IMAGING OF PHANTOM

Experimental methods employed are described in References 9 and 10. In order to simulate the effects of having a bone in the image plane next to soft tissue, the phantom pictured in Figure 4a was developed for scanning in a water tank. A cross-section of the phantom is shown in Figure 4b. A 2.5 cm diameter aluminum rod was placed next to two balloons filled with approximately tissue equivalent liquids. The velocity of ultrasound in the silicone fluid and castor oil was 1370 and 1500 m/sec, respectively; and the acoustic absorption in both liquids was approximately 2.7 dB/cm. Although the aluminum has a lower absorption coefficient than bone, its much higher acoustic impedance means that the fraction of ultrasound penetrating the aluminum rod will be comparable to the fraction penetrating a bone of similar dimensions. Thus with the higher velocity and impedance of the aluminum, artifacts due to reflection and refraction in the aluminum should be larger than the artifacts encountered in UTTAR imaging of a relatively gas-free upper abdomen, neck, infant head, or limb.

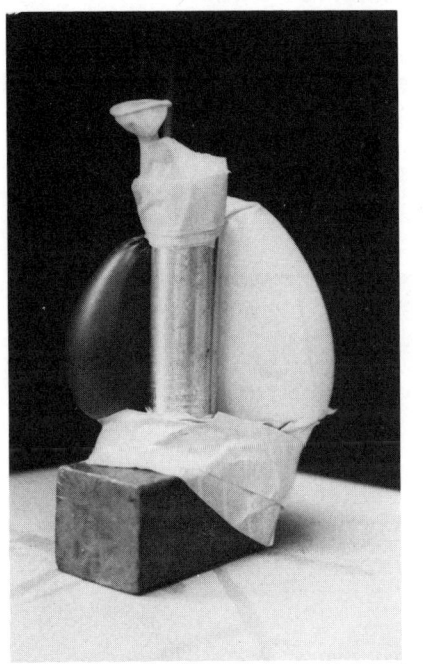
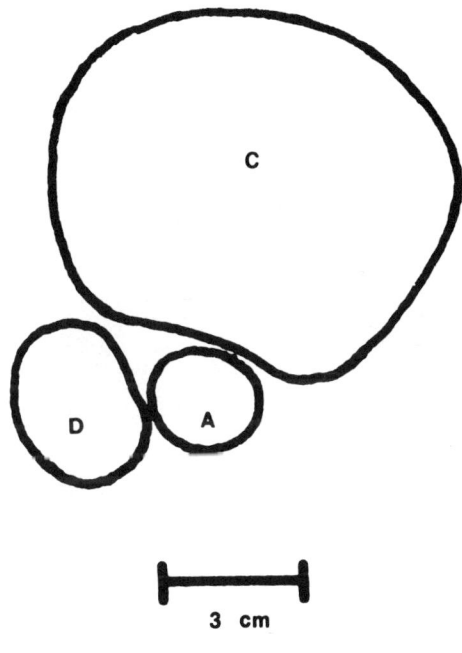

Figure 4. Photograph (a) and cross-sectional sketch (b) of phantom employed in this study. Shown are the aluminum rod A, and balloons filled with castor oil C, and Dow-Corning 710 Silicone fluid D.

Shown in Figure 5a is one of the first reconstructed attenuation (UTTAR) images of the phantom depicted in Figure 4. Figure 5b is a similar reconstruction in which the same transmission data was manipulated to remove both the circular rim around the reconstructed area and the bright straight lines caused by loss of a few transmission data points. The images in Figures 5a and 5b both were reconstructed with the convolution reconstruction method described in Reference 6. The more rigorous, but probably more time consuming, reconstruction method of Reference 8 yielded the image in Figure 5c from the same manipulated data reconstructed in Figure 5b.

All three objects and the water may be recognized in the image in Figure 5, in which higher attenuation is indicated by greater brightness. Of most importance is the fact that the reconstructed attenuation throughout most of the large castor oil-filled balloon appears reasonably uniform, and approximately the same as the reconstructed attenuation in the silicone fluid balloon. Thus, the vertebral body may not prevent diagnosis of lesions in organs such as the liver. Note, also that even the inner portion of the aluminum rod shows up as providing less attenuation than the interfaces at the surface of the aluminum. A characteristic feature of UTTAR images is that the surfaces of the balloons stand out as regions of high attenuation due to reflection and refraction of the sound where the beam is incident at oblique angles. The circular rim in Figure 4a indicates the limits of the reconstruction area. Increasing the length of the linear scan path will remove this rim from the area of interest, and possibly will eliminate other artifacts which, at present, are unexplained.

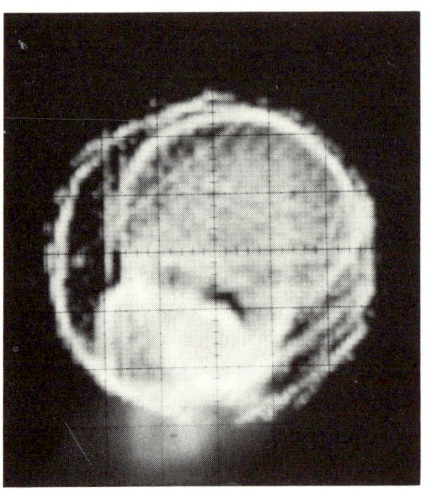

(a)

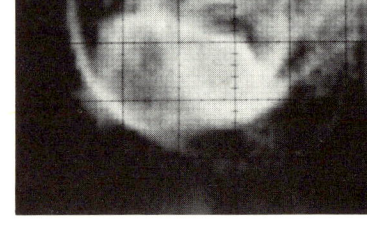

(b)

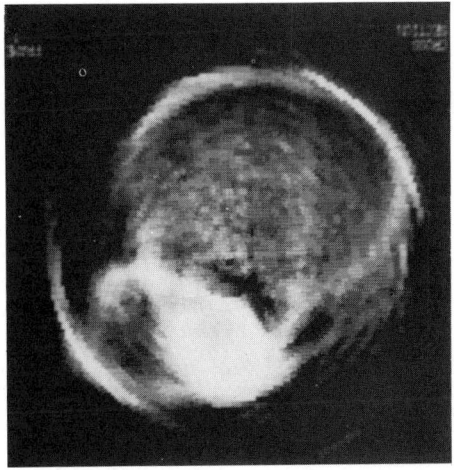

(c)

Figure 5. UTTAR (Ultrasound Transaxial Tomography of Attenuation by Reconstruction) images of the phantom depicted in Figure 4. All three images were reconstructed from the same raw transmission data. The convolution program was utilized for images (a) and (b). Additional "water only" data points and smoothing were introduced prior to reconstructing images (b) and (c). Image (c) was reconstructed by Altschuler and Perry.

UTTVR IMAGING

Initial UTTVR images of the phantom depicted in Figure 3 have not yielded the same geometrical accuracy as did the UTTAR images. In essence, the aluminum rod, with a high velocity of ultrasound, was reconstructed as being larger than its actual size, while the silicone fluid, with a low velocity of ultrasound, was reconstructed as being smaller than its actual size. Two experimental conditions will explain the source of this image distortion:

1. In order to reduce the effects of multiple scattered ultrasound, the received pulses were amplified very strongly so that the very first arrival of the pulse could be detected;

2. The transmitted beam pattern was wider than typical pulse-echo transducer sensitivity patterns.

Therefore, when the central axis of the beam was in a low velocity material, even a weak edge or sidelobe of the transmitted beam could pass through a high velocity material and be refracted toward the receiver. In this case, a short transit time could be recorded as if the whole ultrasound beam had passed through the high velocity material which, in actuality, was located to one side of the ultrasound beam axis.

DISCUSSION

The experiences with UTTVR imaging described above do not mean that meaningful velocity images cannot be obtained in planes containing bones or fat-tissue interfaces. The current experiments indicate only that resolution in UTTVR imaging is limited to the width of relatively low level edges of the transmitted beam. In comparison, amplitude transmission for UTTAR imaging is affected most strongly by the narrow, intense portion of the ultrasound beam. This effect will tend to give attenuation images somewhat higher resolution then velocity images.

As noted in References 1 and 2, refraction and reflection of the ultrasound beam at interfaces may cause most of the transmitted beam to miss the receiving transducer. These effects cause the interface to appear highly attenuating in an UTTAR image. To minimize the resultant overestimation of interface attenuation and thickness, a wide aperture system, such as that diagrammed in Figure 6, should be useful. Sophisticated design will be necessary, however, to assure that a refracted wave front does not interfere with itself at the transducer face, thereby producing an aritificially low signal.

Potential benefits of both UTTAR and UTTVR imaging should not be overlooked. Many important tissues appear to vary more in their attenuation properties than in their reflection properties; and UTTAR imaging should be quite sensitive to variations in attenuation, even though UTTAR images will probably continue to enhance interfaces. UTTVR on the other hand, will be primarily a fat, or fat content, imaging modality. In addition, an UTTVR image should make it possible to correct UTTAR and pulse-echo images for refraction. The potential of UTTVR and UTTAR for imaging accessible soft tissues such as the female breast is quite promising; but UTTR may also provide significant new information in body planes containing some bone.

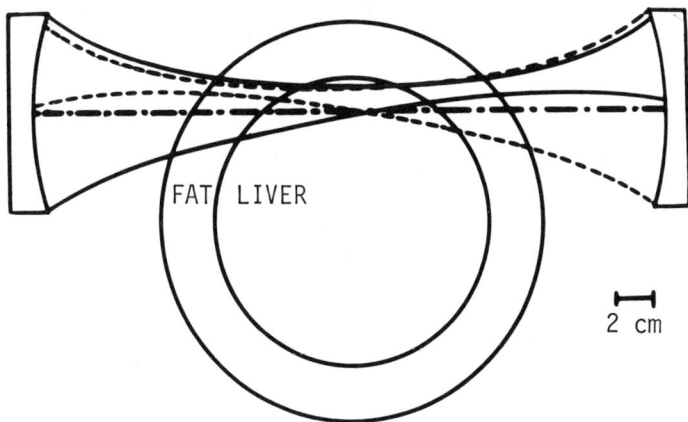

Figure 6. Refraction of transmitter and receiver beam patterns in a realistic situation. Without refraction at the fat-liver interfaces, the beam patterns would be symmetrical about the line shown connecting the centers of the transducers. The transducer diameters and focal zones have been sketched to approximate a geometry providing minimum amplitude loss due to refraction.

The authors are grateful to Thomas Taylor for technical assistance, and to M. D. Altschuler and R. M. Perry for the reconstruction presented in Figure 5c.

REFERENCES

1. Greenleaf, J. F., Johnson, S. A., Lee, S. L., Herman, G. T., Wood, E. H., "Algebraic Reconstruction of Spatial Distributions of Acoustic Absorption within Tissue from their Two-Dimensional Projections," Acoustic Holography 5, Plenum Press, New York, 591-603, 1974.

2. Greenleaf, J. F., Johnson, S. A., Samayoa, W. F., Duck, F. A., and Wood, E. H., "Albegraic Reconstruction of Spatial Distributions of Acoustic Velocities in Tissue from their Time of Flight Profiles," Acoustic Holography 6, Plenum Press, New York, in press.

3. Gordon, R. and Herman, G. T., "Three-Dimensional Reconstruction from Projections: A Review of Algorithms," Internat. Rev. Cytology, 38, 111-151, 1974.

4. Ramachandran, G. N., "Reconstruction of Substance from Shadow: I. Mathematical Theory with Application to Three-dimensional Radiography and Electron Microscopy," Proceedings of the Indian Academy of Sciences, 74, 14-24, 1971.

5. Ramachandran, G. N. and Lakshminarayanan, A. V., "Three-dimensional Reconstruction from Radiographs and Electron Micrographs: Application of Convolutions Instead of Fourier Transform," Proceedings of the National Academy of Science, USA, 68, 2236-2240, 1971.

6. Theime, G. A., Hendee, W. R., Ibbott, G. S., Carson, P. L., and Kirch, D. L., "Cross-Sectional Anatomical Images by X-ray Transmission Scanning," Acta Radiologica, Ther, Phys. Biol., 14, 81-112, February, 1975.

7. Theime, G. A., Ibbott, G. S., and Hendee, W. R., "Cross-Sectional Anatomy Reconstruction and Applications to Radiation Therapy Treatment Planning," Application of Optical Instrumentation in Medicine-III, ed. Carson, P. L., Chaney, E. L., and Hendee, W. R., Soc. Photo-optical Instru. Engrs., Palos Verdes Estates, Calif., 52-59, 1975.

8. Perry, R. M., Altschuler, M. D., and Altschuler, B. R., "Medical Image Reconstruction: Multiangular Sectional Roentgenography by Computer," NCAR TN/STR-108, National Center Atmospheric Research, Boulder, Colorado, 1974.

9. Carson, P. L., Oughton, T. V., Hendee, W. R., Altschuler, M. D. and Perry, R. M., "Phantom Studies of Imaging Soft Tissue Through Bone with Ultrasound Transaxial Tomography," Applications of Optical Instrumentation in Medicine-IV, ed. Hendee, W. R. and Gray, J. E., Soc. Photo-optical Instru. Engrs., Palos Verdes Estates, Calif., in press.

10. Carson, P. L., Leung, S. S., and Hendee, W. R., "Constant Depth Ultrasound Imaging Using Computer Acquisition, Display and Analysis," Ultrasound in Medicine, White, D. N., ed. Plenum Press, New York, 509-517, 1975.

RAYLOGRAPHY, A PULSE ECHO TECHNIQUE WITH FUTURE BIOMEDICAL

APPLICATIONS

I. Beretsky, M.D.; G. Farrell, M.S.B.E.:
B. Lichtenstein, B.E.E.
Technicon Instruments Corporation
Tarrytown, NY 10591

Pulse echo acoustics after many years, has become an accepted clinical modality as a non-invasive medical diagnostic tool. In recent years, the emergence of various display techniques and other electronic improvements have improved the utilization and understanding of the echo patterns. However, the major emphasis in development has been directed towards means which enhance the visual presentation of the processed echo. Traditionally, physicians utilize images to evaluate the presence of "non-normal" tissue. More recently, in the area of echocardiography, investigators utilize acoustically obtained dimensional information referenced to the heart cycle to obtain measures of physiological abnormalities of the heart. Other investigators have recently advocated the use of amplitude color coding as a substitute for gray scale presentation to help interpret "abnormalities" of tissue structure.

We believe a plateau has been reached in biomedical applications using present pulse echo acoustics. While near future applications and instrument modifications may produce additional improvements with contemporary equipment, it is unlikely that a major breakthrough in the technology will occur without fundamental changes in the present technology. The reason for this belief stems from basic fundamentals related to the extraction of the information bearing attributes of echoes.

All contemporary ultrasound systems, used for imaging purposes to produce "B scans", have a common characteristic, in that the acoustic echoes are processed by envelope detection. This processing, falls into the broad category called energy detection. The methods used to produce images from these processed signals

are derived from general principles of light optics. The
processing associated with envelope detection, or energy detection,
while simple to perform, utilizes only a small portion of the
information bearing attributes of the original echo, thereby
limiting the extraction of the potential information of the
acoustic echo. There exist alternatives to this form of signal
processing, which although more tedious and expensive to perform,
will enable a more thorough utilization of the echo information.
This paper is concerned with this problem. The authors will
attempt to define the necessary pathway to gain the additional
information, which, as will be shown in this report, should
result in markedly improved imaging and a means for characterizing
tissue structure.

The common pathway necessary to accomplish this task is to
utilize the raw echo waveforms in a coherent manner and process
the signals to produce an estimate of the impulse response of the
tissue. The definition of impulse response for a linear acoustic
system is the response of the media to an acoustic impulse. The
acoustic echoes produced from the unknown media, are related to
the acoustic interfaces where impedance discontinuities occur. The
various echoes are impulses and contain amplitude information
relating the magnitude of the impedance change and may be either
plus or minus, corresponding to the local gradient of the impedance
discontinuity. Thus the impulse response contains both <u>magnitude</u>
and <u>phase</u> information.

System Concept

The frequency content of a transmitted pulse must be thoroughly
understood and preserved in proper fashion when acoustic focusing
is used. The finite diameter, or aperture, creating the impulse
source can only focus frequencies in a limited band. Frequencies
below a critical frequency determined by optical considerations
related to the transmitter diameter will not focus and, therefore,
distort the acoustic information at the focal point. Similarly,
the spectral characteristics of the transmitted pulse and received
echoes must not be degraded by narrow band receivers and preampli-
fiers.

Application of the Impulse Response

Raylography is the acoustic generation of an axial relative
characteristic impedance profile. Raylography is a term coined by
Technicon and is similar to Impediography as reported by
J. P. Jones[1]. The Raylogram is a form of information extractable
from echo trains which can be calculated after establishing

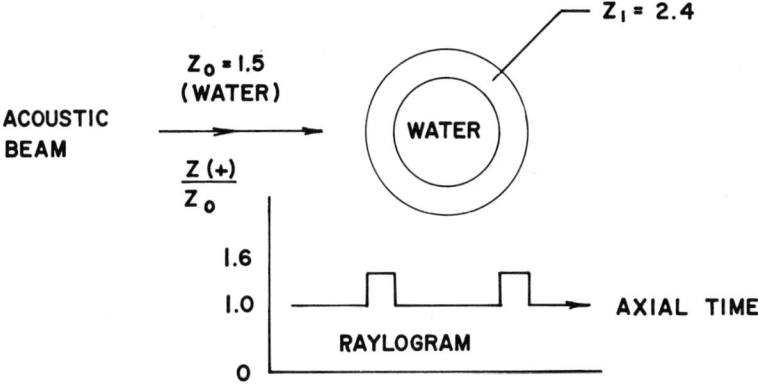

Fig. 1: Theoretical Raylogram of cylinder whose acoustic impedance is greater than that of water.

impulse response. In particular, for certain simplifying assumptions, probably consistent with tissue macrostructure, one can show that the relative acoustic impedance is related to impulse response by

$$\frac{Z(t)}{Z_o} = 2 \int h(t)dt + 1$$

where $h(t)$ = impulse response
        $Z(t)$ = acoustic impedance at time t
        Z_o = reference acoustic impedance

This relationship can be easily derived under the assumption of a multilaminate, linear structure with low values of reflection coefficients.

An example of a theoretical Raylogram of a cylinder with homogeneous walls immersed in water when interrogated by an acoustic beam perpendicular to its axis is shown in Fig. 1.

The Raylogram baseline is the impedance of the water and the Raylogram peaks represent the change in impedance introduced by the cylinder walls. Thus assuming that the characteristic impedance of water is 1.5 gm-cm^{-2}-sec^{-1} and that of the cylinder wall is 2.4 gm-cm^{-2}-sec^{-1} the impedance ratio at the cylinder water boundary is 1.60 and that is what the Raylogram would indicate.

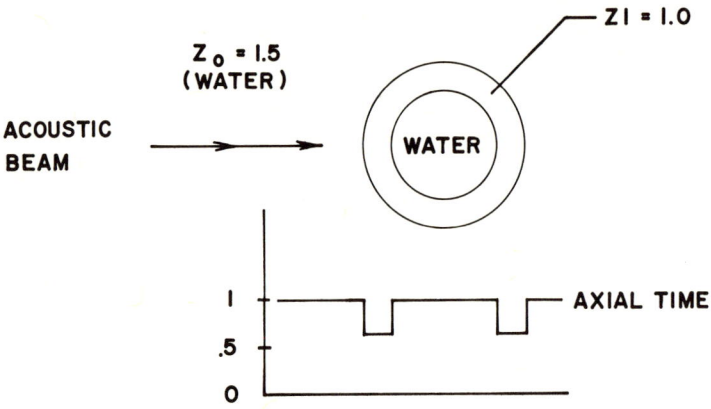

Fig. 2: Theoretical Raylogram of cylinder whose acoustic impedance is less than that of water

If the cylinder were made of a material whose acoustic impedance were less than water, the Raylogram would appear as in Fig. 2. Thus the Raylogram peaks would be oppositely polarized compared to the case shown in Fig. 1.

In the case of a structure as complex as an arterial wall, the Raylogram would look like Fig. 3.

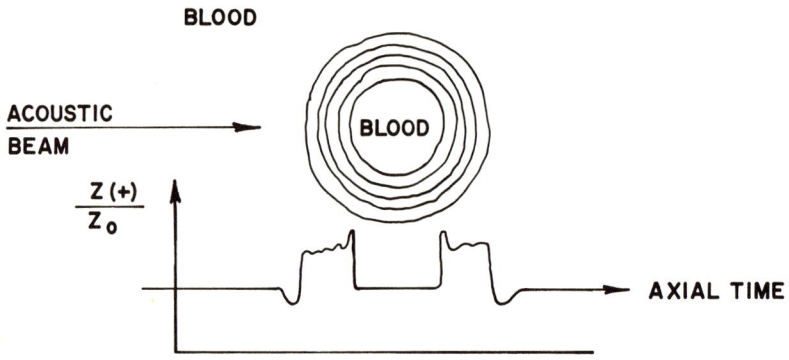

Fig. 3: Theoretical Raylogram of an aorta.

Here we note an initial negative excursion due to the fatty adventitial outer layer followed by a positive excursion at the fat boundary with a distinct indication of the intimal lining.

Similar patterns could be achieved in the A scan mode using conventional energy detection but important information would be lost. Fig. 4 shows what the A scan would look like for the three models when imaged by an energy detector.

What is apparent when comparing the A scans of Fig. 4 to the Raylographs of Figs. 1, 2 and 3 is that:

1. Impedance polarity is lost in energy detection and is maintained in Raylography.

2. Fine boundary detail can be lost in energy detection as a function of integration time constant. Thus dimensional detail can be lost.

3. The relative impedance reference keeps shifting under energy detection but is fixed in Raylography.

The relative impedance information inherent in Raylography becomes the all important ingredient that enables a more complete characterization of the tissue property and thus enables a higher probability of detection of the presence of a pathologic condition.

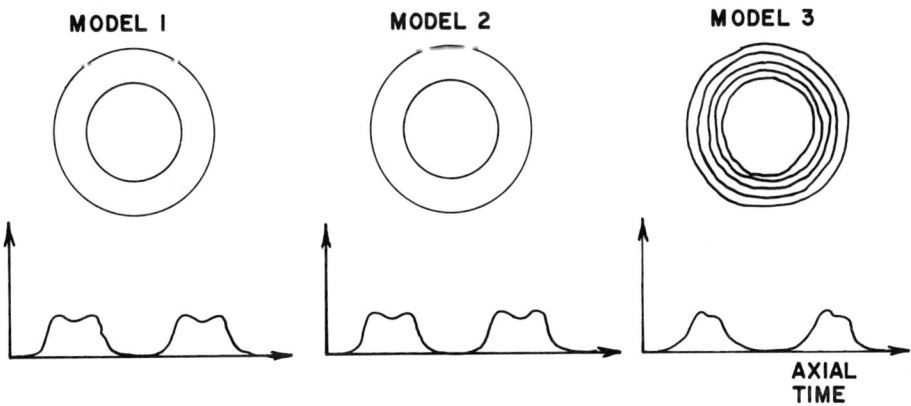

Fig 4: A scan display of cylinders and aorta of Figs. 1, 2 and 3 obtained by envelope detection.

Preliminary Results

A planar section of freshly excised beef aortic wall was mounted on a cylindrical ring with the planar section perpendicular to the acoustic beam. The tissue was positioned such that the acoustic waves insonified the intimal or internal surface first. A section of the aorta was removed after testing, fixed and stained for elastic fibers.

In Fig. 5 is shown the oscilloscope tracing of the aorta echoes ($Y(t)$), together with a computer plot of the echo obtained by hand digitization of several oscilloscope tracings, using expanded time scales. A reference signal ($X(t)$) is also shown, obtained by reflection from a piece of acrylic. The third plot is the computed "impulse response" ($H(t)$) of the aorta.

Fig. 6A is a low power photomicrograph of the aortic wall. The thickness of the wall was approximately five (5) mm. The intima appears to be predominantly elastic tissue. The media is a mixture of muscle and elastic tissue, with collagen at the media/adventitia interface.

Below the photomicrograph, Fig. 6B, is the computed Raylogram for this aorta. At the intimal side is a narrow layer of large acoustic impedance, which probably represents the internal layer composed of dense elastic tissue. The impedance profile then appears to decrease somewhat in the muscular section of the media, with undulations about the lower impedance level. This characteristic is consistent with a complex structure composed of muscle fascicles lined by variable thicknesses of fascia. Exiting from the muscle layer an increase in impedance is associated with the collagenous, layer between the adventitia and media layer. The impedance then decreases below the reference (water) value through the adventitia, consistent with the presence of fatty tissue. The various peaks in the adventitial impedance profile may be due to blood vessels or other fascia covered structures in the adventitial layer.

Note that the Raylogram does not return to the reference impedance (e.g., H_2O), since no correction was made for attenuation loss of the distant echoes.

Conclusions

1. Within the large, but finite, bandwidth of our preliminary test system, the <u>impulse response</u> from a complex biological tissue structure can be derived and further processed to obtain a display of the relative acoustic impedance.

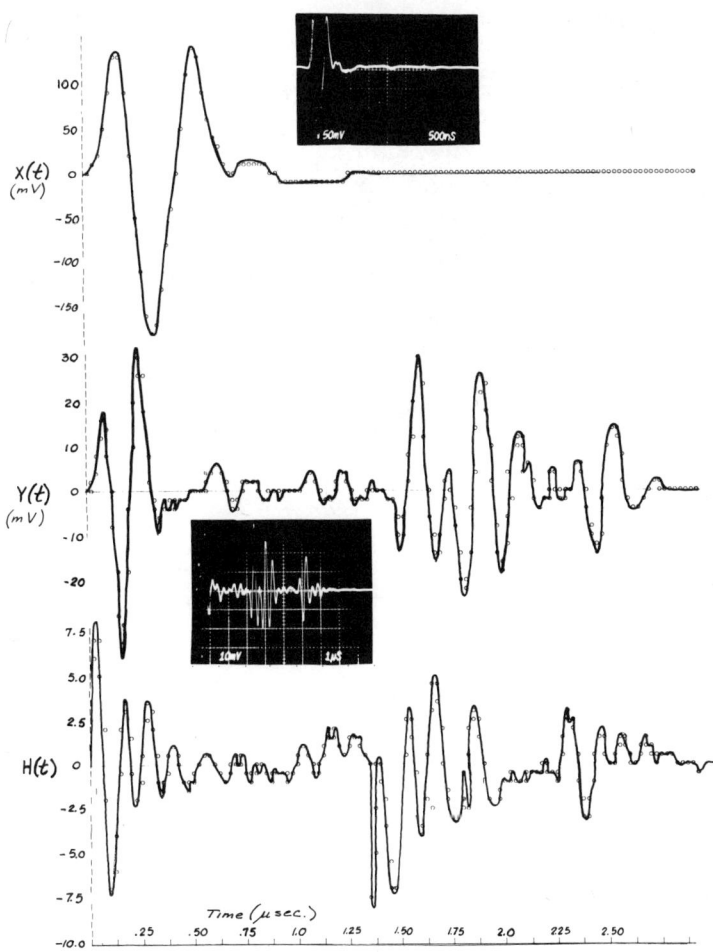

Fig 5: Data from ultrasonic interrogation of fresh beef aorta. The first waveform (X, (t)) is an echo from a flat piece of acrylic used as the reference waveform. The second line (Y(t)) is the echo train from the beef aorta. The third line (H(t)) is the impulse response of the beef aorta obtained by deconvolution

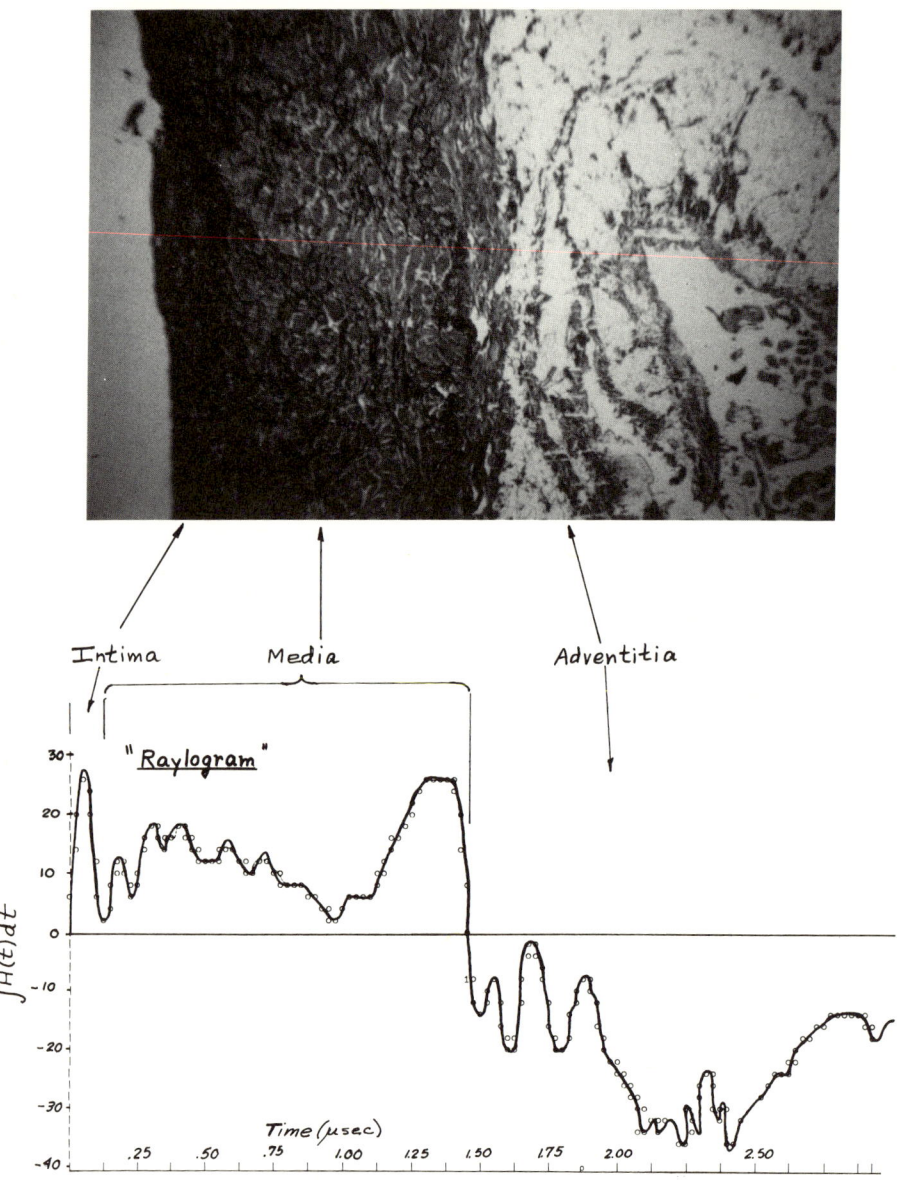

Fig. 6: (A) Photomicrography of beef aortic wall (25X) showing intima, media and adventitia.
(B) Acoustic impedance profile, or "Raylogram", of the aorta wall.

2. Using the deconvolution techniques developed, consistent with deconvolution theory, it is also evident that echoes may be resolved from tissue layers having thicknesses less than the wavelength of the original, transmitted source function.

Summary

The results of this preliminary work suggest that an impulse response estimate can be obtained from tissue. This technique improves resolution of acoustic boundaries by its ability to resolve echoes from tissue structure that is substantially thinner than the wavelength of the transmitted pulse. The impulse response estimate simultaneously provides a means of tissue characterization through Raylography. While much more work is needed in this area before clinical advantage can be realized, there appears no fundamental limitations to this approach and therefore suggests that this area be pursued with great vigor.

[1] Jones, J.P., Further Experiments with Impediography, JASA, 53, 343(A), 1973.

MEDIUM CHARACTERIZATION BY THE APPLICATION OF A DECONVOLUTION
TECHNIQUE IN AN ACOUSTIC PULSE ECHO SYSTEM--RAYLOGRAPHY

B.Lichtenstein,B.E.E.; I.Beretsky, M.D.;
G.Farrell, M.S.B.E.; A. Winder, M.S.E.E. *
Technicon Corporation
511 Benedict Avenue
Tarrytown, NY 10591

The non-invasive assessment of material acoustic properties by acoustic interrogation is known to be based upon the relationship of echo structure to the variation in acoustic impedance at the boundaries of change.

Most often the measurement of reflected acoustic energy is made which enables a determination of the location of acoustic impedance change along the axis of interrogation. More recently, in the field of non-invasive assessment of tissue by diagnostic ultrasound, efforts are being made to utilize reflected/absolute energy levels as a measure of tissue impedance variation and thereby enhance tissue characterization (Gray Shade techniques). Although energy detection techniques produce a measure of impedance change at a given boundary, they are incapable of determining the direction of that change, i.e., impedance polarity, an extremely useful parameter for assisting in medium characterization.

It is known that acoustic echoes bear impedance gradient and therefore impedance polarity information within their phase structure which can be derived from the impulse response of the target material. Additionally, the impulse response enables a unique measure of the target material characteristic impedance variation (ρC variation). We refer to the display of characteristic impedance as a Raylogram after the MKS unit of acoustic impedance, the Rayl. This is similar to the Impedogram described earlier by J. P. Jones [1].

*MSB, Inc., Consultant to Technicon

The Raylogram is a display of relative characteristic
impedance along the axis of acoustic interrogation much like the
A scan but, unlike the A scan, includes acoustic impedance polarity
information and, unlike the A scan, maintains a fixed impedance
reference.

The objective of our work has been the derivation of a good
estimate of impulse response and from this a meaningful Raylogram.
An additional benefit which derives from the measurement of
material impulse response, is a significant improvement in axial
resolution over the limitations of source function pulse width.
This can be achieved only when a good estimate of impulse response
is obtained. A good measurement of impulse response in the limit
is a train of infinitely narrow impulses whose epoch times coincide
with detected boundaries, thus negating the commonly accepted
resolution limitations of pulse width. (Resolution $\geq$ CT/2,
C = velocity of propagation, T = pulse width.)

Theoretical Considerations

As a first approximation, the medium we wish to consider is
modeled as a multi-laminar material, homogeneous between layers
and infinite in extent in a direction parallel to the boundaries.
We wish to interrogate this material with acoustic energy
propagated in a direction perpendicular to the boundary direction
and determine the characteristic acoustic impedance of each layer.
This relative impedance, when plotted, constitutes a Raylogram
which should provide significant material characterization information.

Our initial goals focused specifically on the non-invasive
monitoring of material characteristic impedance, under the
assumption that this would provide a worthwhile characterization
parameter. The ρ C product is, however, the real part of the
complex specific acoustic impedance in a non-dispersive medium
and is essentially frequency invarient. These characteristics
therefore define a processing need to separate the ρ C product
from the frequency sensitive complex impedance.

One approach to this is to utilize an approximation to the
integral of the impulse response which reduces to a frequency
invariant expression and, for our model, can be shown to relate
to <u>relative characteristic acoustic impedance</u> (ZR), i.e., the
ratio of the density, velocity of propagation product, $\rho_i C_i$, at
any layer to some reference $\rho_o C_o$ product (ZR = $\rho_i C_i / \rho_o C_o$).

Since the impulse response of any material is defined as the
output of that material when its input is a pure impulse, the
impulse response of our multilaminate model can be defined by the
non-dispersive echo train resulting from insonification by a

MEDIUM CHARACTERIZATION AND RAYLOGRAPHY

perfect impulse. This echo train would be seen to consist of a series of elementary impulses each associated with a boundary and weighted by its reflection coefficient. This can be approximated mathematically by

$$h(t) = r_o \delta(t) + r_1(1-r_o^2)\delta(t-t_1) + r_2(1-r_1^2)(1-r_o^2)\delta(t-t_2)$$
$$+ \cdots r_n(1-r_{n-1}^2)(1-r_{n-2}^2)\cdots(1-r_o^2)\delta(t-t_n) \quad (1)$$

where: $t_i = 2\sum_{i}^{i}(\Delta l_i / c_j)$
Δl_i = layer thickness
c_i = layer velocity of propagation

Equation (1) assumes zero attenuation loss, perpendicular ensonification by a plane propagating wave plus no multiple reflections between layers (no material reverberation). By discrete summation of both sides of (1) we get

$$\sum_{t=0}^{t=N} h(t) = r_o + r_1(1-r_o^2) + r_2(1-r_1^2)(1-r_o^2) + \cdots + r_N(1-r_{N-1}^2)\cdots(1-r_o^2) \quad (2)$$

from which

$$\sum_{t=0}^{t=N} h(t) \cong \sum_{i=0}^{N} r_i \quad (3)$$

for $r_i \ll 1$

From consideration of the basic properties of the acoustic propagation of plane waves and assuming $\omega = 0$ it can easily be shown that a good approximation to the relative impedance ratio (ZR) of a multilaminate model is

$$ZR = \frac{Z_N}{Z_c} = \frac{(1+r_o)(1+r_1)(1+r_2)\cdots(1+r_N)}{(1-r_o)(1-r_1)(1-r_2)\cdots(1-r_N)} \quad (4)$$

which may be generalized to

$$ZR = \frac{Z_N}{Z_o} = \frac{1+\sum r_i}{1-\sum r_i} \cong \frac{1+\sum h(t)}{1-\sum h(t)} \quad (5)$$

A display of (5) is the Raylogram and can be seen to depend upon the detection of the impulse response h(t).

Since insonification by an impulse source function is not practical, the impulse response estimate may be derived from the Fourier transform of the transfer function, $H(\omega)$, of the model assuming that the medium behaves linearly.

The complex transfer function of the medium is the ratio of the echo to source function Fourier spectra, i.e.,

$$H(\omega) = Y(\omega)/X(\omega) \tag{6}$$

where $Y(\omega)$ = Fourier spectra of the echo train
$X(\omega)$ = Fourier spectra of the source function
$H(\omega)$ = transfer function of the medium

which suggests the process of frequency deconvolution for its derivation. Deconvolution, whether carried out in the time or frequency domain, is a noisy process and the simple operation suggested by (6) is not stable and, by itself is not realizable. Therefore, before the process becomes usable, coherent techniques for enhancing echo processing gain must be added as well as filtering of deconvolution noise. Additionally, the impulse response estimate trades off with source function phase characteristics and spectral shape.

We have had good results by preprocessing with an extraction filter whose processing gain improves inversely to input signal to noise level. Our deconvolution technique was programmed and the functional algorithm is shown in Fig. 1.

The algorithm is written to enable tests of hypothetical models and signals perturbed by assumed levels of random noise and, to accept real digitized data obtained from the acoustic interrogation of real models.

Observation of Fig. 1 will show that processing takes place in both the frequency and time domains and includes both pre and post deconvolution filtering in the frequency domain. The transfer function $H(\omega)$ once determined, is Fourier transformed to obtain the impulse response which is summed and converted to equation (5) for final printout as the Raylogram.

Synthetic Signal and Model Tests

The algorithm was tested assuming a bipolar source function (Fig. 2a) and a multilaminar model producing the echo train shown in Fig. 2b. The theoretical Raylogram is shown in Fig. 3a. This model was chosen to examine the detectability of 30 db of reflectivity variation (30:1) under various conditions of minimum echo signal to noise ratio (MSNR). The model also was used to test the algorithm's capability of resolving overlapped signals and detecting small signals in close time proximity to large signals.

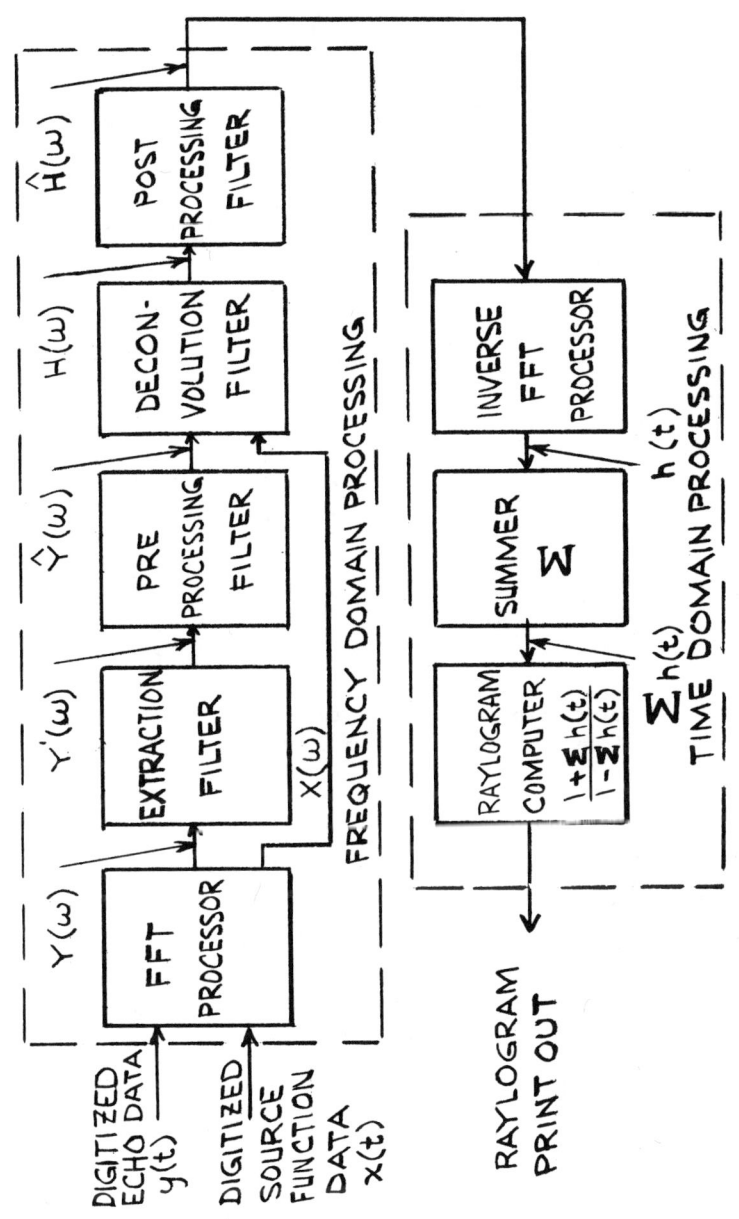

Fig. 1 - Signal Processing Algorithm Functional Description

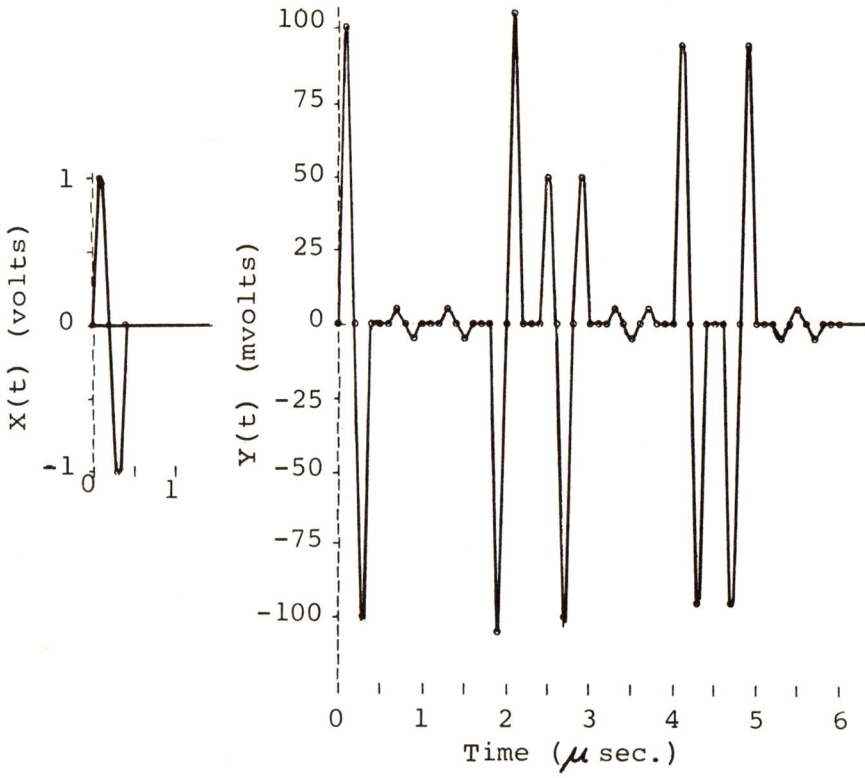

Fig. 2(a) - Synthetic bipolar source function
(b) - Resulting echo train from assumed multilaminate model

Figs. 4, 5 and 6 show the resulting impulse response and Raylogram under conditions of +30 db, +20 db and +10 db MSNR, respectively. Observation of the impulse response in Figs. 4 and 5 (30 db and 20 db cases) shows that boundaries are identified within one time scale division (100 nsec). The lower reflectivity boundaries are not seen in the impulse response printout because of amplitude scale selection. However, observation of the Raylograms of Figs. 4 and 5 on an expanded (vertical) scale shows detection of all the low reflectivity boundaries. We might consider the 20 db MSNR as the threshold of detection since we begin to see the last low reflectivity thin layer (layer 11) become base line distorted. Observation of Fig. 6, the +10 db MSNR case, shows excessive Raylographic distortion making low reflectivity boundaries and the impedance pattern essentially unrecognizable. Thus, we consider an MSNR of +10 db as below the threshold of detection and we conclude that the algorithm's minimum detectable MSNR is conservatively 20 db for a 30 db (30:1) reflectivity range.

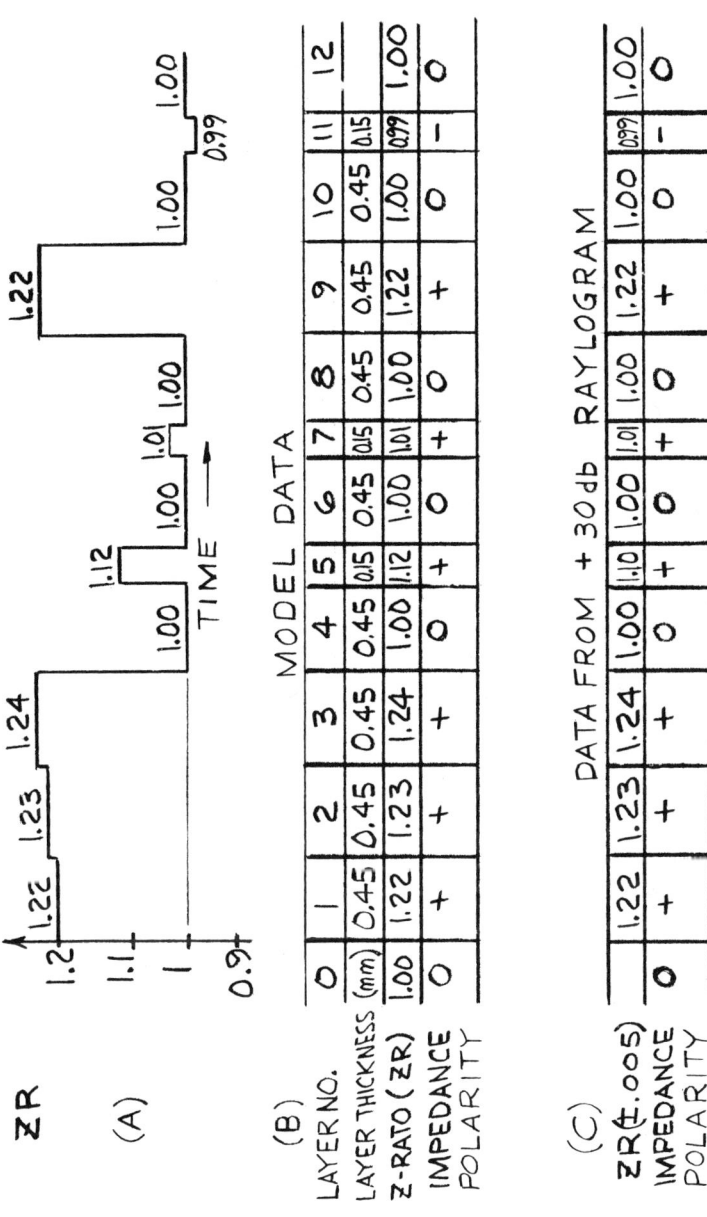

Fig. 3 - Data summary of synthetic model. A is the theoretical Raylogram, B is the material characteristics, C is data from an algorithm-computed Raylogram.

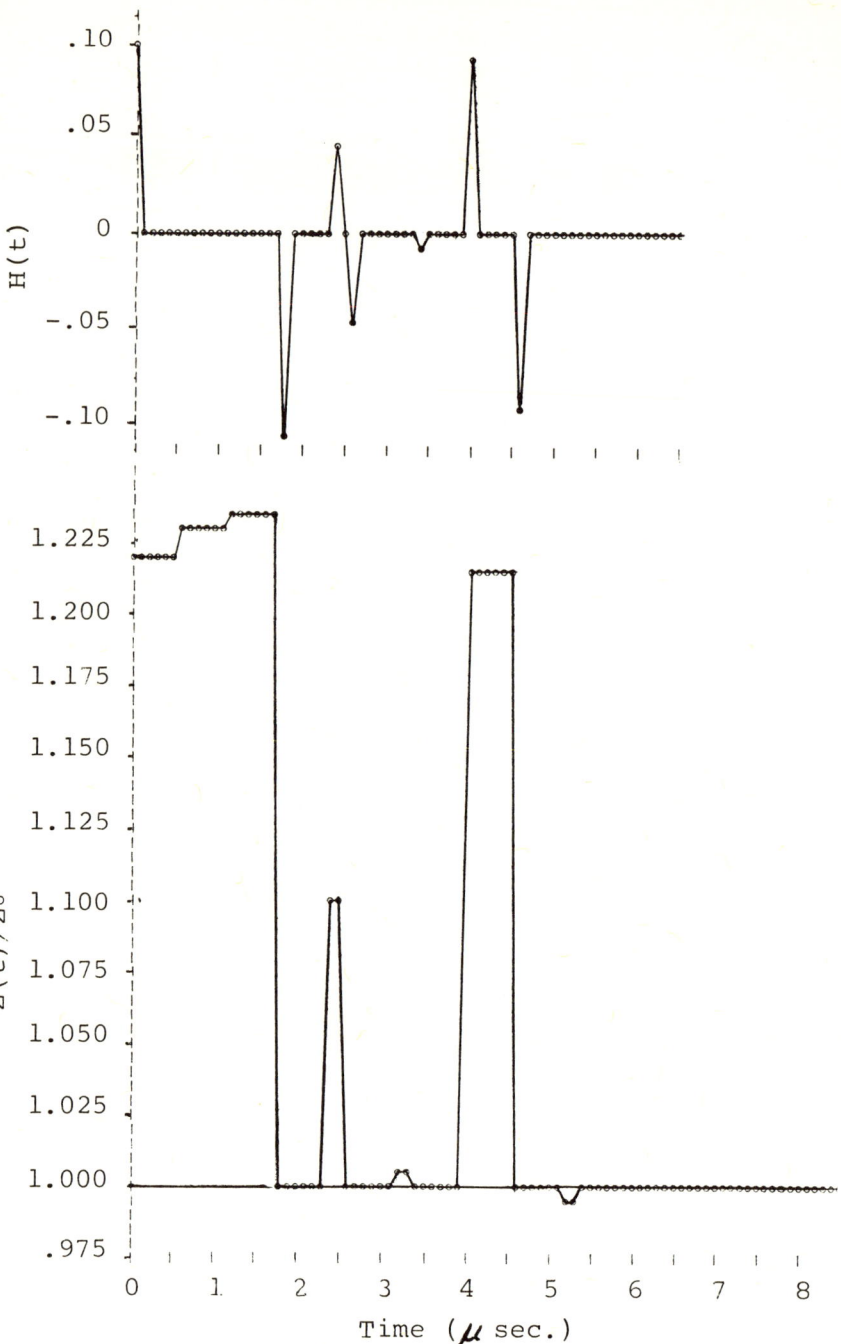

Fig. 4 — Synthetic model processed results for +30 db MSNR
(a) Impulse response, (b) Raylogram

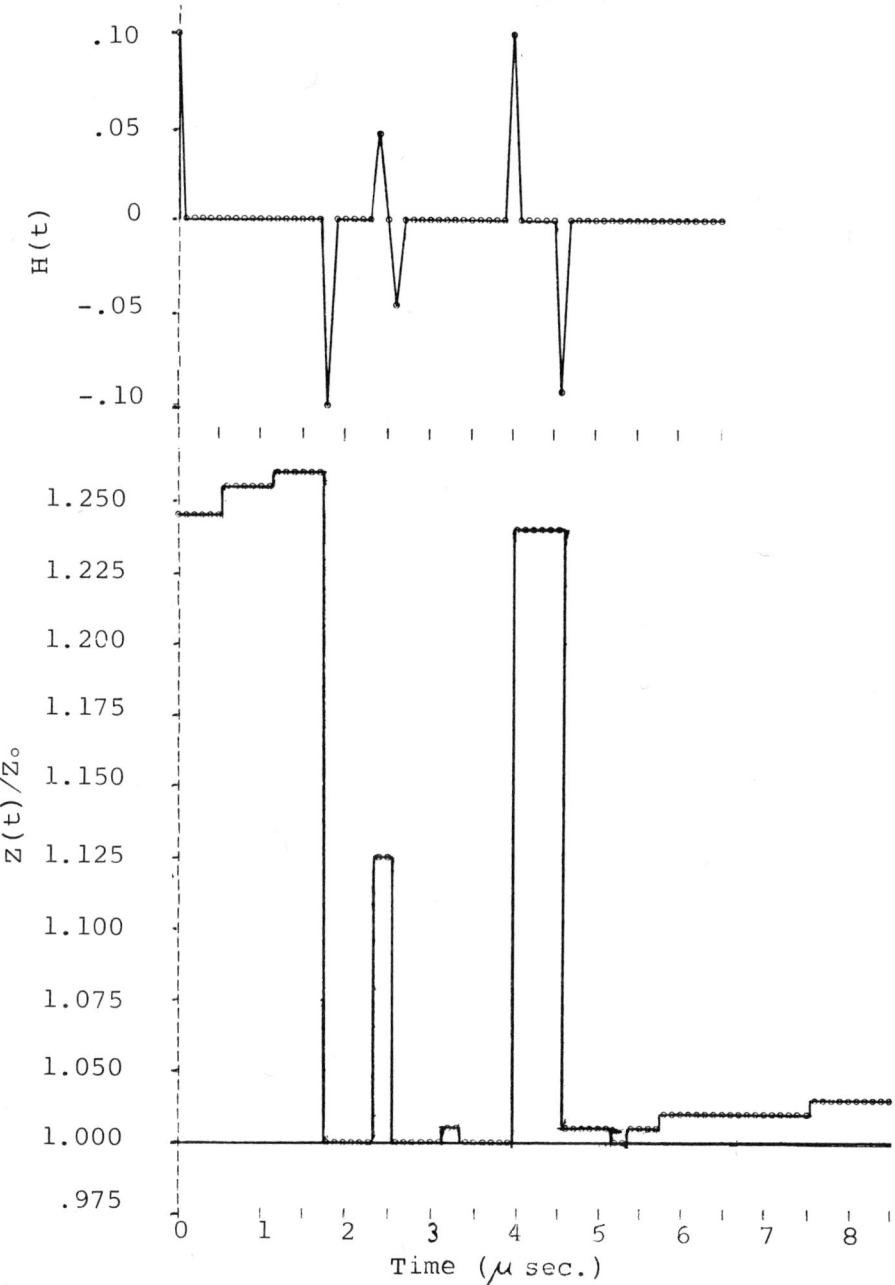

Fig. 5 - Synthetic model processed results for +20 db MSNR
(a) Impulse response, (b) Raylogram

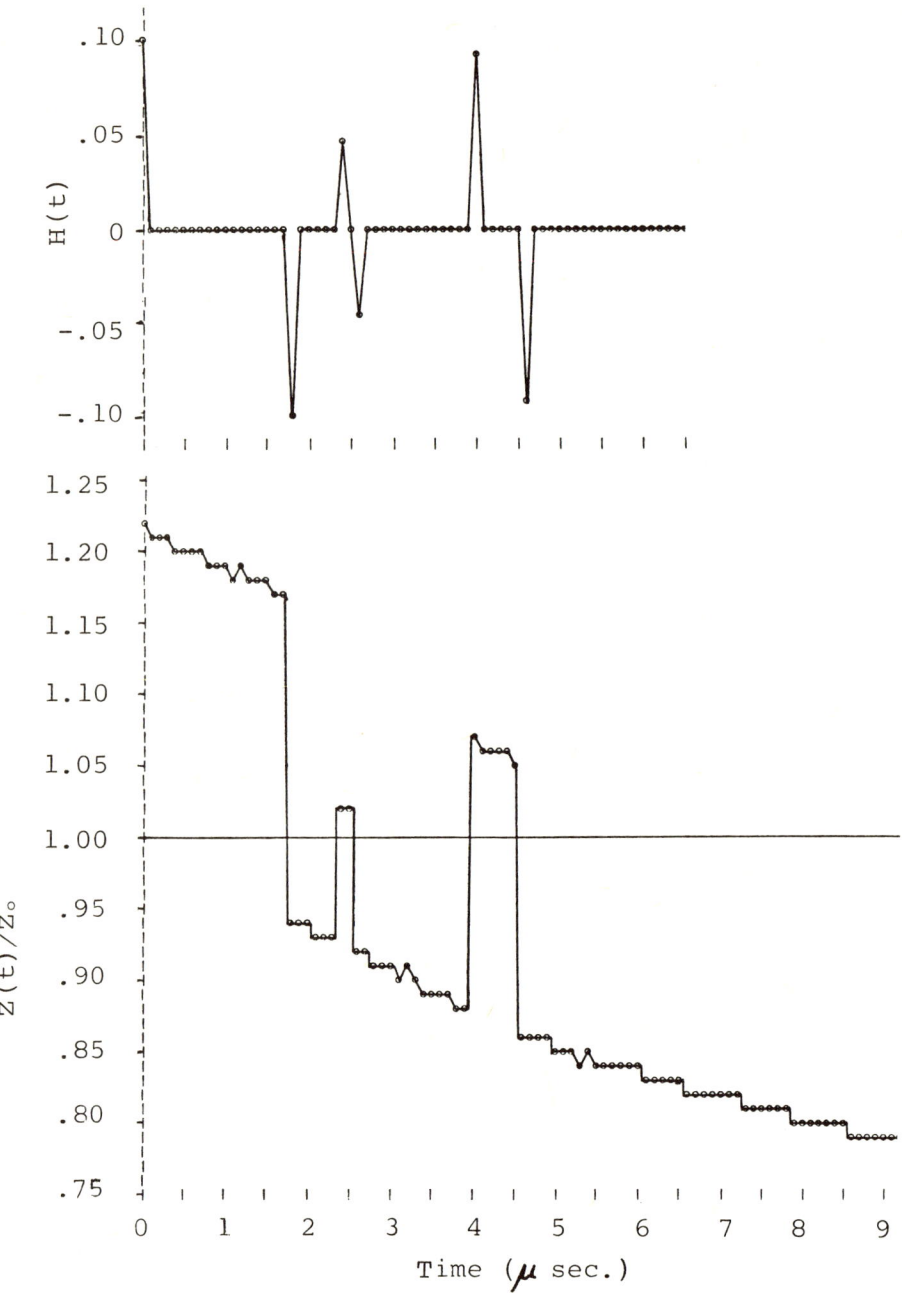

Fig. 6 - Synthetic model processed results for +10 db MSNR
(a) Impulse response, (b) Raylogram

The model laminate thin layers were adjusted so that reflections from consecutive boundaries would overlap. The source function pulse width is spatially equivalent to 0.6 mm while as shown in Fig. 3(B) the thin layers are 0.15 mm thick thus, producing one-half pulse width overlap. Note from the Raylograms in Figs. 4 and 5 that these thin layers (5, 7 and 11) are all resolved. Axial resolution turns out in fact to be limited by the accuracy of the impulse response estimate and the size of the Fast Fourier Transform computational matrix and not by source function pulse width.

Figs. 3(B) and 3(C) summarize the results of this test of the interrogation of a known synthetic laminate with a bipolar source function. The table shows good agreement between the theoretical values of ZR implied by the synthetic echo train and the values obtained from the Fig. 4 Raylographic printout. Also, the table shows complete correlation between assumed and Raylographically displayed impedance polarity even at low reflectivity boundaries in close proximity to high reflectivity boundaries.

Experimental Acoustic Interrogation System

An acoustic interrogation system is being built to incorporate some of the more important operating specifications which we consider necessary for a good match between the interrogated material and the computer. A functional illustration of this system is shown in Fig. 7.

Our work is done in a 2 x 2 x 3 foot acoustically damped tank fitted with spatial manipulators having 4 degrees of freedom. The system front end includes a well focused ($F \approx 1$) reflector-spherical transducer combination designed to produce a focal dimension of approximately 7 by 20 mm at 0.75 MHZ. This provides reasonably good spatial coherence over these interrogated volume dimensions for most of our usable bandwidth. The reflector is elliptical thus enabling acoustic interrogation at the far focal point by a transducer at the near focal point. The transducer is excited by a controlled ramp, which enables stepless source function shape control. The receiver can be seen to include a broad band, high impedance preamplifier and range gate working into a coherent noise cancellation circuit. This circuit monitors transducer second order modes and reduces them by a factor of approximately 20 db.

Raw echo signal information from the noise cancellation circuit is displayed on the oscilloscope and recorded on Polaroid R_* film. Values are then hand digitized for manual entry into the computer terminal.

*Registered trademark of Polaroid Corporation

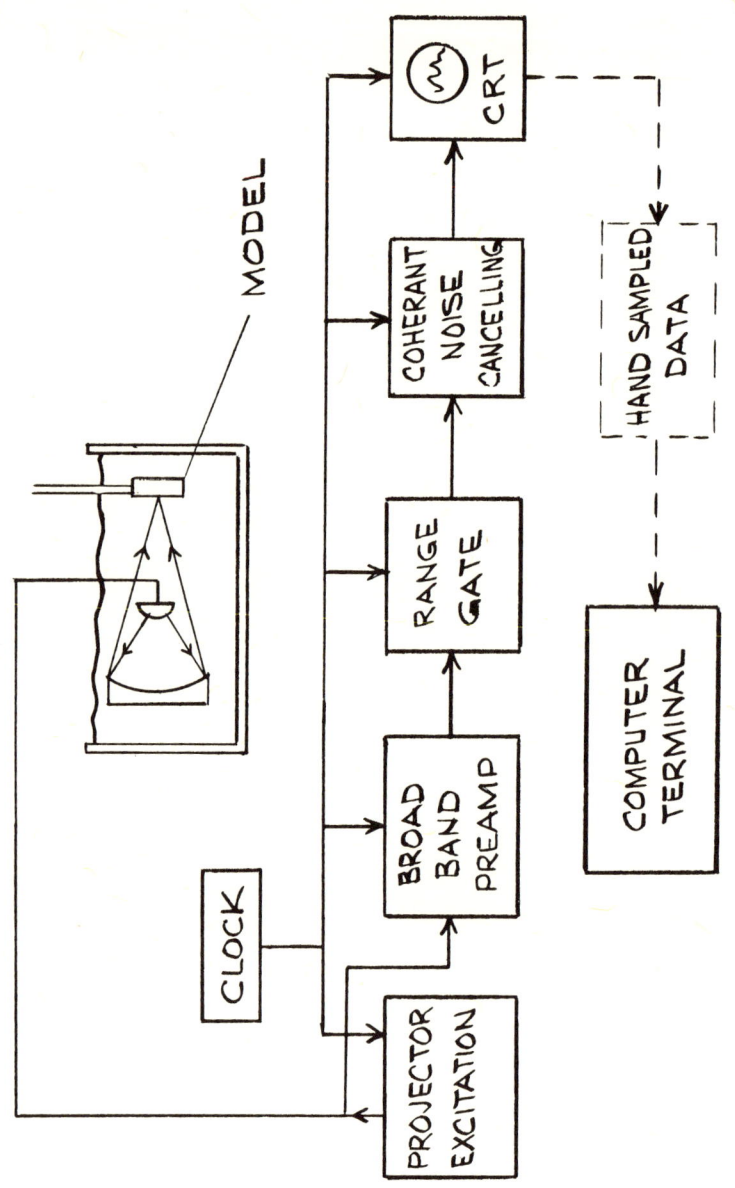

Fig. 7 - Experimental Acoustic Interrogation System

Real Model Tests

Tests were performed with laminates chosen to evaluate the system's capability of deriving good estimates of impulse response under conditions of overlapped signals. A 100 mm by 100 mm by 2.10 mm laminate consisting of a polyethylene layer 0.60 mm thick followed by 1.5 mm butyl rubber layer was placed in our test tank and insonified with the focused reflecting system. The insonifying source function and resultant echo wave forms are shown in Fig. 8, while Fig. 9 shows the deconvolved impulse response estimate and Raylogram. Observation of the Raylogram shows first that the impedance polarity with respect to water is clearly detected, i.e., the polyethylene polarity is positive, and the butyl rubber polarity is negative. Secondly, we note that the thin 0.60 mm layer is resolved and thirdly, that the average ZR values agree fairly well with the separately measured values (see also Fig. 10).

The tables in Fig. 10 summarize for comparison the essential, separately measured, parameters and the Raylographically derived characteristics of the model laminate. Note that the ratio of layer thicknesses as shown by the Raylogram (Fig. 9) are in error by the ratio of propagation velocities in each material thus creating some imaging distortion. Note also, from Fig. 9 that Raylographic values are equal ahead of and behind the model material (Z_o = 1 in both places) indicating that model and medium distorting effects on the impulse response (such as attenuation) for this case were negligible.

Discussion

Thus far, work with simple models confirms our system capability of achieving good estimates of impulse response with signal to random noise ratios of +20 db or more. Raylograms derived from this impulse response do enable a reasonably good measure of ZR and impedance polarity both of which should prove to be useful medium characterization parameters. The ability to resolve layers which produce overlapped echoes, achieved as a spinoff of the good impulse response estimate, represents a significant potential for detection of fine tissue detail. This too could prove to be an important characterization tool. Observation of Fig. 9 shows that the real data taken with the laminate model at a 40 db MSNR produces more distortion and noise in the Raylogram than the synthetic model at +30 db MSNR. This indicates that the threshold of detection, although conventionally a function of perturbing noise power, is limited in our coherent detector by both random noise amplitude and signal phase distortion. Phase distortion could be caused by factors in the medium such as multipath, reverberation, non-longitudinal mode conversion (shear), surface curvature and texture, etc. Further work with this

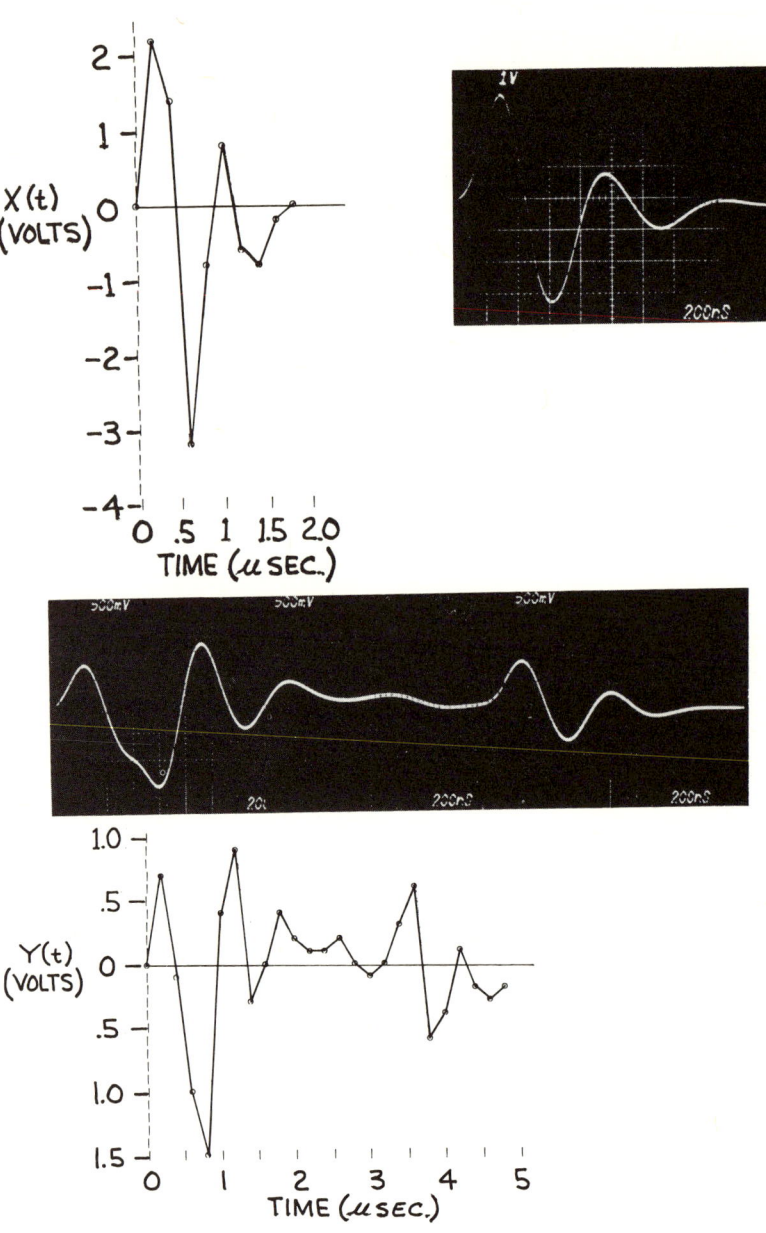

Fig. 8 - Raw Wave Forms

MEDIUM CHARACTERIZATION AND RAYLOGRAPHY 425

deconvolution technique remains to minimize these effects as well as to compensate for the effects of absorption.

Data collected to date shows reasonably good agreement with theory and strongly suggests further pursuit of development of impulse response detection for tissue characterization.

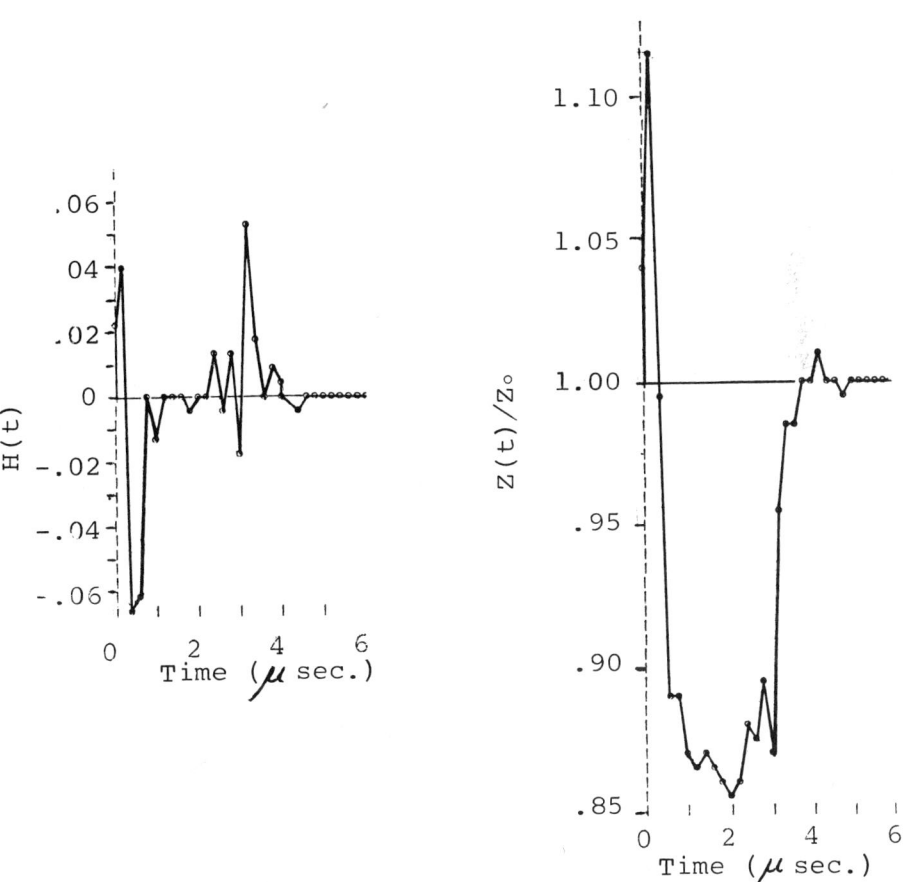

Fig. 9 - Real model derived (a) Impulse response, (b) Raylogram

(A)　　　　　　Real Model Measured Pertinent Data

Measured Values	Polyethylene	Butyl Rubber	Water
2-way propagation time (us)	0.6	2.80	
layer thickness (mm)	0.6	1.50	
speed of sound, C (mm/us)	2.00	1.07	1.55
density, ρ (g/cm^3)	0.88	1.12	1.00
acoustic impedance = ρC	1.76	1.20	1.55
ZR = $\rho C/1.55$	1.14	0.78	1.00
impedance polarity	+	−	0

(B)　　　　　　Real Model Data from Raylogram

	Polyethylene	Butyl Rubber	Water
2-way propagation time (us)	0.6	3.4	
ZR	1.12	0.86	1.00
impedance polarity	+	−	0

(C)　　　　　　Real Model Cross Section

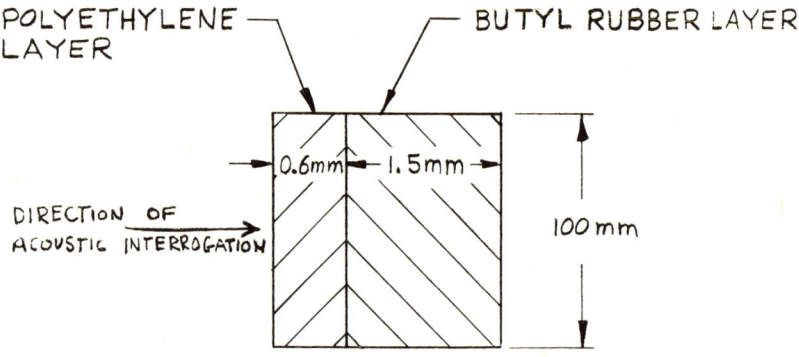

Fig. 10 - Real Model Summary Data

---

[1] Jones, J.P., Further Experiments with Impediography, JASA 53, 393 (A), 1973.

ULTRASONIC SPECTRAL INVESTIGATIONS FOR TISSUE CHARACTERIZATION

F.L. Lizzi; M.A. Laviola

Riverside Research Institute

New York, New York 10023

The spectrum analysis system described in this paper has been integrated with a clinical ultrasound system, used for ophthalmic examinations at the ultrasound laboratory of Dr. D.J. Coleman at the Harkness Eye Institute. Three papers discussing various clinical results from this ultrasound system are reported in the Ophthalmology Session.(1,2,3)

The main objective of this paper is to describe the characteristics of the spectrum analysis system and the calibration procedures used to insure data quality and repeatability. The paper (4) following in this session discusses the theory involved in making tissue measurements and some of the in vivo results obtained to date on clinical subjects.

The spectrum analysis system has been designed for ease of operation so that it can be routinely included in the diagnostic procedures during clinical examination. As a consequence, the system is currently yielding spectral data on a large number of patients thus permitting study of a wide variety of ocular and orbital disorders. An important benefit attending this clinical application is that the high-resolution A- and B-mode diagnostic displays can be used to advantage to assist in the accurate placement of the spectral-gating window which selects tissue segments for spectral examination.

The spectrum analysis system is instrumented with

a digital averager to perform real-time smoothing of the characteristically random spectra obtained from certain types of heterogeneous tissue. Hard-copy strip chart plots of the averaged spectra are available for immediate diagnostic interpretation and for subsequent digital processing.

Particular care has been taken in incorporating several types of system calibration to insure data accuracy and to permit normalization of the spectral results so that they are independent of system parameters. Software has been developed for computer post-processing of the hard-copy data and currently is being used to digitize the data, perform normalization procedures and organize a cross-indexed data file of tissue pathology as collected.

SYSTEM DESCRIPTION

Figure 1 presents a simplified blocked diagram of the spectrum analysis and clinical systems. The components of the clinical system are enclosed within the dashed lines. The major components of the clinical system include the transmitter/receiver, transducer with encoder trigger generator, and A- and B-mode displays. The RF signal required for the spectrum analysis is tapped from the RF output of the receiver. Preparatory to the spectrum analysis, the RF signal is summed with a frequency calibration standard and then gated in time to obtain that portion of the echo upon which spectrum analysis is to be performed. Simultaneous with the gating operation, RF signals are modulated with a time-weighting function to suppress spectral sidelobes. The spectrum analyzer output is then digitally averaged in a special purpose computer; typically, 100 independent spectra are collected to compute each average. The output from the average is available in real-time from a strip chart recorder. Subsequent data analysis is performed via computer.

Figure 2 presents a detailed timing diagram of the intertransmission interval illustrating the operations, that are performed after a single transducer excitation. In Fig. 2a, the typical A-mode display of the signal echo complex is depicted. Transducer excitation occurs at a 1 KHz rate. In Fig. 2b, the weighted gating function is shown; during system operation the position of this gate can be continuously controlled in range utilizing the A-mode display as a monitor. When collecting data the position of the spectral-gating window

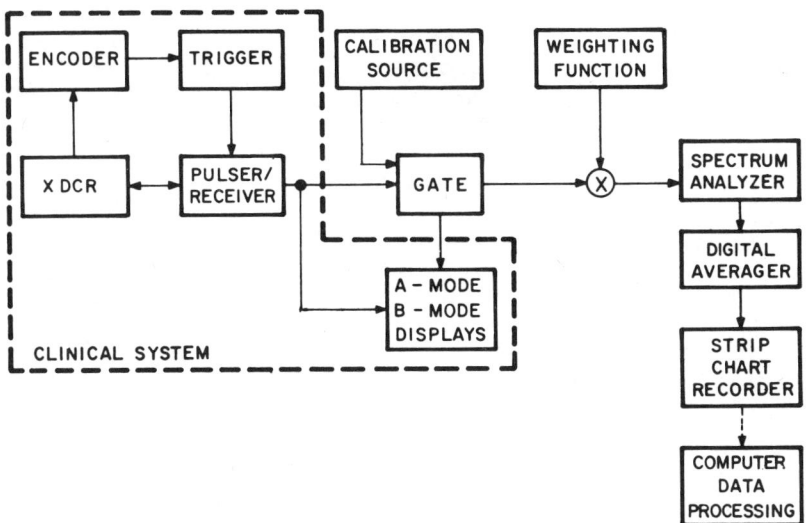

Fig. 1   Spectrum Analysis System Configuration

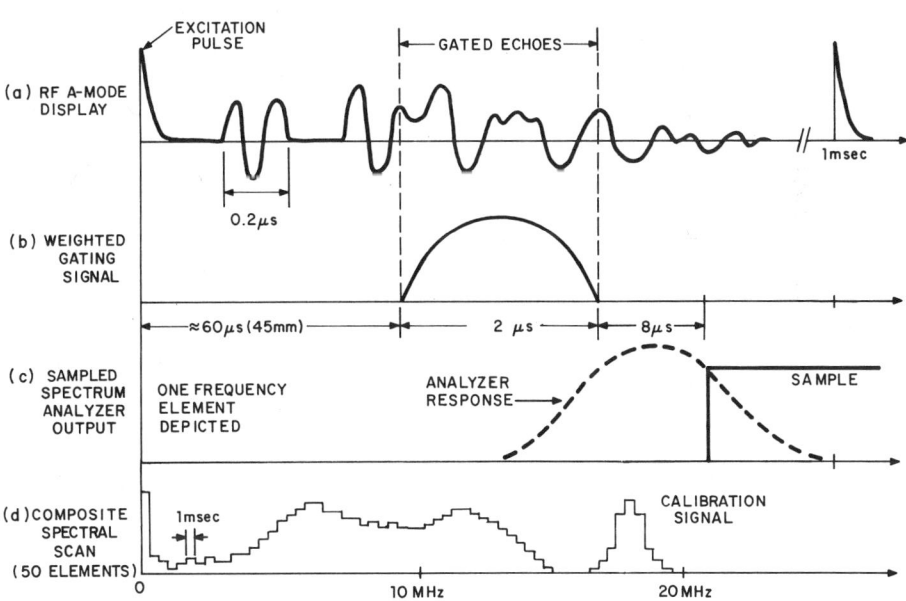

Fig. 2   Detail of Inter-Transmission Interval

is confined within the depth of focus of the transducer to assure adequate data calibration and avoid complex Fresnel beam patterns. Line (c) of Fig. 2 demonstrates how one spectral element at a single frequency in the spectral scan of 50 elements is generated by sampling the output from the spectrum analyzer. The sampled signal is held for a full interpulse period until the next spectral sample is available. A complete spectral scan of 50 frequency elements (Fig. 2d) is generated by sequentially advancing the spectrum analyzer center frequency by an increment equal to an analysis resolution element. Figure 3 depicts system timing in the generation of complete spectral scans. The system is capable of approximately 10 complete spectral scans per second. Spectral scanning triggers, generated by system timing, generate a burst of 1 KHz excitation pulses which lasts for 50 msec, the interval during which the spectral scan is generated. A short receiver off time is necessary to permit analyzer recovery.

Before discussing system parameters, a word is necessary concerning the distinction between frequency coverage and resolution. Frequency coverage is dependent on the combined transmitter/receiver and transducer bandwidths and represents the range over which the system provides sufficient radiated power to permit meaningful measurements. Frequency resolution strictly is determined by the duration of the spectral-gating window and is proportional to the reciprocal of the gating-window length; i.e., the longer the temporal gating waveform, the narrower will be the frequency resolution. The frequency coverage obtainable with the system can be selected by using transducers with center frequencies as high as 25 MHz. Each transducer provides about a 60-per cent fractional bandwidth. By sequentially using transducers of differing center frequency on a test subject, a large composite frequency coverage can be achieved. Table I lists the typical system parameters used for most of the clinical measurements being made. Most frequently, a 10 MHz transducer has been used with a 2-μsec spectral gate, corresponding to a 1.50-mm range window. The choice of range window was predicated on several factors including the relatively small range extent of some of the pathologic structures encountered in the eye.

SYSTEM CALIBRATION

In the implementation and the routine operation of

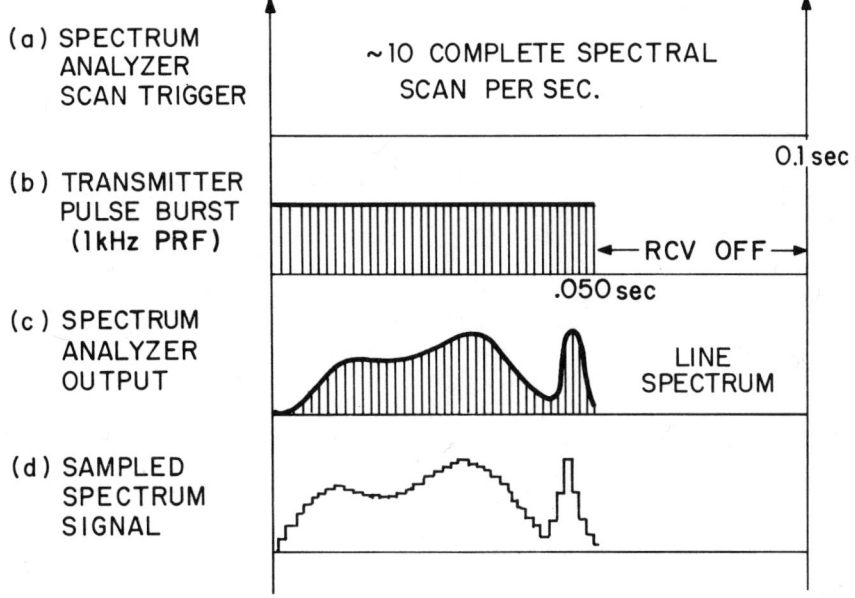

Fig. 3 Spectrum Analysis System Waveforms

this system, particular emphasis has been placed on the development of reliable calibration procedures. Figure 4 depicts the various calibration signals used. Figure 4a shows a typical tissue spectrum as obtained from the strip chart recorder. To calibrate the frequency axis,

TABLE I. TYPICAL SYSTEM PARAMETERS

Range Gate Duration	2 μsec (1.5 mm)
Center Frequency	10 MHz
Frequency Coverage	7 - 14 MHz
Frequency Resolution	0.5 MHz
Number of Resolution Cells	14
Number of Averaged Spectra	100

frequency marker signals are placed at both zero frequency and the high end of the frequency band. Figure 4b depicts the step frequency and amplitude calibration performed before and after each data collection session. Note from this figure that the system produces in excess of 40 dB of dynamic range. The bottom line (Fig. 4c) presents typical reference spectra which are obtained to develop the z-axis spectral profiles used in the normalization of data to remove system spectral-shaping. The reference spectra are obtained by analyzing the echo derived from a glass-plate target situated at range positions equal in delay to those at which the tissue measurements are performed.

The spectrum analysis system was thoroughly checked out utilizing a variety of test targets preliminary to its utilization in clinical examinations. Essentially, these measurement targets fall into two categories: planar targets such as glass or lucite plates and distributed targets such as sponges. Representative of the measurements made with planar targets is the propagation loss experiment performed on various fluid media including milk, propanol, castor oil, and acetone. In these experiments comparative spectral measurements are taken between propagation in water and the lossy fluid using a glass plate reflector positioned to yield the same round-trip delay in each case. To obtain the propagation loss of the medium under test, the spectrum is normalized with respect to the spectrum obtained with water. Figure 5 presents the results measured for milk for the stated experimental conditions. The measured loss is in close agreement with published data.(5)

Measurements were made on distributed targets to

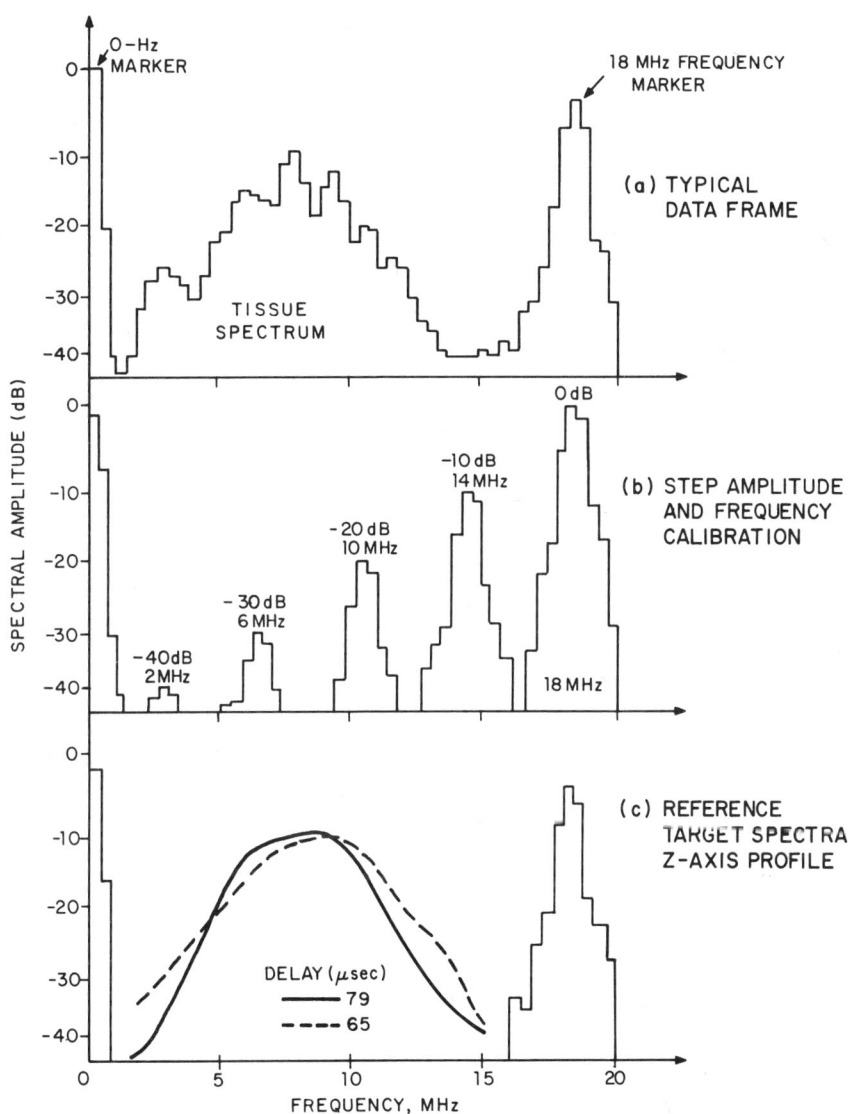

Fig. 4 Data Calibration

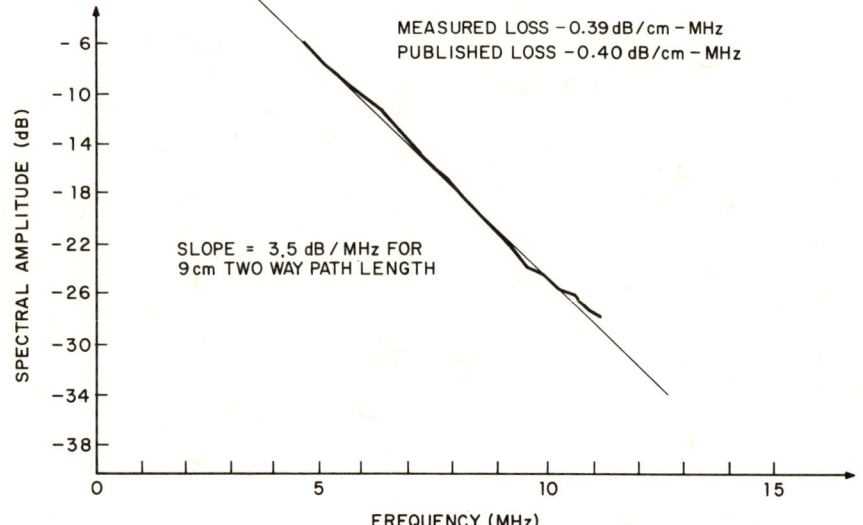

Fig. 5 Propagation Loss in Milk

verify the concepts used in spectral averaging procedures. A distributed target, such as a sponge yields a random type spectrum for any given aspect since its acoustically heterogeneous structure consists of large numbers of randomly positioned scatterers. To obtain any definitive structure characterization it is essential to remove by spatial averaging the random spectral fluctuations and obtain the power spectral density function of the material reflectance. The spectra to be averaged are obtained at a sequence of transducer illumination angles relative to the target. Spatial averaging can only be effective if the individual spectra are statistically independent. Spectral independence is achieved by incorporating within the transducer mount an encoder which provides a spectral scan trigger only at angular intervals commensurate with transducer displacements on the order of a beamwidth.

A demonstration of the averaging of sponge spectra is shown in Fig. 6. The top spectrum (a) was obtained without averaging. The wide variance and the random quality of the spectra are demonstrated on the second line (b) by superimposing a number of single-look spectra. Note an apparent 20-dB peak-to-peak spread in spectral power at any given frequency; a range of this order is consistent with a Rayleigh distribution. The third line (c) depicts the result of averaging 100 independent spectra. The great reduction in spectral variance is demonstrated on the fourth line (d) by superimposing the averages obtained from independent groups of averaged spectra. Note the apparent peak-to-peak deviation has been reduced to approximately 4 dB. Theoretically, the spread in spectral amplitude should be reduced by the square root of the number of independent spectra which in this case would amount to a reduction by a factor of ten. The fact that the spread of the averaged data is not reduced by this factor indicates the presence of redundant data in the acquired RF signals.

COMPUTER POST PROCESSING

The averaged spectra depicted in (c) of Fig. 6 is representative of the data from the spectrum analysis system. Further analysis of such data is performed using computer post-processing which includes the following operations: digitization and editing, normalization with respect to the reference target, and least-square computation of spectral slopes with statistical confidence limits. Data so processed by the computer

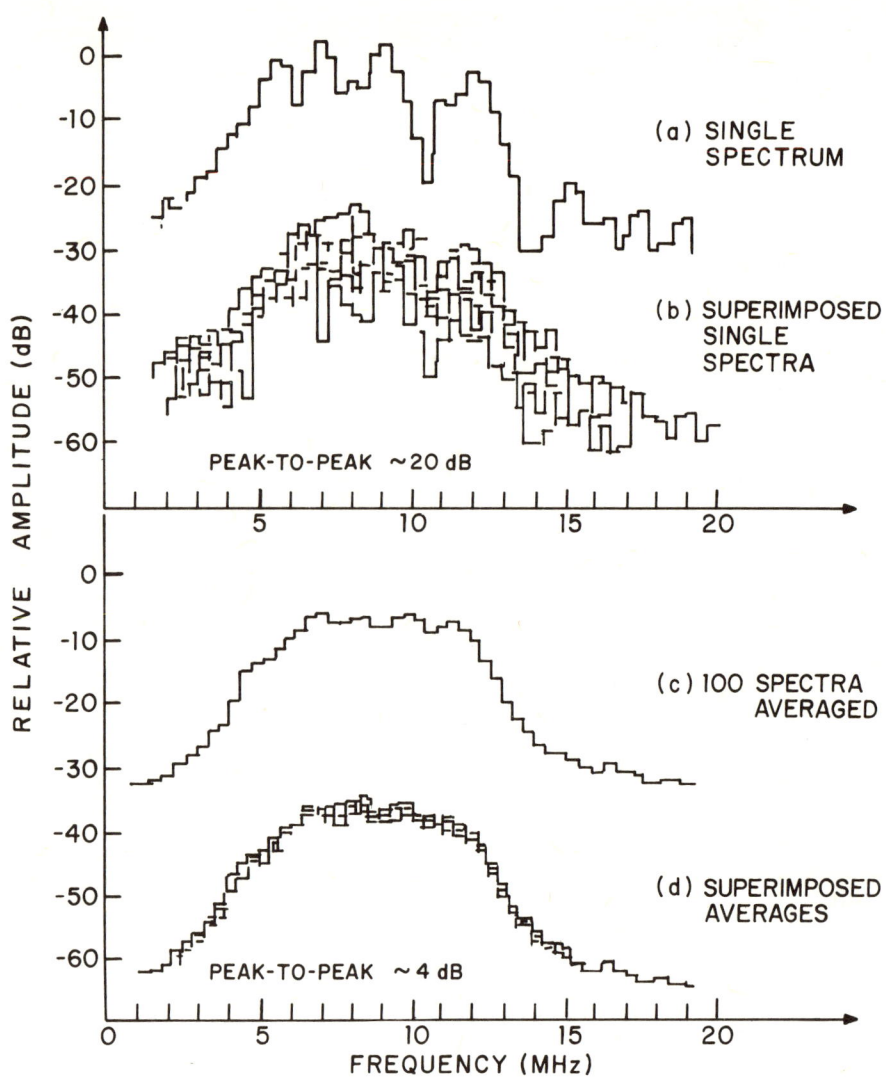

Fig. 6 Demonstration of Spatial Averaging Sponge Spectra

is being stored in files cross-indexed accoding to pathology so that once sufficient data has been collected, studies of tissue characteristic can be readily implemented utilizing computer sorting and pattern recognition procedures.

Figure 7 presents an example of orbital fat data which has been processed by computer. This spectrum was obtained by averaging 200 individual spectra from a region of orbital fat situated 6 mm behind the sclera. It has been normalized to remove system spectral shaping and gain factors. As a consequence, the spectral amplitude is given in terms of "dBr" units which references the echo return relative to a glass plate target standard. The dBr level so designated is a measure of tissue "reflectance." Reflectance as measured by this procedure includes the combined effects of both the tissue scattering properties and the propagation losses incurred along the illumination path through the eye anterior to the examined region of orbital fat. Calibrated reflectance data obtained in this manner can be very useful in predicting echoing properties of specific tissues. For example, in the case of orbital fat 6 mm behind the sclera, one can expect a return signal level approximately 60 dB below a glass plate target at an illumination frequency of 10 MHz. Repeated measurements of orbital fat on a number of clinical patients have yielded similar results confirming the reliability of this measurement.

Included in the computer post-processing is a least-square estimate of the spectral slope which in the case of Fig. 10 was computed as being 3.3 dB/MHz. Since These data were obtained without transmission through the lens, the spectral shaping with frequency can be assumed to be the result of a true backscatter spectra weighted by overlying fat. Other intervening tissues (i.e., the vitreous humor, retina, choroid and sclera) are known not to introduce any significant spectral shaping. Computed also by the least-squares procedure is the statistical uncertainty of spectral slope corresponding to the residual ripple about the fitted line. The computed slope uncertainty of 0.07 dB/MHz is representative of the present capability of the system as imposed by the spatial volume of tissue that can be averaged in realistic circumstances.

This paper has reviewed the characteristics and calibration of the system presently being used routinely

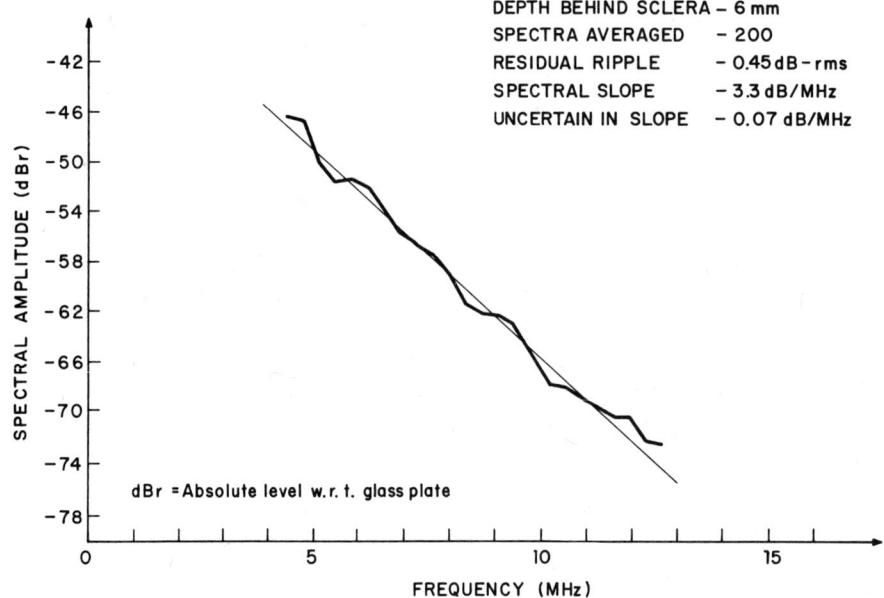

Fig. 7 Typical Spectrum of Orbital Fat

to collect spectral data from a clinical ultrasound system engaged in ophthalmic examinations. The paper (4) following this describes the various types of tissue results obtained. Representative examples on clinical data obtained for a variety of normal and abnormal tissue can be found in a paper (1) presented in the Opthalmology Session and in other publications.(6)

References

1. Smith, M.E., Franzen, L.A., Lizzi, F.L., Coleman, D.J. "Power Spectral Resonance Analysis in the Evaluation of Vitreous Pathology. Ultrasound in Medicine. Edited by D.N. White and R.W. Barnes, Plenum Press, New York pp. 255-256 1976

2. Sterns, G.K. and Coleman, D.J. "The Ultrasonic Characteristic of Orbital Dermoid Cysts,". Ultrasound in Medicine. Edited by D.N. White and R.W. Barnes. Plenum Press, New York. pp. 259-260 1976

3. Franzen, L.A., Smith, M.E., Coleman, D.J. and Jack, R.L., "Ultrasonographic Diagnosis of Tumors of the Anterior Choroid and Ciliary Body", Ultrasound in Medicine. Edited by D.N. White and R.W. Barnes, Plenum Press, New York pp. 257-258 1976.

4. Lizzi, F.L., Laviola, M.A. and Coleman, D.J., "Clinical Results Obtained with an Ultrasonic Spectral Analysis Syst m," Ultrasound in Medicine. Edited by D.N. White and R.W. Barnes. Plenum Press, New York. pp. 507-509 1976

5. Kelly, E., "Ultrasonic Energy" University of Illinois Press, Urbana, Illinois, 1964

6. Lizzi, F.L., and Laviola, M.A., "Power Spectrum Measurements of Ultrasonic Backscatter from Ocular Tissues," Ultrasonic Symposium Proceedings of the I.E.E.E. Group on Sonics and Ultrasonics, 1975.

Acknowledgement

This investigation was supported by Public Health Service grants EY-01212-02 and EY-01218-02 from the National Eye Institute.

EFFECT OF DRUGS ON MOUSE EMBRYO HEARTS IN ORGAN CULTURE VISUALIZED

BY ACOUSTIC MICROSCOPY

R. C. Eggleton*, L. W. Kessler**, F. S. Vinson* and G. B. Boder†; *Fortune-Fry Research Labs of the Indianapolis Center for Advanced Research and Indiana University School of Medicine, Indianapolis; **Sonoscan, Inc., Bensenville, Ill., and †Lilly Research Laboratories, Indianapolis

A method has been developed for sustaining 12-day mouse embryo hearts (approximately 2mm diameter) in organ culture for extended periods of time on the stage of an acoustic microscope. A culture chamber (Fig. 1) was fabricated to supply the hearts with a continuous flow of oxygenated culture medium to maintain contractile function. Simultaneous acoustic and optical viewing[1] of the hearts permits more complete observation of the contractile events than heretofore possible. Anatomical features of the heart such as atria, ventricles, coronaries and valves have been observed. A group of hearts has been maintained simultaneously in the chamber for several days. The hearts may be in various physiological conditions, e.g. synchronous, asynchronous, rhythmic or arrhythmic. Drugs are introduced into the chamber either by pulsing (as short as 5 sec. exposure) or using a continuous perfusion. The effectiveness of these agents in restoring normal behavior can be evaluated. A videotape will be presented to describe the method and results.

The only other successful organ culture method, described by Wildenthal[2], was not a continuous flow system and required a gaseous interface which is not compatible with acoustic microscopy. In this experiment the culture medium is oxygenated, brought to temperature, pumped through a 30µl chamber, and returned to the reservoir bottle (see Fig. 2). The culture medium consists of Grand Island 199, 10% newborn calf serum, 1% L-glutamine, 50mg/l insulin and an antibiotic. The circuit is made up of disposable administration sets. The oxygenator is an inverted separatory funnel packed with stainless steel wool. The tube running from the heat exchange bath to the stage is a disposable sterile cannula with a 0.030" lumen. The flow is 260µl/min. resulting in a complete change of fluid within the chamber every 7 seconds. The return is by gravity feed back

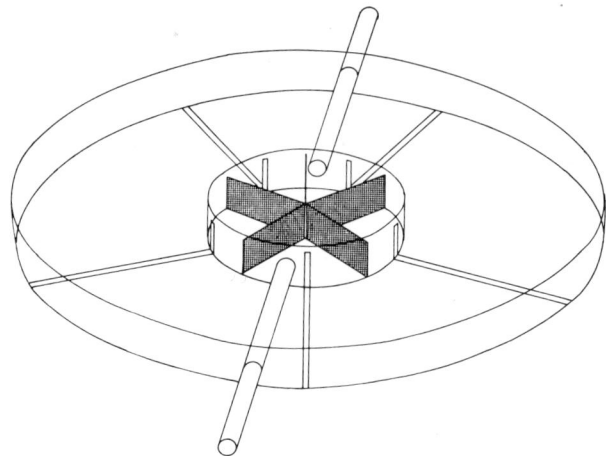

Fig. 1 - Lucite culture chamber for 5 mouse embryo hearts. The screen divides the 5mm diameter (30μl) chamber into 5 pie-shaped compartments and also serves as ground electrode for ECG recording. 5 foil active leads provide the other contacts. Tubes are provided for in- and out-flow of the culture medium.

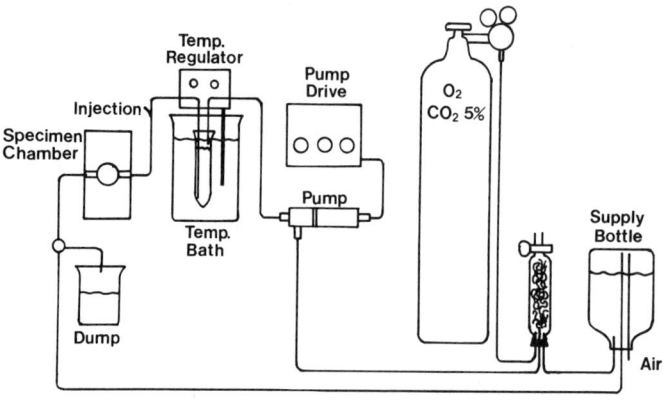

Fig. 2 - Schematic drawing of the culture medium flow circuit. Flow progresses from the supply bottle to the oxygenator and is then pumped through the heat exchanger to the stage, where it passes through the culture chamber and returns to the supply bottle by gravity feed. The valve is provided to dump the culture medium during drug administration.

to the reservoir bottle. A three-way valve on the chamber output permits diverting the outflow to a dump when the drugs are being administered.

Three methods of introducing drugs are used. The first method involves placing a drop of the drug on the stage; the material is introduced into the chamber by capillary action. Because the new material is likely to have a different index of refraction (either optically or acoustically), it is possible to see the drug on the screen as it is introduced and as soon as it clears the stage. Short pulses on the order of 5 seconds are possible by this method. The second method involves injecting the drug through an injection port in the administration set. This method provides for longer exposure of the heart to the drug (30-60 sec.). Prolonged exposures can be achieved by mixing the drug with the culture medium, thus adequate controls over the experimental environment can be achieved.

The functional activity of the heart can be recorded by two methods: placing ECG electrodes in the chamber to record electrical activity of the heart, or placing photocells on the television display tubes over the regions of the atria and ventricles. The brightness modulation of the display due to the motion of cardiac structures is converted to electrical signal and the relative phases of the cardiac activity can be determined. Thus by appropriate positioning of the photocells on the acoustic image display of the heart, a means of recording the integrity of the conduction pathways is provided. Synchronous, asynchronous, rhythmic and arrhythmic patterns are easily recognizable. The records of the acoustic and optical images are readily stored on magnetic tape. Because the data is already in TV format, commercial television or recorders may be used for this purpose. A tape will be presented in which a 2mm mouse embryo heart exhibits only atrial activity. The drug (Levophed) is introduced, and within a few seconds contractile activity is noted near the AV node. Within a short time activity commences at the apex and progresses up over the ventricles, restoring full contractile activity. The escape takes place over a number of cardiac cycles. This preparation constitutes a model which can be used effectively for evaluating cardioactive drugs.

This work is supported by Grant Number HL 16311 and the Indianapolis Center for Advanced Research.

REFERENCES

1. Eggleton, R. C. and Kessler, L. W.: Mouse Embryo Heart in Organ Culture Visualized by the Acoustic Microscope. In <u>Ultrasound in Medicine, Vol. 1</u>, ed. D. White (Plenum Press, NY 1975) pp. 537-542.
2. Wildenthal, K.: Long-term Maintenance of Spontaneously Beating Mouse Hearts in Organ Culture. J. Appl. Physiol. 30(1):153, 1971.

FIELD EVALUATION OF THE AIUM STANDARD 100 mm TEST OBJECT

AIUM Standards Committee
K. R. Erikson,[1] Chairman; P. L. Carson,[2] Vice-Chairman and H. F. Stewart[3]

INTRODUCTION

As instrumentation and diagnostic ability improves the need for quality control and standardization also increases. The AIUM Standards Committee has developed the 100 mm Test Object to partially fulfill this need. This test object, adopted by the AIUM in 1974, is shown in Figure 1. It is used for aligning, calibrating, and measuring the performance of pulse-echo diagnostic apparatus, including B-scanners. The standard defines geometrical arrangement and diameter of the stainless steel rods, but does not require a particular method of construction. The test object is to be immersed in a degassed aqueous solution whose velocity of sound is 1540 $\pm$ 10 meters per second.

In developing this standard over the past four years, two different construction methods have evolved. The simplest requires a seperate water container, which is inconvenient, but offers the best measurement flexibility. The second version with a self-contained solution is easier to use in many ways. While it is more costly and limits some measurements, this approach decreases "set-up" time significantly for routine tests, while still providing key information.

[1] Rohe Scientific Corporation, Santa Ana, CA 92705
[2] University of Colorado Medical Center, Denver, CO 80220
[3] Bureau of Radiological Health, Rockville, MD 20852

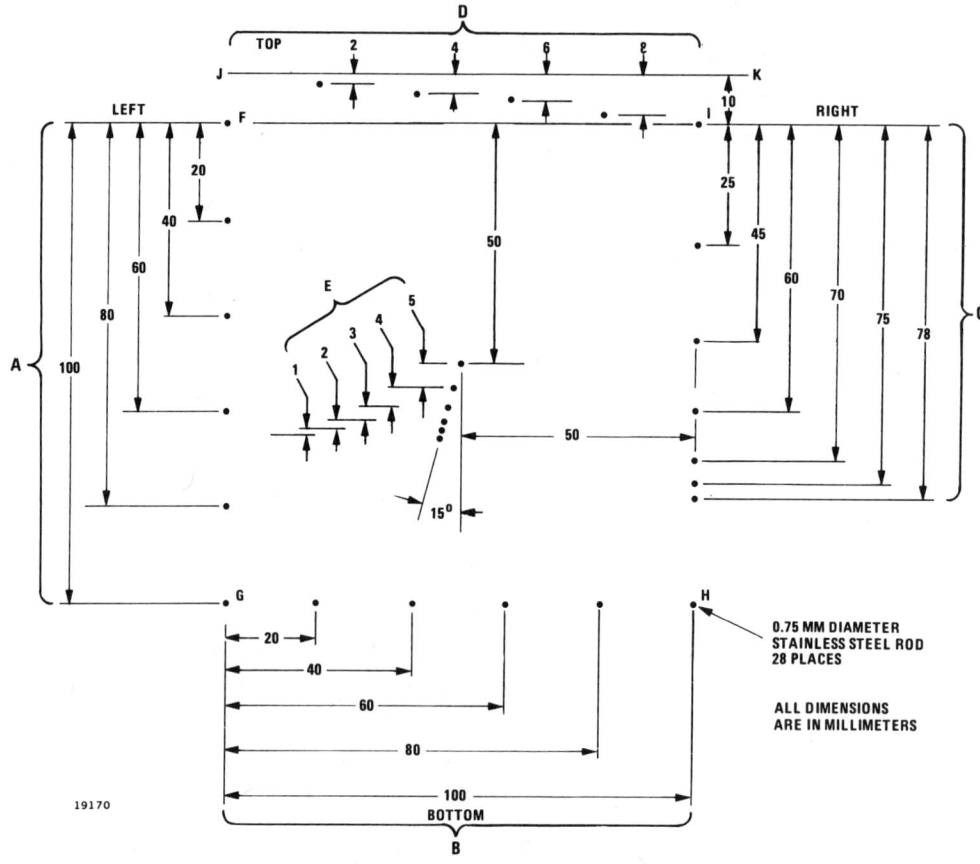

Figure 1. The AIUM 100 mm Test Object

Along with the definitions of the standard is a protocol for measuring depth calibration (rod group A in Figure 1); horizontal calibration (B); lateral resolution or beamwidth (C); dead zone or "ring down" distance (D); axial resolution (E) and scanned B-mode alignment (groups A-D). Procedures for measurement of gray scale and TGC parameters are also included.

When the test object was adopted at the 1974 AIUM meeting it was felt that a formal field evaluation of its usefulness was required. Evaluators were solicited at the meeting and over 50 laboratories, hospitals, and manufacturers responded. Dr. Harold Stewart and his group at The Bureau of Radiological Health have been kind enough to assist the standards committee in this project by providing test objects and by handling the mailing and calibration of the test objects. At the time of this meeting the first results of the evaluation are being compiled. Additional evaluations have been performed by Paul Carson and Steven Christenson of the University of Colorado. To date approximately 30 systems have been evaluated using the test object.

THE AIUM 100 mm TEST OBJECT

A brief review of the test object will be included here to familiarize the reader with its properties. This will make the initial results of the survey more understandable. For those wishing more details regarding the standard and the protocol please write to the Executive Secretary of the AIUM (Appendix I).

Figure 2 is a scan of a test object in a water tank made in a single pass. Note that the rods are displayed as horizontal smears due to the beamwidth of the transducer. The center group of rods is useful for measuring axial or depth resolution. The rods are inclined to 15 degrees to decrease acoustical shadowing. The rods on the left side are useful for depth calibration and also provide some indication of beamwidth with depth. The rods at the right side are useful for beamwidth measurement when scanned from the right side. The rods at the top can be used to measure the dead zone or ring down of the transducer when the transducer is scanned in a straight line 2 mm above the upper most rod. By adding two scans to Figure 2 (one scan with the transducer angled left at 45 degrees and the other right at 45 degrees) Figure 3 results. A perfectly aligned B-scanner will show symmetric asterisks. This particular scanner was quite well aligned.

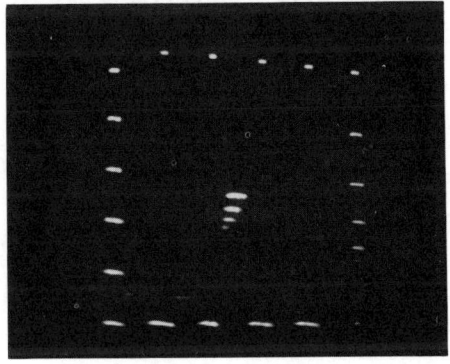 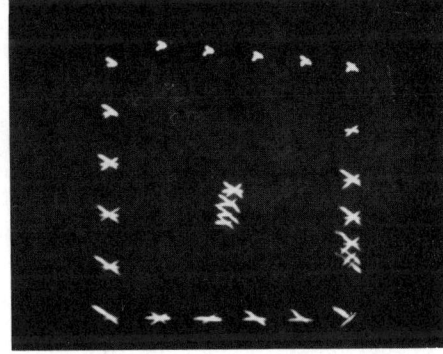

Figure 2. Single pass scan of test object showing beamwidth artifact.

Figure 3. Scan made in three passes.

An enclosed version of the test object is shown in Figure 4. The enclosed style is very convenient and is recommended for routine use. Commercial versions of both styles are available (Appendix I).

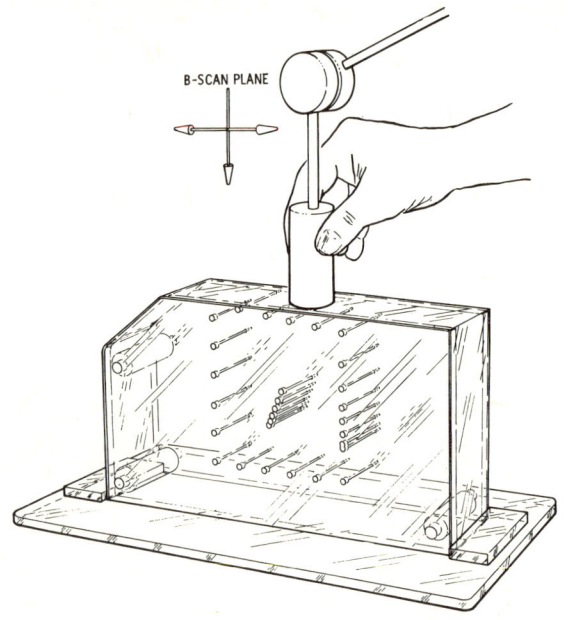

Figure 4. A version of the 100 mm Test Object with self-contained medium.

The present scanned B-mode alignment criterion requires that the centers of each of the displayed beamwidth smears fall within a 7 mm diameter circle for the outer rods in the test object. This criterion is one of the items to be checked in the evaluation program and should not be construed as a performance specification. It is rather an upper limit of alignment. Misalignment greater than this should be corrected by a service call.

SELECTED INITIAL RESULTS

Depth calibration is one of the easiest measurements to make with the test object. Figure 5 shows that many A-mode and B-mode depth calibrations were significantly in error, which could lead to errors in measurements of biparietal fetal head diameters, for example. Scanned B-mode alignment is the most dramatic and most important use of the test object. Four of the worst systems encountered are shown in Figure 6. We have reasonable certainty that such misaligned systems are being used daily in hospitals. Service can easily correct such problems once they are identified. Weekly scans of the test object are an easy way to verify proper operation.

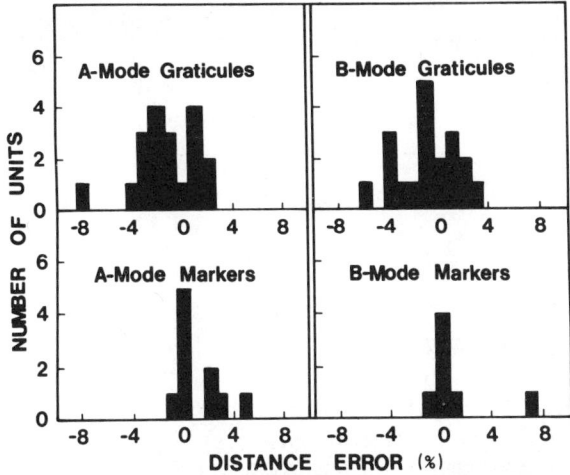

Figure 5. Depth calibration errors found in survey.

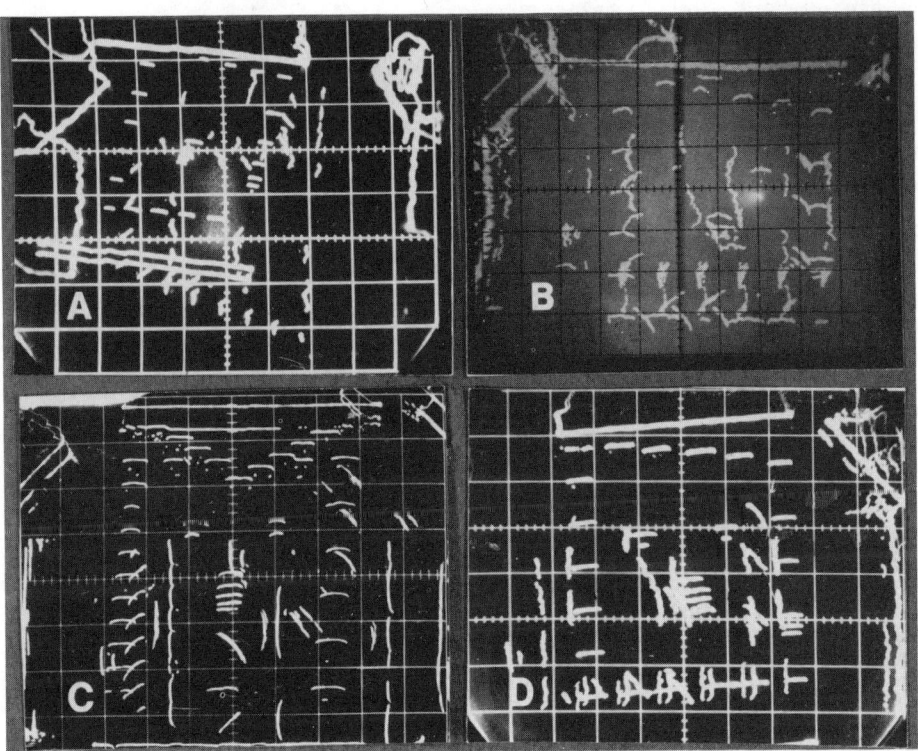

Figure 6. Four systems with the worst scanned B-mode alignment encountered. These scans were made with an enclosed test object which produces continuous lines at the top and sides of the scan, analogous to the "skin line" artifact in a human scan.

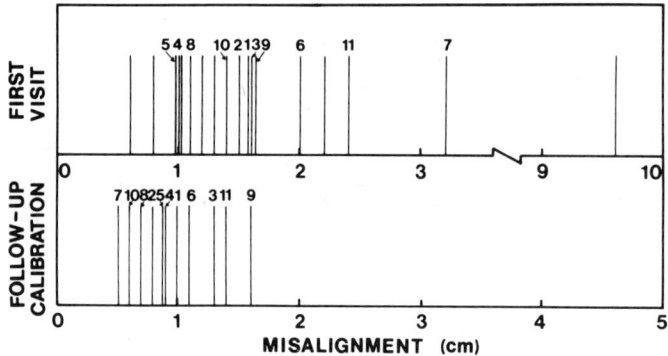

Figure 7. Scanned B-mode misalignment found in survey. The cm scale is correct. The upper chart summarizes misalignments initially found. After service some of these systems (denoted by the numbers) were remeasured.

Figure 7 demonstrates that service improved all the systems, although only a few actually improved to meet the 7 mm criterion. This is an area which warrants the immediate attention of manufacturers.

CONCLUSIONS

Although the survey is only partially finished at this time, some conclusions can be drawn. The test object is a rather rigorous test for many portions of an echoscope. Regular use is very important for establishing accurate system operation and preventing use of a degraded system. This can improve the confidence level of everyone involved.

In the evaluation itself, many expected problems are occurring. Enclosed test objects have been received through the mail in damaged condition. In the open test object, the water/alcohol solution must be prepared at the site. The use of tap water or water which was not degassed has led to bubbles formation on the rods. In one case, lack of correlation to a manufacturers test object was noted. In several instances portions of the protocol could not be performed due to lack of flexibility in some manufacturers instruments.

One comment made by several evaluators is that the test object procedures are difficult to follow and that simplification would be useful. This is planned, however, a short training course seems to be indicated for proper use of the test object. After such a course, ultrasonic technical specialists have used the test object successfully with repeatable results. We feel that this should be part of the training provided to such specialists. In addition, training sessions should be provided at annual meetings of the AIUM and AUSTS.

Experienced users have found that the enclosed version has many advantages. As one evaluator put it, "the closed model was a pleasure to use. In fact, during the evaluation I used the model in lecturing in physics and instructing technicians in scanning techniques. This was the most useful device I have yet seen for this purpose".

APPENDIX I

AIUM Executive Secretary, Box 26901, Oklahoma City, OK 73190

The AIUM Standards Committee has verified that the samples submitted by the following manufacturers meet the requirements of the standard. Any other manufacturer who wishes to use the AIUM name or test procedures must first submit a sample for such approval.

(Listed Alphabetically)

Anderson Technical
3350 Stuart Street
Denver, CO 80212
(303) 458-5872

Fred S. Dunning Company
2910 Franklin Blvd.
Sacramento, CA 95818
(916) 451-4259

Modern Electronic Diagnostics Corporation
820 West Hyde Park Blvd.
Inglewood, CA 90302
(213) 673-2201

Ross Chemical Associates
4237 Baldwin Avenue
El Monte, CA 91731
(213) 579-5880

TECHNICAL CONSIDERATIONS OF ULTRASONIC PHOTOGRAPHY:
CHOOSING THE RIGHT FILM AND PHOTOGRAPHIC PAPER FOR
YOUR PRESENT ULTRASOUND CAMERA SYSTEM

H. Walter Pepper, M.D. and Stefan Arnon, M.D.

Downey Park Radiology Medical Group, 1213 Coffee Road, Modesto, Calif. and University of California, Sacramento Medical Center, Davis, Calif.

The rapid growth and development of diagnostic ultrasound is best evident in the significant technical advances apparent in instrumentation and its resultant increased capabilities. Unfortunately parallel advances in camera systems and photographic systems have not as yet been as apparent. At the present time, Polaroid film is most widely used in diagnostic ultrasound because of its easy access and convenience. The rapid growth of ultrasonic units utilizing photographic film for permanent recording of images necessitates a reassessment of available films and photographic papers for this purpose. In an attempt to establish the most desirable film and photographic paper for ultrasonic purposes, evaluation of currently available photographic materials were reviewed. Before such a review is presented a brief summary of some basic photographic and ultrasonic principles is necessary.

Conventional echotomography generally utilizes a green phosphor oscilloscope. The actual phosphor of the oscilloscope may vary with the manufacturer, however, in all instances the image is predominantly green. For this reason, a highly orthochromatic (green sensitive) photographic film is somewhat helpful in photographing the resultant image. Orthochromatic film need not be less sensitive to other colors in the visible spectrum but is highly sensitive to the green band in the visible spectrum. It should also be noted that most green phosphor oscilloscopes produce a relatively low output of light necessitating a rather high speed photographic film. Conventional (bi-stable) ultrasonic images are inherently of high contrast. This does not mean that high contrast film is necessary in photographing conventional echotomography but rather resultant images will contain a high degree of contrast.

Gray-scale ultrasonography, on the other hand, utilizes a video type image built up by the scan converter and presented on a video monitor. This image is presented in a gray scale. Filming of gray scale images requires a low contrast film. Low contrast can be best explained by the quantity of gray tones which are visible on the film. Low contrast film is essential in photography of gray scale ultrasonography. It is also somewhat desirable in gray scale photography to choose a film with an acceptable latitude. This feature will allow accurate or acceptable exposure in view of minimal differences in available light.

After acceptable ultrasound photographic images are available the necessity for representing these images on photographic paper becomes necessary. The characteristics of contrast and latitude are then to be considered once more. One would prefer to use photographic paper with low contrast and acceptable latitude for reproducing these images. Low contrast qualities are essential in gray scale ultrasonography. The inherent high contrast of conventional ultrasonography can adequately be presented on low contrast film and photographic paper.

With these basic principals in mind, evaluation of several films was performed:

A. <u>Kodak Panatomic X</u>: This 7 mil, panchromatic acetate based film, although not specifically designed for rapid processor development, is easily handled in your radiographic rapid processor. Manufacturer estimation of photographic speed is 25 ASA. Development in the rapid processor at temperatures between 90 and 100° F necessitates readjustment of this rating. When developed in the rapid processor this film has a relative rating of approximately 400 ASA. As previously described the film is panchromatic and is sensitive to the full spectrum of visible light. It shows no specific sensitivity which would be advantageous in ultrasonic photography. The fact that this film is highly panchromatic and sensitive to red light necessitates absolute darkness in the dark room, unless appropriate safe lights are available. Processing of this film through the rapid processor imparts a pink tinge to the developed film. This is due to the slight incompatibility of the film with the rapid processor. The fact that this film is 7 mil as opposed to the 4 mil films described below makes it somewhat more difficult to work with. This film will produce a negative image of the oscilloscope or TV monitor. The latitude of the film is quite acceptable.

Development in the typical radiographic rapid processor at 90-100° F will significantly increase the inherent contrast qualities of the film. For these reasons listed above Panatomic X appears to be a less desirable film for ultrasonic use. It is included in this summary only in a classical sense.

   B. Kodak CFA 1530, RP/F: This 4 mil, orthochromatic estar based film, is specfically designed for development in rapid processors. Although no relative ASA rating is recommended by the manufacturer the relative speed of this film approaches 800 ASA. Since this film is highly orthochromatic the speed will vary somewhat depending upon which colors of the visible spectrum are present in the object to be photographed. This orthochromatic quality makes CFA 1530 quite desirable in photography of green phosphor oscilloscopes (conventional ultrasonography). Its high speed is likewise desirable in photography of low intensity green oscilloscopes. Although the film is highly orthochromatic it does exhibit some sensitivity to the red spectrum and therefore appropriate safe lights are necessary in the darkroom. The 4 mil estar base makes this film somewhat easier to work with when compared to the 7 mil base of Panatomic X. CFA 1530 is minimally blue tinted. When cleared through the processor this imparts a slight blue tinge to the base. This quality does not interfere with the image. The images are negative of the oscilloscope or TV monitor. The latitude of this film is excellent and its low contrast makes it quite desirable for gray scale photography. The combination of high sensitivity to green light, low contrast and relatively high speed makes this film an excellent choice fo both conventional and gray scale ultrasonic photography.

   C. Kodak CFV 1541, RP/FC: This 4 mil, orthochromatic, estar based film is quite similar to CFA 1530, RP/F. It differs slightly in its sensitivity to the green spectrum. Although slightly more sensitive to green light, its relative speed is slightly less. Its relative speed is approximately 600 ASA. Contrast of this film is slightly higher and its latitude slightly less than the CFA 1530 film. It is also slightly sensitive to red light and a Wratten 6-B Filter can be used in the dark room to provide adequate safe light. The image is again reversed, as this, like other films is a negative. For the reasons described above including slightly high contrast, decreased latitude, and slightly diminished speed, this film is somewhat less desirable for conventional and gray scale ultrasonic photography.

   D. Kodak Linagraph Shellburst 2476: This 4 mil,

orthochromatic, estar based film is likewise designed for rapid processor development. It is highly sensitive to green light but also slightly sensitive in the blue spectrum. This added quality does not detract from its ultrasonic purposes. Relative ASA rating of this film is approximately 1600 which makes it approximately 1f stop faster than the CFA 1530 film. The latitude of this film is excellent for ultrasonic photography. Its low contrast makes it extremely desirable for gray scale echotomography filming. The developed film is virtually totally transparent. This quality minimizes the apparent chemical and background fog on the film. The qualities of high speed, 4 mil estar based, low chemical and base fog but most of all its desirable latitude and contrast makes this film the most desirable for conventional and gray scale photography.

All of the films described above are available in 35 mm, 70 mm, and 90 mm sizes for application to various camera systems. The relative cost per frame will vary between 1.5 cents per frame for 35 mm film to approximately 14 cents per frame for 90 mm film. This compares quite favorably to the cost of comparable photographic or hard copy systems.

E. <u>Photographic Paper Evaluation</u>: Now that you have an accurate photographic negative of your conventional and gray scale ultrasound study, how can suitable prints or copies of this negative be made? It is obvious that photographic copies can be made utilizing the same type negative films or direct positive films. However, another alternative is available. Kodak Kodabrome RC Photographic Paper and Kodak Linagraph 1930 RC Photographic Paper are excellent alternatives in this regard. The Kodabrome RC photographic paper is easily available through retail photographic outlets and will allow you to make a print of suitable negatives. This may be accomplished by means of contact prints or 90 or 70 mm negative as well as enlargements of 35 mm negatives. These resin coated (RC) photographic papers may easily be developed in your rapid processor. Photographic enlargements comparable to Polaroid images may be made at a cost of less than 5 cents per print. Kodak Linagraphic 1930 RC photographic paper appears better designed for development in the rapid processor. The contrast and latitude of these photographic papers lend themselves excellently for reproduction of conventional as well as gray scale echotomographic images. These photographic papers are insensitive to normal darkroom safe lights and excellent enlargements may be reproduced in your darkroom utilizing inexpensive enlargers, contact printers or available duplication and subtraction material in your Radiographic Department. These techniques may be utilized in making copies or photographs to send to referring physicians or to affix as a permanent record on the patient's chart. Contact printing of the entire ultrasonic study provides an excellent copy of the study with the originals remaining in the Ultrasound or Radiographic Department.

It has been our purpose to describe several photographic systems which lend themselves excellently to conventional and gray scale ultrasound photography. Kodak Linagraph Shellburst 2476 film appears to be the most desirable film of the group described for this purpose. Its relative speed, sensitivity, latitude, contrast and cost make it quite desirable in this regard. We have also described a convenient alternative which will allow accurate photographic prints to be made of the resultant negatives.

A NEW MECHANICAL REAL TIME ULTRASONIC SCANNER

H.H. Holm; J. Kvist Kristensen; J.F. Pedersen; S. Hancke; A. Northeved; F. Jensen

Ultrasonic Laboratory, Department of Surgery H
Gentofte Hospital, DK-29oo Hellerup, Denmark

It is the aim of the paper to present a new mechanical contact scanner which is able to produce real time sector images as well as total sectional static images in gray scale.

The new mechanical dynamic contact scanner consists of a unit with a rotating wheel with a diameter of six cm. The wheel contains four identical two MHz transducers with a diameter of two cm. The transducer are placed radially at 9o degree intervals with their fronts at the periphery of the wheel. The wheel, partly encapsulated is, via a Bowden cable and a chain, driven by an asynchronic motor with an infinitely variable gear. The use of a chain drive makes it possible to displace the connection of the Bowden cable off the axis of the transducer wheel. This allows for a larger degree of tilting of the unit. The repetition frequency of the pulsgenerator is 2ooo per second.

The rotating scanner can be used handheld or mounted on a conventional scanning arm. The scanner is held with a slight pressure of the transducer wheel against the skin using abundant contact oil. With more than four revolutions per second of the transducer wheel real time 5o degree sector images are produced.

When mounted on the scanning arm one movement of the transducer unit across the abdomen in the sectional plane chosen will automatically produce a total compound scan. The scanning unit is especially designed for the production of gray scale scans.

With an open camera the scanning unit is moved across the body in approximately four seconds with about four revolutions of the transducer wheel per second.

The scanner presented seems to possess certain qualities:

1. The scanner can be used handheld. It can thus be moved freely in the area of interest which is easily and rapidly examined while observing the dynamic image on the oscilloscope.
2. The unit can be mounted on the rod system of a Gentofte-scanner (Mediscan, Copenhagen), but in principle it can be used in combination with any type of rod system.
3. High quality dynamic sector scans are produced.
4. The total cross sectional scans possess high degree gray scale characteristics with a special "soft" appearance.
5. Cross sectional scans are obtained rapidly.
6. Relative operator-independency of cross sectional scans.
7. The dynamic sector imaging guides appropriate cross sectional scans and saves time and film.
8. The scanner can be used for heart imaging.

ABDOMINAL SCANNING WITH A ROTATING TRANSDUCER

J. Kvist Kristensen; Fl. Jensen; H.H. Holm

Ultrasonic Laboratory, Department of Surgery H

Gentofte Hospital DK-2900 Hellerup Denmark

It is the aim of this paper to present the results obtained in practical use of a new mechanical real time contact scanner.

The scanner consists of a unit with a rotating wheel with a diameter of six cm. The wheel contains four identical two MHz transducers with a diameter of two cm. The transducers are placed radially at 9o degree intervals with their fronts at the periphery of the wheel. The wheel can rotate at a speed of one to five revolutions per second.

The unit can be used handheld, in which case a 5o degree sector will appear with a fixed orientation on the oscilloscope. With more than four revolutions per second of the transducer wheel real time images are produced.

When used handheld the unit can be moved freely and a 5o degree real time sector of any part of the abdomen can be obtained. It must, however, be admitted that the flat fronts of the transducers make the passage across ribs a little unpleasant. This type of scanning has the advantage of a quick orientation in the anatomy of the region to be examined. For example the longitudinal, possibly tortuous, orientation of the aorta is easily established so that correct transverse scans can be obtained. It may also be possible using only this type of imaging to exclude aneurysmatic dilatations of the aorta, whereas the sector is too small for a detailed outlining of a large aneurysm. Normal kidneys can be outlined satisfactorily with this type of sector scanning, possible pathological lesions are quickly demonstrated so efforts can be concentrated on detailed scanning of the lesions. Foetal movements and foetal heart movements may be more convincingly demonstrated than in conventional A - and TM - modes.

The unit can also be used mounted on a conventional scanning arm, and the potentiometers of the rod system will ensure a correct positioning of the dynamic sector on the oscilloscope. When the conventional scanner is automatically moveable in all planes the unit produces sector images with the same advantages as when used handheld.

When mounted on a scanning arm one movement of the transducer unit across the abdomen in the sectional plane chosen will automatically produce a total compound scan in gray scale, either with an open camera technique or by means of a scan converter. In this way total cross sectional scans are obtained in 3-4 seconds and the scans are relatively operator independant because of the automatic transducer angulation. Scans will be presented to illustrate the usefullness of this special type of gray scale scanner.

THAUMASCAN: IMPROVED IMAGE QUALITY AND CLINICAL USEFULNESS

Olaf T. von Ramm and Fredrick L. Thurstone

Departments of Medicine and Biomedical Engineering

Duke University, Durham, North Carolina 27710

During the past year of clinical evaluation, several modifications have been made to the two-dimensional, real time, high resolution ultrasound imaging system known as the Thaumascan system. These modifications were designed to improve the final image quality as well as to enhance the clinical usefulness of this imaging system in assessing various cardiac disorders.

In improving image quality, the inherent flexibility of the digital computer which controls the entire scan sequence was exploited in generating a non-sequential scan format. The transmit and receive phasing for this scan format is such that consecutive line images are generated at significantly different azimuth angles rather than at small incremental azimuth angles in a sequential manner from one extreme of the sector scan to the other. The result of such a non-sequential scan is to reduce the apparent flicker in the final image and, more importantly, to reduce reverberant artifacts. In addition, several transmit focal points were incorporated in the scan generation in an effort to further improve the depth of field of this system as well as to diminish the effect of coherent speckle.

The clinical usefulness of this system has been extended by the addition of an EKG display which appears on the same primary oscilloscope monitor used to display the acoustic images. In this way, both the EKG and the acoustic image can be recorded simultaneously onto video tape so that electrical and mechanical events of the cardiac cycle can be analyzed. A T-M mode feature which can be used in conjunction with the two-dimensional scan formation has also been incorporated into this system. The orientation of the T-M mode is selectable by means of a potentiometer and this orientation appears as an intensified line on the two-dimensional sector image.

REAL-TIME ULTRASOUND ABDOMINAL IMAGING

Michael L. Johnson, M.D., Olaf T. von Ramm, Ph.D.,
Joseph A. Kisslo, M.D. and Frederick Thurstone, Ph.D.
Depts. of Medicine, Radiology and Biomedical Engineering
Duke University Medical Center   Box 3373
Durham, North Carolina   27710

The application of the Thaumascan imaging system has been described in cardiology. This system can also be utilized in producing high quality images of abdominal structures. High resolution, real-time, tomographic images are generated at the rate of 30 frames/sec. in a circular sector format by electronically phasing a linear array of ultrasound transducers. The small, hand held transducer can be placed on any portion of the abdomen and various tomographic sections can readily be obtained. The real-time feature of this imaging system aids in localizing specific anatomic structures by providing immediate visual feedback.

The system has been used in obstetric patients for the rapid localization of the placenta and exclusion of placenta praevia. In addition, measurements of bi-parietal and transthoracic diameters are rapidly obtained. The real-time aspect allows detection of fetal heart and limb movement.

It has been useful in the evaluation of the jaundiced patient as the gall bladder, cystic duct, and biliary ducts can be localized and the transducer easily manipulated to follow their anatomic path. Gall stones have been demonstrated and this technique may prove useful in the patient with a non-visualized gall bladder.

Because of the real-time operation of the system, intra-abdominal vascular structures such as abdominal aortic aneurysms can be easily identified. The hepatic veins, inferior vena cava, portal vein, superior mesentery vein, abdominal aorta, superior mesentery artery, and renal arteries can be dynamically visualized.

It has been found that this system can be used diagnostically in all areas which are currently evaluated by the conventional compound B-mode scanning techniques. This real-time, two-dimensional ultrasound imaging system provides two unique advantages in visualizing intra-abdominal structures. First, the high resolution images allow accurate measurement and differentiation of two closely adjacent structures. Second, the real-time feature and ease of transducer manipulation allow rapid integration of spatial relationships.

CONTINUOUS CONTACT B ABDOMINAL SCANNING WITH PHOTOGRAPHIC

RECORDING FROM A NON-STORAGE OSCILLOSCOPE ON 70 MM FILM

M. Leon Skolnick, M.D.

University of Pittsburgh, Presbyterian-University Hosp.

Pittsburgh, Pennsylvania

This presentation will describe and illustrate a technique for improving the resolution of abdominal contact B scanning and decreasing time required for the examination. In brief, the technique is as follows: the transducer is manually rapidly moved in a linear motion back and forth over the abdominal region being examined while the entire scanner arm is continuously moved to the right or left by the motor operated traverse mechanism. The resultant scanning pattern is a raster arrangement with each scan being produced in 1-2 seconds, and separated by approximately 3-5 mm from the adjacent scan. Two oscilloscopes are employed; a non-storage one for image recording upon which a 70 mm hand operated camera is mounted, and a storage scope for image viewing. With the camera shutter kept open during the entire scan sequence, the film is rapidly advanced at the end of each transducer pass over the abdomen. At the same time the image on the storage scope is erased. Thus, as the operator rapidly views a series of images briefly on the storage scope, the images are recorded on the 70 mm camera from the non-storage scope. This procedure requires the coordinated effort of two persons, one to perform the scanning and erasing of the storage oscilloscope and the second person to advance the 70 mm camera.

Improved resolution results from this technique because: (1) more scans per unit area are produced -- approximately each scan is 3-5 mm apart, (2) each single sweep scan takes 1-2 seconds to perform, thereby eliminating organ unsharpness from respiratory motion or vascular pulsations, (3) the slight lateral variability in transducer position that can occur during compound scanning when using an arm that has several mm of lateral instability (as the Picker scanner arm has) is eliminated since only a single sweep is made to produce each scan.

This technique is best applied to areas in which the scan can be limited to an approximate length of 10-20 cm, and which can be examined using a simple linear or arcuate scanning motion. The upper abdomen, especially the pancreatic and hepatic areas, and the kidneys lend themselves best.

Examples of the application of this technique to the study of upper abdominal organs will be presented.

HIGH RESOLUTION ULTRASOUND MAMMOGRAPHY

G. Baum

Department of Ophthalmology, Albert Einstein
College of Medicine, Bronx, New York 10461

Ultrasound mammography has been carried out in over 100 patients. From the data produced by these studies, special equipment for ultrasound mammography has been designed and will be described.

From these studies, the range of normal ultrasonographic breast patterns have been determined and will be described.

The ultrasonographic characteristics of fibrocystic disease, lipomas, fibroadenomas, ductal hyperplasia, adenosis, and breast cancer will be described. These studies show that ultrasound mammography can correctly determine the benignity or malignancy of a breast mass in 86.7% of the cases examined with a false positive rate of 18.5% and a false negative of 7.6%.

The need for supplemental data processing will also be discussed.

Ultrasound mammography is a more effective medium for the early detection of breast cancer because it is capable of displaying structural changes which are invisible on x-ray mammography as well as the features displayed by x-ray mammography. Whereas x-ray mammography outlines the lesion, ultrasound mammography both outlines the lesion and produces a cross sectional view through the lesion. Structures as small as 1 mm in size may be resolved and the grey scale exceeds two density units. Ultrasound mammography produces a planigram or tomogram, so that there is no superimposition of structure. The exact plane and extent of the lesion may be determined in altitude, azimuth and depth. This makes it possible to measure the effects of surgery, radiation and chemotherapy on the breast in vivo, painlessly and without modifying the observed tissues in any way.

In addition, ultrasonographic radiation at the energy levels used for diagnostic purposes is painless, safe and does not have any immediate, delayed or cumulative injurious effect in contrast to x-ray radiation. Hence, this examination may be repeated at very frequent intervals.

This paper will present the specialized instrumentation and techniques that have been developed at this laboratory to cope with the unique properties of breast tissues.

The two breasts of a given patient are symmetrical organs when viewed at corresponding levels of observation. Even minor disease processes disturb this symmetry. Breast cancer produces a marked distortion of both the anatomical and amplitude symmetry of the two breasts.

This paper will also demonstrate a "staining" technique that we have developed to facilitate the localization and differential diagnosis of breast lesions. Thus, the problem at the present time is the problem of interpretation, rather than ultrasonographic visualization of breast lesions. Successful ultrasound mammography will require the use of high resolution extended dynamic range ultrasonographic equipment with a constant velocity arc scanner and supplemental data processing, such as that which we have developed.

Ultrasound and x-ray mammography are mutually complementary and supplemental techniques where the results of one form of examination can be used to enhance the findings of the other.

CLINICAL FINDINGS WITH REAL-TIME COLOR B-SCAN ULTRASONOGRAPHY

N. R. Bronson II; N. C. Pickering

Ophthalmological Electronics Laboratory
Southampton Hospital
Southampton, N. Y.   11968

At the past two meetings of the American Institute of Ultrasound in Medicine, the Ophthalmological Electronics Laboratory of Southampton Hospital has reported on the development of a real-time color B-scan ultrasonoscope using analog to digital conversion to supply color coded amplitude information and improved resolution. This paper will describe the clinical findings using this equipment, which improves the quality of the information presented without sacrificing any of the original objectives of ease of operation, simplicity of controls, real-time display, and low cost.

The original Bronson-Turner contact B-scan unit which was designed in this laboratory has been in production by a commercial company for nearly three years. This instrument has always displayed a gray scale equivalent to that discernible on a television picture tube. When it was introduced about three years ago, most other B-scan equipment was using storage tube displays which suppressed gray scale. General agreement now seems to have been reached on the importance of gray scale, and much of our work has been focussed on increasing the number of visible steps of amplitude information. Since only a few steps of gray can be distinguished by a viewer, and those few subject to visible error, it was believed that color-coding of amplitude information can provide many more unambiguous steps of information. This has proven to be the case. Furthermore, digitizing of the amplitude information has resulted in elimination of "blooming" caused by bright parts of an analog picture display. This feature alone has resulted in much improved resolution. Wide-band amplification, and circuits to produce short pulses have contributed to improved axial resolution.

The purpose of this paper is to present clinical results based on direct comparison of essentially simultaneous examination of patients with a production Bronson-Turner B scan and the new color B scan. The work is being done to establish the usefulness of color-coding in actual diagnosis, and to determine whether the improved resolution and dynamic range really give the doctor more useful information on which to base his clinical diagnoses.

Note: The acoustic power density of this equipment is approximately 1.5 milliwatts/cm^2 at the focal point of the transducer.

STUDIES WITH A REAL-TIME

ACOUSTICAL HOLOGRAPHY SYSTEM

Walter W. Taylor, M.D.

Holosonics, Inc.

2950 George Washington Way, Richland WA   99352

The system described operates on the principle of acoustical holography and allows the operator to display and record soft tissue information in real-time. By interchanging transducer assemblies, the system can function in any one of three different frequency ranges to best accommodate imaging of various tissues and tissue path lengths.

The transducers are 4" x 4" in size and operate in such a manner that multiple frequencies are emitted within each frequency range. Frequency ranges which may be selected for specific imaging are 1.5MHz to 2.3MHz, 2.1MHz to 3.1MHz, and 3.5MHz to 4.4MHz. The ultrasound passed through the subject, is pulsed 143 times per second having a pulse duration of 200 microseconds and a duty factor of about 3%. The average power density ranges between 5 and 50MW/cm^2.

The ultrasound is transmitted horizontally through the patient Coupling is accomplished with neoprene bags, attached to the water tanks, which contact the patient's skin surfaces. The ultrasound which has passed through the patient is focused on a liquid surface using an acoustic lens and a reflecting surface. A reference transducer emits the same frequencies to the liquid surface. This liquid surface is illuminated by an Argon laser and the reflected light is used to form an optical presentation. This presentation can be photographed directly with single frames, movies, or a television camera can be used and the images viewed in real-time. If videotape recordings are made, the images may be reviewed in real-time, slow motion, or single frames. This provides a variety of methods for recording dynamic information and the operator has an important advantage viewing dynamic information in real-time during the study.

One of the major problems encountered in through transmission holographic imaging has been diffraction effects and small "lines" which degrade image quality. By using five discrete frequencies, each 200 microseconds in duration, pulsed sequentially from the lowest frequency to the highest frequency at 143Hz rate, the diffraction lines are swept from the image. The frequencies utilized are determined for the best efficiency of each transducer. The transducer (frequency image) chosen for any given study was selected, primarily, on the tissue path length and, secondarily, on the type of tissue or structure being imaged.

The examples of imaging listed illustrate some of the areas of potential clinical use. Soft tissue orthopedic information includes structures such as tendons, muscles, vessels, etc., as well as dynamic information. Tumors, breast studies, observations in fetal activity, and other examples are also presented.

TRANSSKULL ULTRASONIC IMPEDIOGRAPHY

Joie Pierce Jones*; Francis J. Fry**

*Bolt Beranek and Newman Inc.; **Fortune-Fry Res. Lab.

*Cambridge, Mass.; **Indianapolis, Indiana

Ultrasonic impediography (see papers presented by J.P. Jones at 1974 AIUM meeting) offers a means, at least in principle, for quantitatively and noninvasively measuring tissue acoustical properties at appropriate anatomical sites within the body. Such measurements are of diagnostic value since many types of normal and abnormal tissues can be uniquely classified in terms of their acoustical properties. Impediography involves (1) a processing operation upon both the incident and reflected acoustical signals to obtain a time-domain characterization of system dynamics known as the system impulse response, and (2) a processing operation upon the system impulse response to obtain physical properties as a function of acoustic travel time. In present implementations, the impulse response is obtained by time-domain deconvolution of short duration deterministic incident and reflected waveforms. A profile of specific acoustical impedance vs acoustic travel time (or position) is generated through analytical relationships involving the integral of the impulse response.

The measurement of attenuation is intimately and irrevocably tied to the measurement of impedance. In fact, in many cases, knowledge of the attenuation may be more important to tissue identification than knowledge of the impedance. Impediographic determination of attenuation requires either the _a priori_ knowledge of the impedance, measurement of both the transmitted and the reflected waves, calibration of the system using a known internal reflecting interface, or the use of more sophisticated signal processing techniques.

Present impediographic processing schemes are capable of generating impedance profiles for simple physical models and soft tissue structures where simple absorption is the only mechanism producing attenuation. More complex situations require alternate approaches. For example, transskull impediography is difficult because of aberrations introduced by the presence of skull bone. An analysis of the propagation of sound through skull shows that the spatial waveform, at least for focused beams, remains virtually unchanged whereas the temporal characteristics are severely altered. Transskull signal degeneration is a result of frequency dependent absorption, multipath reflections, mode conversion, curvature, and scattering. The importance each of these effects plays in altering an acoustic signal propagated through the skull will be discussed in this presentation. Also, a number of transskull experiments will be described and several alternative processing schemes for transskull impediography will be presented.

ACOUSTIC IMPEDANCE PROFILING--AN EXPERIMENTAL MODEL AND ANALYTICAL

STUDY WITH IMPLICATIONS FOR MEDICAL DIAGNOSIS

A. C. Kak, F. J. Fry* and Narendra T. Sanghvi*
Department of Electrical Engineering, Purdue University,
Lafayette, Indiana 47906; *Indianapolis Center for Advanced Research, Indiana University Medical Center,
Indianapolis, Indiana 46202

Acoustic parameter characterization in a quantitative manner of soft tissues in the human body leading to tissue typing is a potentially powerful method for clinical medicine for the identification and differentiation of disease entities in a non-invasive manner. This study is concerned with the determination of acoustic impedance profiles in physical models, some of which have impedance values in the range of body soft tissues. The physical models used are of a plane parallel face multilayer type, and the sound beam is at normal incidence to the plane face. Materials used in the model have been lucite, silastic rubber of varying compositions (to produce acoustic impedance differences of a few percent at a boundary) and ρc rubber. The sound beams used mostly have been those produced by focused transceivers (fundamental frequency 1MHz-2MHz) delivering a damped oscillatory wave. A more nearly unipolar pulse unfocused beam has also been used (supplied by Bolt, Beranek and Newman of Cambridge, Massachusetts under a subcontractual arrangement). The algorithms used for the study involve the determination of the impulse response of the medium; and from this impulse response, the impedance profile is computed.

The algorithm implemented for impulse response determination in this study uses the matched filtering technique, which is applicable to a rather generalized acoustic waveform (damped oscillatory wave). Computations of impedance are made in a stepwise fashion throughout the layered medium based on a priori knowledge of the impedance of the first layer and the determination of the reflection coefficient at the first and subsequent interfaces.

Attenuation in the interrogated model must be included if the impedance values are to be correct. Layer thickness is computed automatically since an acoustic velocity is inserted for each layer. Each layer has inserted an acoustic pressure absorption coefficient (α_n) so that the attenuation per layer is automatically computed from the layer thickness and the α_n.

The first implemented algorithm for impedance profiling is capable of handling twelve discrete layers, although in principle the method can be expanded to include the more medically realistic case of perhaps an order of magnitude larger number of reflection zones.

Experimental data show computed values of impedance profiles for models involving three and five layers (i.e., water-lucite-water-lucite-water) in which reproducibility of the impedance values made on the same target over a number of runs is maintained within a few percent of the average values. The magnitude of the computed impedance values are within 10% of the absolute values, which is considered quite good at this stage of development.

This work is supported in part by National Institutes of Health Contract N01-NS-3-2319, "Study and Test Ultrasonic Technique for Diagnosis of Cerebral Disorders".

COMPUTERIZATION OF MANUAL ECHOCARDIOGRAMS

L. R. Smith, S. E. Wixson

University of Alabama in Birmingham

Birmingham, Alabama 35294

Knowledge of the function of cardiac chambers and related structures is essential in the study of patients with ischemic and valvular heart disease. Furthermore, serial determination of cardiac dimensions from patients in the coronary care unit has become increasingly important in clinical research. Echocardiography is a useful non-invasive tool, but manual reduction of data from a large number of studies is prohibitive. This paper describes a computer system that provides a variety of quantitative measurements from manual echocardiograms.

Echoes are recorded on polaroid film or strip charts from commercially available equipment. Each structure echo is manually traced using a Graf/Pen(R) graphic digitizer. Incoming X-Y coordinates are scanned by computer programs in real time and coordinates which differ from the last saved points by a predetermined distance are saved. The predetermined distance is varied depending on the structure being traced. Structures are traced for 3-4 cardiac cycles, and displayed on a CRT for quality control review. Data is transferred to background processing programs for data editing, resampling, and analysis. Analysis is done asynchronously with the acquisition of subsequent data providing the researcher with results immediately upon completion of digitizing. Data and calculations are stored in disk files, indexed by time and date, for linkage to angiographic and hemodynamic data from the catheterization laboratory. Raw data and calculations can be reviewed on a CRT in the dimensional analysis laboratory for hard copy or at the patient's bedside for physician review.

*Supported in part by Myocardial Infarction Research Unit Program Contract PH 43-67-1441.

Structures studied are left ventricular (LV) posterior and septal wall, mitral valve, and aortic valve. The LV pressure waveform is digitized permitting an estimation of LV mechanical performance. The onset of the QRS, and end of the T wave from the ECG are acquired to provide a cardiac cycle frame of reference. Analysis consists of wall motion, velocity, mass, and stress, LV volume, pressure-volume relationships, mitral valve leaflet velocity, and aortic root movement. Future work will be directed toward serial comparison of LV wall parameters for patients undergoing drug infusion or metabolic studies.

ULTRASONIC VISUALIZATION AND THERAPEUTIC COMPUTER CONTROLLED SYSTEM

F. J. Fry, N. T. Sanghvi, R. C. Eggleton and W. Erdmann

Indianapolis Center for Advanced Research, Indiana University School of Medicine, Indianapolis, Indiana 46202

During the last two years at the Fortune-Fry Research Laboratories of the Indianapolis Center for Advanced Research, a major effort has been applied in developing an automated computer controlled multi-purpose ultrasound system. The system offers multifold advantages since it is potentially useful for real time monitoring and controlling of ultrasound instruments and image information acquisition. Particularly, the automated system provides an easy interaction in real time between a physician and the visualization/therapeutic equipment through the assistance of a minicomputer. Presently the described system is in use on a routine clinical research basis, especially, for brain scanning and some very selective brain irradiation procedures.

The complete system is composed of a DEC PDP-11/45 computer running under a Real-Time Executive Operating System, a three-dimensional programmable coordinate scanning device, an IFI M469 5-KW wideband amplifier for high intensity irradiation, an ultrasonic visualization system and a Biomation high-speed digitizer.

The ultrasound visualization system consists of a focused wide aperture transceiver, a wideband linear/logarithmic amplifier and a PEP-400 video-graphic scan converter and associated electronics. The visualization system can be used for B-mode display presentation in linear mode of scanning in x or y coordinate, or in 45° sector scan mode. The echogram displaying appropriate soft tissue details is received on-line and stored on the video-graphic system. The stored echogram can be recorded on a video tape for future usage or these video analog signals can be digitized selectively at a 10 or 20 nsec sampling rate using the Biomation high-speed digitizer. The digitized signals can be fed to the computer via a direct memory access interface to the computer for processing to determine acoustic parameters which can be utilized in a quantitative evaluation for diagnostic purposes.

The therapeutic system is a closed loop fail-safe unit and contains a focused high intensity ultrasonic lesioning transducer, a 5-KW wideband amplifier, a frequency synthesizer, a programmable attenuator and the feedback circuitry. From the received echogram information a physician can localize the area for high intensity ultrasound treatment and can decide the dosage of high intensity irradiation. The dosage parameters (time duration and intensity) and coordinates information are fed to the computer via a CRT terminal. The computer then presets a programmable counter, and the programmable attenuator with appropriate values, and opens the gate of a frequency synthesizer to feed the sinusoidal signal to the 5-KW amplifier through the programmable attenuator for high intensity irradiation. Also, the same signal is fed to the programmable counter which in turn is incremented at each cycle, and at the end of the preset count, it gives an interrupt signal to the computer, and the computer closes the gate of the frequency synthesizer that in turn stops the source signal to the 5-KW amplifier.

This system is a further evolution of the systems approach to ultrasonic diagnosis and surgery followed in our laboratories for the past two decades.

HOW TO SELECT TRANSDUCERS TO ACHIEVE BEST CLINICAL RESULTS BY USE
OF TRANSDUCER BEAM SENSITIVITY PROFILE DATA

R. E. Hileman, Ph.D.

Unirad Corporation
4765 Oakland Street
Denver, Colorado 80239

Transducers can now be selected to achieve optimum clinical results by using beam sensitivity profile graphs. Each organ being examined may require different transducer focus, diameter and frequency. With unfocused transducers now being abandoned in favor of a range of focused transducers, it is important to have an accurate understanding of what each transducer beam pattern actually looks like to know when to use it and when not to use it. The beam sensitivity profile is a graph showing how the beam sensitivity varies both with depth from the transducer face and how it varies with lateral alignment. Beam sensitivity profiles give a clear indication of the zone of optimum sensitivity and optimum focus. To examine a particular organ, it is important to select a transducer whose focal zone covers this depth.

Most transducers used in the past were specified by giving frequency, diameter and radius of curvature. The clinician was expected to figure out how these influenced beam profile or accept someone's word for what he should use. Many users believe that a 13 mm diameter, 2.25 MHz frequency and a 10 cm radius of curvature transducer gives best focus at 10 cm when, in fact, it gives best focus in the 4 to 8 cm zone and is rather poor at 10 cm depths. This misconception is avoided when focal zone is specified from a beam profile graph. Presently, many transducers are labeled as having been "focused at so many cm" and a single number given, that number really being a radius of curvature. This practice is misleading and should be stopped since radius of curvature and best focal point are not the same number.

The text book explanations of transducer patterns presented to ultrasound seminars are couched in terms of near fields, transition zones, Y0+ points and far fields, or even worse, as Fresnel zones and Fraunhofer zones. Usually some rather involved mathematical formulas are given. These are the last things a doctor trying to establish what is wrong with a patient should worry about. A beam sensitivity plot removes this difficulty and gives full scale graphs of actual patterns with no mathematics or arm waving. Another textbook misconception often shows the on axis sensitivity going through several humps and nulls near the transducer face implying inability to detect objects in the null region. The error here is the mathematics is for continuous sinusoidal excitation while the diagnostic ultrasound transducers are driven by very short pulses which avoid such nulls. The beam profile plots are made using the same pulse as the diagnostic ultrasound system so the plots show what really goes on. Still another misconception is side lobes which occur with continuous excitation, but do not exist with medical transducers driven by short pulses.

The talk will cover the following items:
1. Transducer beam measurements
2. How a beam sensitivity profile is obtained
3. How to interpret beam sensitivity profiles in relationship to clinical applications
4. Profiles of commonly used transducers
5. Examples of scans showing transducer effects
6. Optimization of TGC and gain with different transducers to get the best results
7. Common myths about transducers (aging, variation from transducer to transducer, fragility, etc.)

A CHOPPED ULTRASONIC RADIOMETER OPERATING IN THE MILLIWATT

ACOUSTICAL POWER LEVELS WITH DIGITAL READOUT

T. Matzuk, Ph.D., P.E., W.A. Lindgren, M.S.

Carnegie-Mellon University and Xenotec Ltd.

Pittsburgh, Pennsylvania

An ultrasonic power radiometer working on the radiation pressure principle utilizes the chopped-beam principle to extend the sensitivity of direct radiation pressure measurements into the range of ultrasonic power emission levels commonly associated with diagnostic medical instruments.

In the chopped-beam radiometer, a novel mechanical chopper means is described wherein the acoustical field under test is periodically and quietly interrupted at a slow mechanical rate. Behind the chopper is located a mechanically resonant radiation-pressure sensor that converts acoustical energy into a frequency-modulated electrical detection signal.

By so deriving this frequency-modulated signal from an acoustical field on a totally broadband basis, the opportunity for signal-to-noise ratio enhancement and final display readout entirely via digital signal-processing means is realized, and the need to rely upon conventional piezoelectric field mapping transducers is eliminated.

Several different types of resonant radiation-pressure sensors are shown, and several types of mechanical chopper designs are discussed. Through transmission images depicting beam pattern diffractions, attenuations, and beam-spreading through the chopper geometrics illustrate the development of the acoustical beam progressing through the mechanical pathway of the radiometer mechanism in both the open and closed positions.

By scanning the acoustical opening of the radiometer with a small search transducer probe, the effective acoustical aperture is determined, and contour plots are presented to show the effect of tapering of acoustical sensitivity, otherwise known as "crowning", across the axis of the aperture.

Insonification tests done at several frequencies show that the cumulative effects of mechanical devices in the radiometer lead to a broadband frequency dependence describable largely in terms of acoustical absorption versus frequency in the constituent materials. The effects of standing waves, such as experienced when testing C.W. doppler instruments, are discussed, and special contouring of the radiometer geometry is proposed to minimize standing wave effects.

Tissue Interactions

THE THERAPEUTIC EFFICACY OF ULTRASOUND IN TREATMENT OF AUTOIMMUNE

DISEASES

J. A. Roseboro[*]; A. Norman[**]; H. I. Machleder[**]; H. Paulus[**];
R. Stern[**]
[*]Department of Environmental Sciences and Engineering
University of North Carolina, Chapel Hill, N.C. 27514
[**]University of California, Los Angeles, Calif. 09924

The elimination of circulating lymphocytes by thoracic duct (TD) cannulation and drainage has shown to be a effective treatment for some patients suffering the debilitating effects of autoimmune diseases.[1-5] It was desirable to eliminate the thoracic duct cannulation procedure and its associated lengthy hospitalization. Therefore, we undertook an experimental investigation of the feasibility of using an ultrasonic transducer for the destruction of TD lymphocytes in vivo. In addition we investigated potential hazards to the patient associated with this method of lymphocyte destruction. Finally, we made some measurements on the ultrasonic destruction of red blood cells and Hela cells in order to determine whether there were qualitative or quantitative differences among different cell types in their response to ultrasound. In this article we present data showing that it is feasible to destroy lymphocytes by ultrasonic irradiation (US) of the thoracic duct fluid and that it may be feasible to destroy lymphocytes by the ultrasonic irradiation of peripheral blood. In addition data is presented which show that red cells and Hela cells exhibit similar sensitivities to that shown for lymphocytes following ultrasonic irradiation.

MATERIALS AND METHODS

Thoracic duct lymphocytes (TDL) were obtained from patients undergoing thoracic duct drainage. Peripheral blood lymphocytes (PBL) and red blood cells (RBC) were obtained from normal donors. The PBL were separated from the whole blood by standard methods.[6] Gey's strain Hela cells were obtained from commercial sources. For irradiation and culture the cells were suspended at concentrations of 1-5 x 10^6 per ml in a tissue culture medium consisting of NCTC-109, 80%, and fetal calf serum, 20%, together with penicillin and streptomycin. The suspensions were cultured at 37°C in a 5% CO_2 atmosphere. Cell concentrations were determined by counting in a hemocytometer. Viable lymphocytes were differentiated from non-viable ones by the exclusion of the vital stain erythrosin B. Hela cell viability was determined by the ability of exposed cells to form colonies.

The experimental arrangement for US is shown in Figure 1. The peristaltic pump drives the cell suspensions at flow rates of about 1 ml/min - approximately the flow rate in the human thoracic duct. The cells pass through a hollow cylindrical PZT4 or PZT5 piezoelectric transducer (Valpey Corp., Holliston, Mass.) of length 2.54 cm and with an inside diameter of 0.64 cm. The transducers were driven at their resonant frequencies of 65 and 52 kHz, respectively by an oscillator (Hewlitt-Packard, Model 650A), a tone burst generator (General Radio Co., Type 1396) and an amplifier (General Radio Co., Type 1233-A). The total power, P, to the transducer was determined by measuring the change in temperature of the fluid as it passed through the transducer. The power determined in this way includes both the acoustic power output and the power that goes directly to heating the transducer. The temperature was measured at the reservoir which was maintained at the room temperature of 20 - 22°C, and by a thermocouple right at the exit of the transducer. As expected the temperature change was directly proportional to the duty cycle, at constant flow rate and voltage, and proportional to the square of the voltage at constant flow rate and duty cycle. For flow rates of 1 ml/min a temperature change of 16°C correspond to a total power input of 1.12 W. At higher power levels the transducer and the cell suspensions were cooled in order to keep the maximum temperature of the lymphocyte suspensions below 41°C.

The mode of oscillation of the transducer at resonance is primarily the circumferential mode. Since the internal diameter of the transducer is too small to permit radial resonant modes to propagate in the fluid, the system must be considered as a lumped parameter. Based on the voltage applied to the transducer at maximum input power of 2.24 W (112 volts rms), the measured Q of the system, 30, the electromechanical coupling coefficient, 0.33, and the appropriate piezoelectric strain constant d_{31} (-122 x 10^{-12} meters/volt), we estimate the pressure amplitude in the transducer was in the range of 1-5 x 10^5 dynes/cm^2. At this power level, but not at lower power, bubbles characteristic of cavitation were observed. The threshold for cavitation in water is conventionally taken as about 10^6 dynes/cm^2, although cavitation at lower pressures has been reported. The two estimates of pressure considering the uncertainties in each are not inconsistent. They are consistent in suggesting that the pressure is too low for cavitation at power levels below 0.5 W, the interesting range for our proposed application.

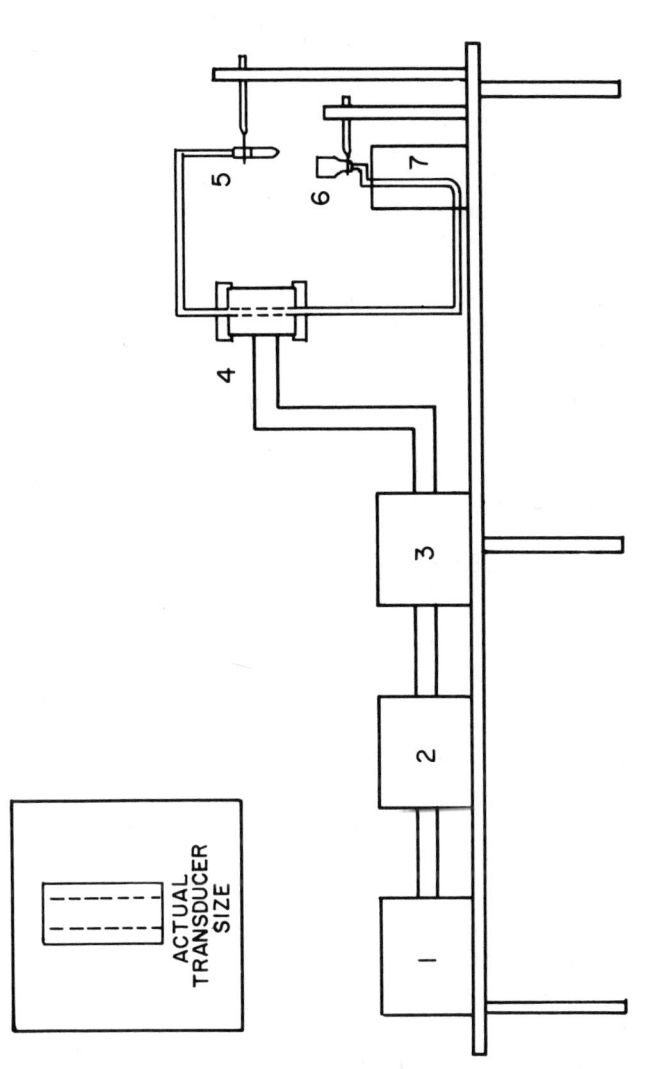

FIG. 1. Experimental arrangement for the exposure of cells to ultrasound: 1) Oscillator, 2) Tone-Burst Generator, 3) Amplifier, 4) Transducer, 5) Specimen Tube, 6) Specimen Reservoir, and 7) Peristaltic Pump.

The cells are exposed to ultrasound for a time, t, that is the product of the residence time in the transducer and the duty cycle (the fraction of the time the transducer is on). The duty cycle was controlled by the tone burst generator. The exposure dose, D, was calculated as D = Pt. To convert to an ultrasound exposure dose it is necessary to multiply by the 0.33 conversion efficiency. All powers given on the graphs are expressed as total power to the transducer.

RESULTS

Figure 2 shows typical results obtained with TDL irradiated at two power levels and assayed either immediately after US or following an eight day incubation after US. The per cent viable cells are plotted on a semi-log plot against the exposure dose which was varied by changing the duty cycle. The results can be represented adequately by the expression $S = \exp(-D/D_o)$ where S is the surviving fraction of cells and D_o is the dose which reduces the survival to 37% of its initial (unirradiated) level. As can be seen the results are independent of power, but strongly dependent on the time after irradiation at which the cells are assayed. The value of D_o appears to decrease from 27J when measured at day zero to 4J when measured at day eight. Figure 3 shows the very similar results obtained with PBL. The D_o changed from 27J at day zero to 8J six days after irradiation.

The results of many runs are summarized in Figure 4 which shows the value of D_o for lymphocytes, both PBL and TDL, as a function of transducer power at zero, 6, and 8 days after irradiation. As can be seen D_o is independent of power over the range of 0.12 to 2.24 watts but decreases by an order of magnitude when the lymphocytes are cultured for one week after US and then assayed.

Similar results were obtained with the RBC. These are summarized in Figure 5 which shows that D_o is independent of power over the range of 0.7 to 2.24 watts. When the power was reduced below 0.7 watts, the RBC were no longer destroyed. This threshold for the destruction of RBC separates sharply the behavior of RBC and PBL. This is illustrated in Figure 6 which show the results of repeated passages of RBC and PBL through a transducer operated at 0.5 watts. As can be seen the RBC are unaffected, whereas the survival of the PBL is reduced by a constant fraction with each pass through the transducer.

Figure 7 shows the effect on colony formation of Hela cells exposed to varying doses of ultrasound. As with the results of other mammalian cell types survival is an exponential function of dose. The D_o value was 18J, not significantly different from that of lymphocytes and red cells.

To examine whether US will alter the thoracic duct fluid in ways

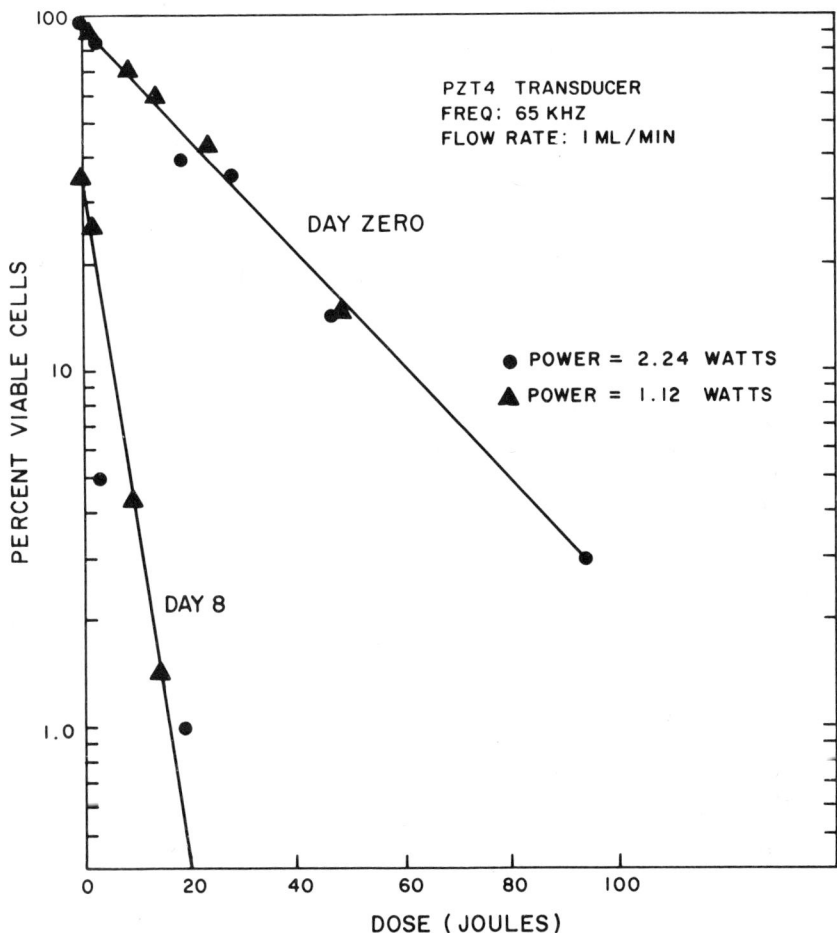

FIG. 2. Survival of TD lymphocytes at two power levels. The cells were exposed to a transducer driven at 65 kHz at an output power of either 1.12 W or 2.24 W.

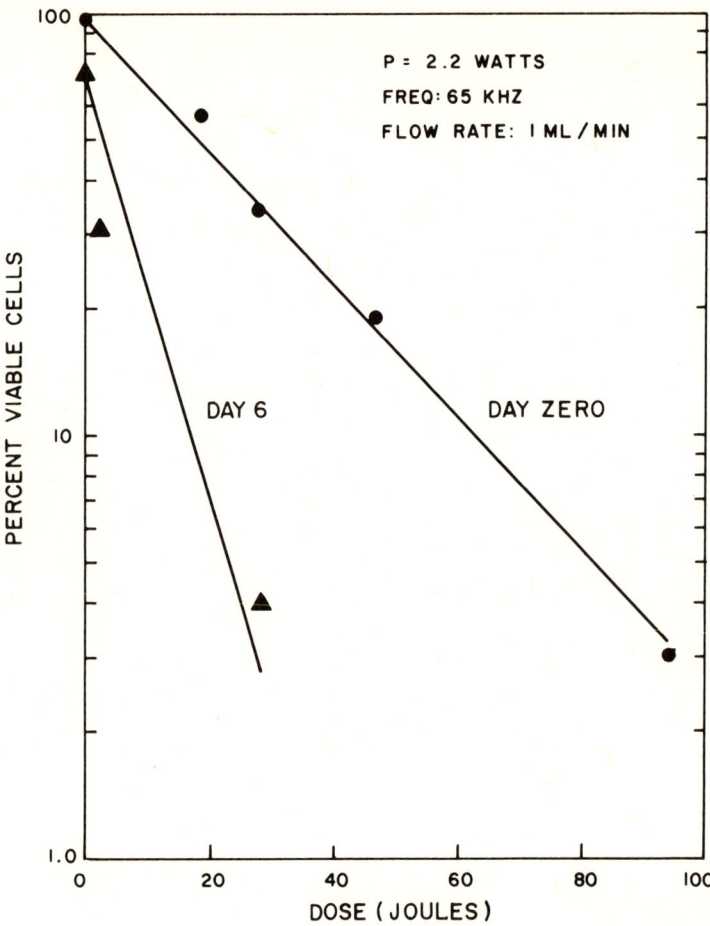

FIG. 3. Survival of human peripheral blood lymphocytes in a varying sonic field of frequency 65 kHz (and power of 2.24 W) and a flow-rate of 1 ml/min. Curves are shown for day zero and day 6 survival.

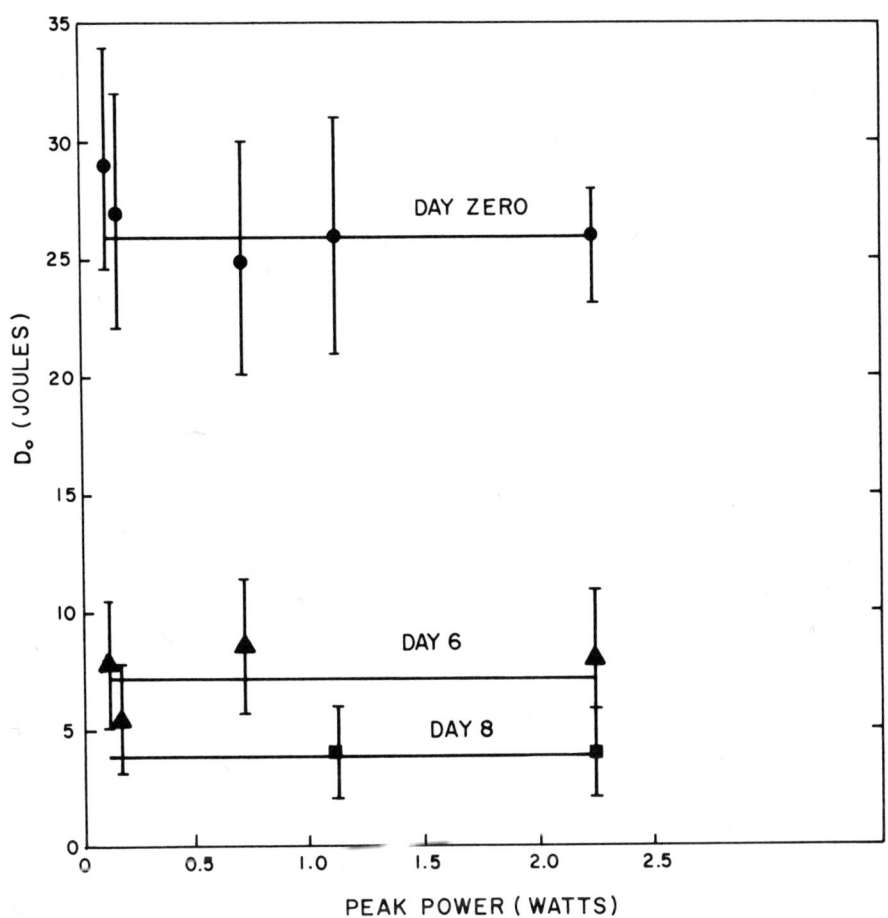

FIG. 4. D_0 values vs peak power for lymphocytes as determined in vitro. Values were measured at a frequency of 65 kHz and a flow-rate of 1 ml/min.

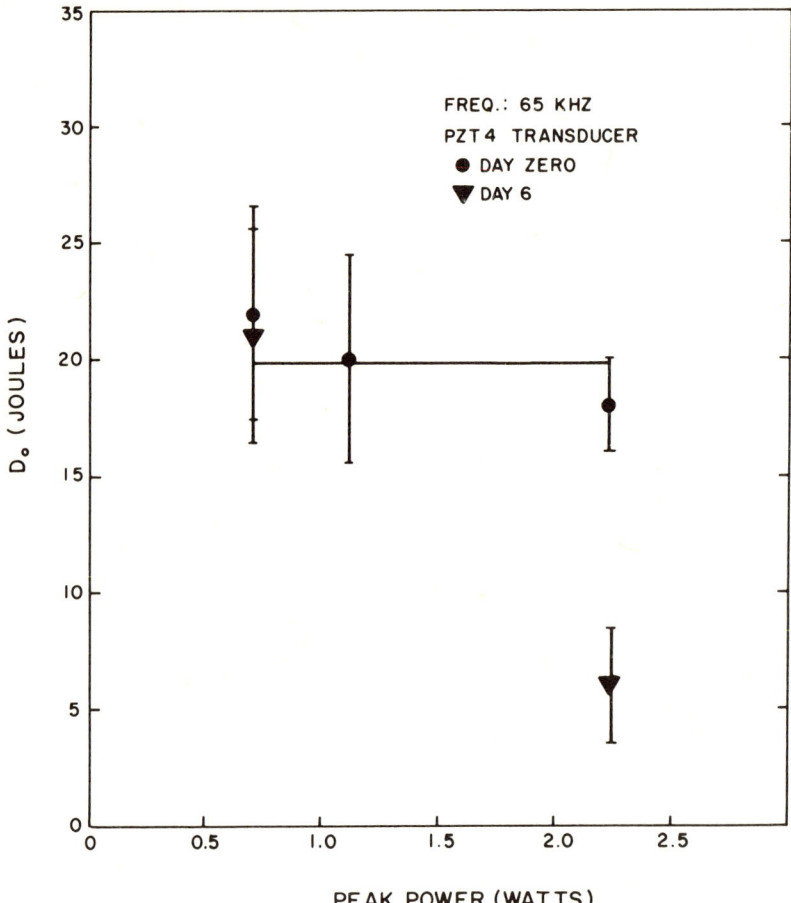

FIG. 5. D_0 values vs peak power for red cells as determined in vitro. Values were measured at a frequency of 65 kHz and a flow-rate of 1 ml/min.

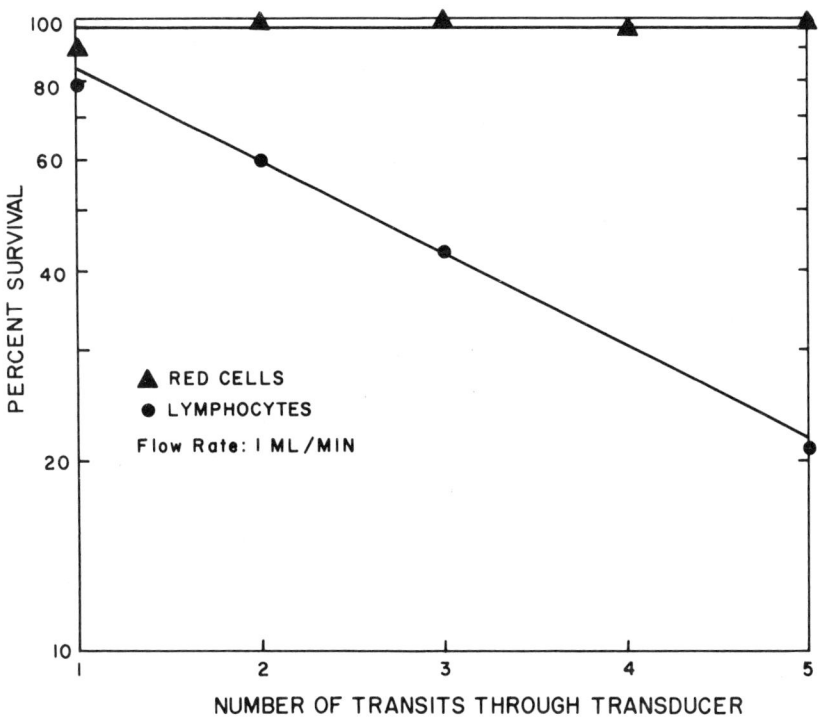

FIG. 6. RBC and peripheral blood lymphocyte survival in suspension after exposure to 0.5 W ultrasonic intensity. At a flow-rate of 1 ml/min and a cylindrical volume of 0.7 cc for the transducer the exposure time for the cells was 42 sec. for each pass through the transducer.

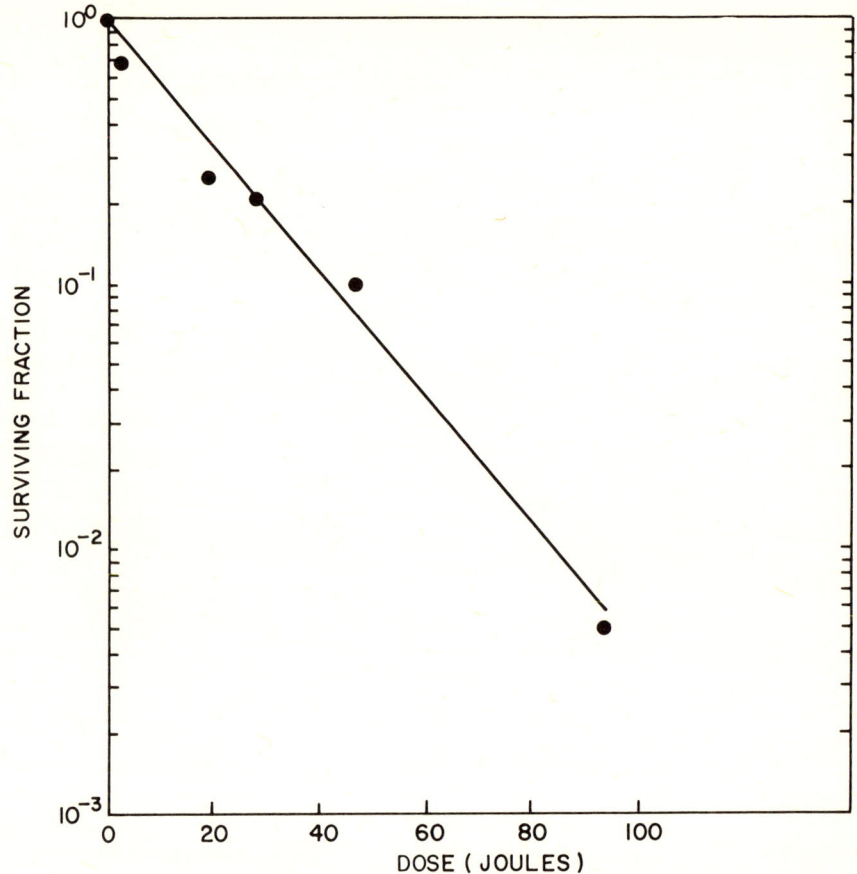

FIG. 7. Survival of Hela cells. Survival was assayed by counting the number of colonies that were produced in 14 days of culture.

that might be harmful to the patient, the cell free fluid was irradiated. Lymphocytes were then suspended in the irradiated fluid and incubated for various times. The results plotted in Figure 8 do not show any deleterious effect of the irradiated thoracic duct fluid on the lymphocytes. To investigate this question further the proteins in the thoracic duct fluid were analyzed by gel disc electrophoresis. The results pictured in Figure 9 fail to reveal any effect of exposing the thoracic duct fluid for one minute to power levels up to 2.24 W. These results suggest that the irradiated thoracic duct fluid will not be injurious to the patient.

DISCUSSION

The survival of TDL, PBL, and RBC following exposure to US decreases markedly with time after irradiation. In this respect the effect of US resembles the effect of ultraviolet and ionizing radiations on lymphocytes.[6,7] Thus we can destroy the bulk of lymphocytes at power levels and doses that are far smaller than those required for the immediate lysis of the cells. These results together with an apparent lack of effect of the US on the thoracic duct fluid suggest that US can be useful for the destruction in patients of lymphocytes circulating through the thoracic duct.

The surviving fraction of lymphocytes is independent of the power to the transducer over the entire range investigated of 0.12 to 2.24 W. For the RBC the survival is independent of power only from 0.7 to 2.24 W. Below 0.7 W the US seems to have no effect on the RBC. It may be feasible, therefore, to eliminate lymphocytes by irradiating the blood of patients at power levels below the threshold for RBC damage.

The presence of a power threshold for RBC destruction demonstrates that peak power as well as average power and total energy is an important consideration in assessing the potential hazards of ultrasonic equipment. The demonstration of delayed effects of ultrasound on the survival of lymphocytes also indicates that estimating the hazards of ultrasonic exposure is a complex undertaking.

The lymphocyte suspensions were heated as they passed through the transducer and exposed to the elevated temperature for about one minute. Lymphocytes can be rapidly heated to 45°C and kept at that temperature for 30 minutes or kept at 42°C for six hours without significant effects on immediate survival.[8] In these experiments the maximum temperature of the lymphocytes did not exceed 41°C. Moreover, for power levels of 1 W or less their temperature was never more than the 37°C at which they are routinely cultured. Thus heat effects cannot account for the observed cell killing. It seems probable that the cell killing is due to the sheer stresses produced in the cell suspensions by US induced microstreaming. It is known that there is a

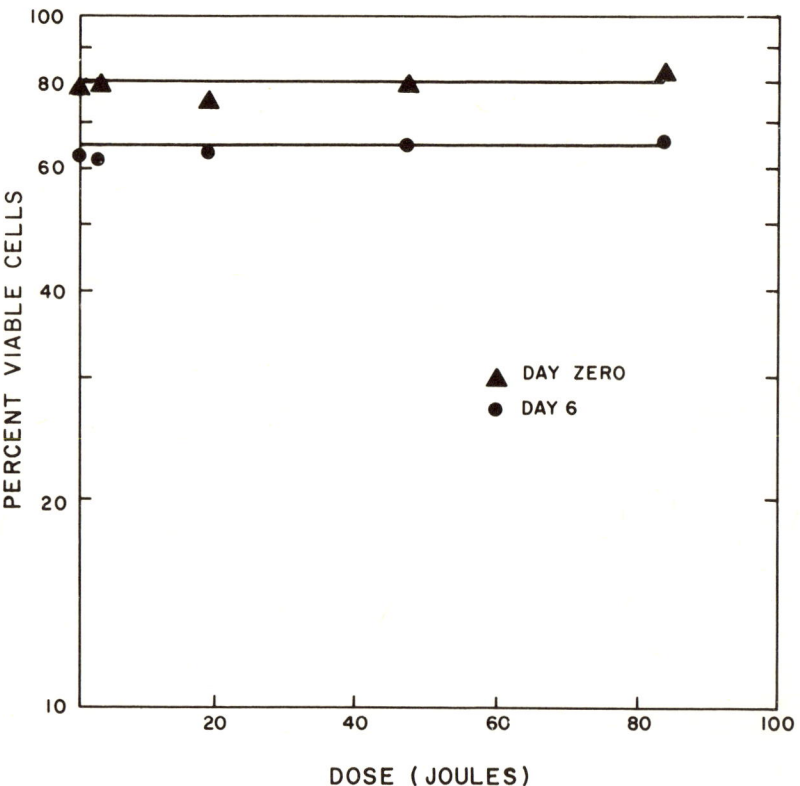

FIGURE 8. Thoracic Duct Lymphocyte Survival in Sonicated Medium.

TREATMENT OF AUTOIMMUNE DISEASES

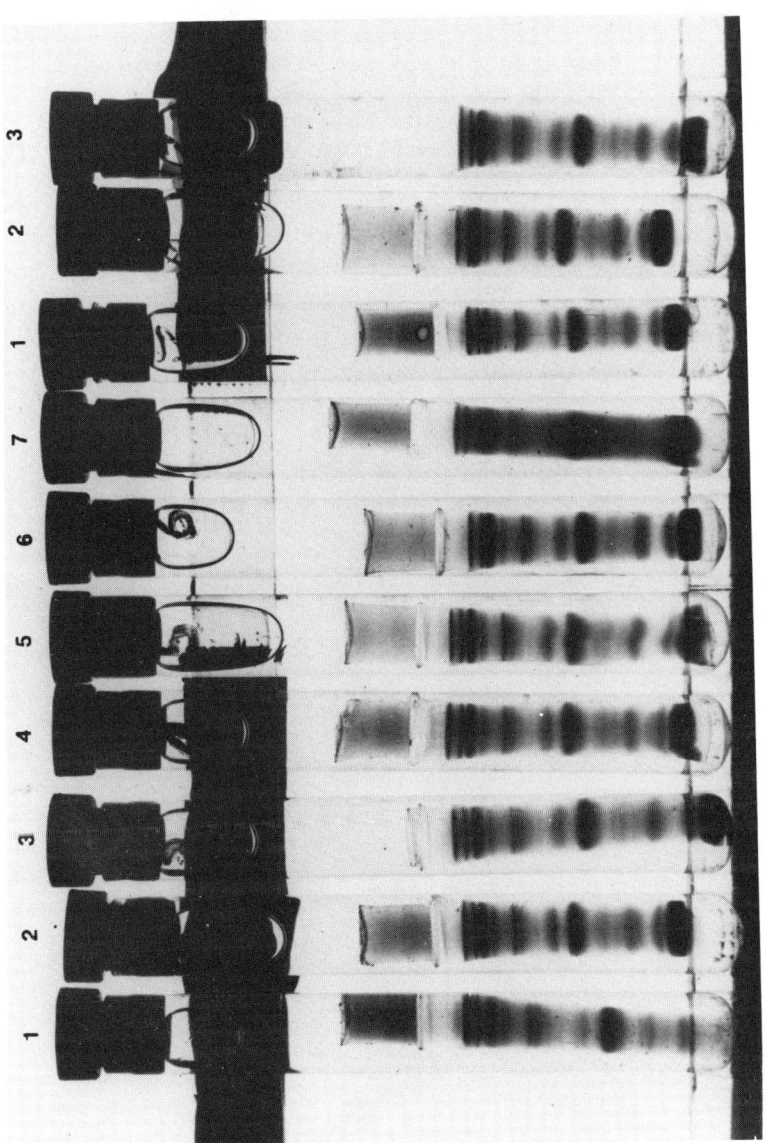

FIG. 9. Electrophoretic gel "disc" patterns of human thoracic-duct lymph. Lymph was collected from patients after introduction of a silastic tube cannula into the thoracic duct during general anesthesia. Note extreme similarity between sonicated (tubes 1 – 5) and non-sonicated (tube 6) lymph patterns. Tube 7 was exposed to 1 Mega-red ionizing radiation for comparison.

threshold for the destruction of RBC by microstreaming.[9] We were surprised, however, not to find a threshold for the destruction of lymphocytes at approximately the same power levels. Thin sections (by transmission electron microscopy) of sonicated Hela cells exhibited some morphological changes in their mitochondria that are commonly found in dying cells almost without regard to the mechanism of killing.[10,11,12] Very likely these mitochondrial changes are secondary to some failure in the cell membrane. Whatever the mechanisms the finding of differential thresholds for the destruction of various cell types opens up the possibility that US can be used for selective cell killing in a number of possible applications. To exploit this possibility clinically will take much work both on the design of appropriate equipment and on experimental investigations of the effects of US on living cells.

REFERENCES

1. A. E. Dumont, J. M. Donald, and J. M. Mulholland, Ann. Surg. 160, 374 (1964).

2. N. L. Tilney and J. E. Murray, Transplant. 5, 1204 (1967).

3. O. Wezelius, V. Laine, B. Lindstrom, and M. Klochars, Acta Med. Scand. 187, 539 (1970).

4. K. Bergstrom, C. Franksson, G. Matell and G. von Reis, Europ. Neurol. 9, 157 (1973).

5. V. Bartos and V. Brzeh, Chirurg. 44, 110 (1973).

6. R. G. Evans and A. Norman, Radiation Res. 36, 287 (1968).

7. R. Santos Mello, D. Kwan, and A. Norman, Radiation Res. 60, 482 (1974).

8. P. Spiegler and A. Norman, Radiation Res. 43, 187 (1970).

9. A. R. Williams, W. L. Nyborg and D. E. Hughes, Science. 169, 871 (1970).

10. D. W. van Bekkum, et al, Transactions of the Faraday Society. 49, pp. 329-334 (1953).

11. Anna Goldfeder, Cellular Radiation Biology, pp. 539-546, The Williams and Wilkins Co. (1965).

12. B. F. Trump, et al, The Role of Energy Metabolism, Ion, and Water Shifts in the Pathogenesis of Cell Injury, Dept. of Pathology, Duke University, Durham, N. C. (1973).

INTERCELLULAR GAS: ITS ROLE IN SONATED PLANT TISSUE

A. Gershoy; D. L. Miller; W. L. Nyborg

Departments of Physics and Botany
University of Vermont, Burlington 05401

INTRODUCTION

Determination of conditions for safe medical use of ultrasound is a difficult task which will probably require a variety of approaches. In one approach, model systems are chosen as test objects, in the hope of gaining insights which are useful generally. Plant tissues have been found suitable as models; with these, bio-effects are found at relatively low ultrasonic levels and can be investigated to determine thresholds. We shall not review previous studies here but note that in recent work a group of investigators at the University of Rochester[1-4] have shown that 2 MHz ultrasound at intensities as low as 1 W/cm^2 causes damage in the form of chromosome anomalies in plant roots. They also have shown that the temperature elevation during sonication is negligible under their conditions, and have suggested that some kind of cavitation might be a mechanism for the sonic effect.

The question of mechanisms for bio-effects at low levels has practical significance. For if the principles were known we should be able to anticipate with greater confidence whether damage would or would not occur in animal tissues at similar low levels. In a previous paper[5] and in this one we present evidence that a special form of cavitation occurs generally in sonated plant tissues, and may be a dominant mechanism for bio-effects at near-threshold conditions.

The term "cavitation" has been used broadly to cover many kinds of activity. Flynn[6] has distinguished between (1) stable cavitation, which occurs at moderate sound levels and involves pulsation of gas bubbles over an indefinite period of time; and (2) <u>transient</u> cavitation, a violent activity which occurs only at relatively high levels. In plant tissues at low and moderate ultrasonic levels our concern is with stable cavitation, involving small gaseous bodies whose dimensions are of the order of microns. When considering very small gas bubbles another distinction should be made: (A) they may be caused by the ultrasound to grow from pre-existing gaseous "nuclei" of even smaller (characteristically invisible) size, or (B) they may already be present in the medium previous to the application of ultrasound. Under condition A, little or no activity is observed until a threshold amplitude is reached which is high enough to cause growth of active (often visible) bubbles from the pre-existing nuclei. The sonically grown micro-bubbles will usually shrink and disappear when the sound field is removed, or its amplitude decreased. In contrast, under conditions B the stresses and movements set up by bubble vibration increase continuously as the sonic amplitude is increased from zero, allowing such bio-changes as can be produced by weak stresses to occur at relatively low amplitudes. It has been realized since the work of Harvey[7] that if statement B is to apply, some means must exist to stabilize the small bubbles against their tendency to dissolve. In plant tissues it appears that conditions B apply very commonly; here gas exists in a ramifying network of narrow channels in intercellular space. It is expected then, that in these tissues, bioeffects should occur at relatively low ultrasonic levels.

INTERCELLULAR GAS IN PLANT TISSUES

The intercellular gas spaces in plant tissues may be found in a wide variety of sizes and shapes, but for our purposes we consider just two classes: Type 1, a ramification of channels following the junctions of three or more enlarged rounded polyhedral cells and Type 2, an array of parallel tubes along the junctions of three or more elongated cells. Where two cells are in direct contact a cemented double wall is formed without any apparent free gas. The Type 1 configuration occurs in some fleshy leaves and in germinating seeds, and looks generally the same regardless of viewing angle; Type 2 spaces are observed in stem and root tissue, and their appearance depends on the orientation of the tissue sample. Examples are shown in Figs. 1 and 2 of gas-filled regions as they appear in thin samples of living plant tissues immersed in water and viewed with transmitted light. Gaseous spaces appear dark in the photographs because the interfaces of gas with water are curved and thus refract the transmitted light.

Fig. 1A shows a section from the interior of a fleshy leaf of Senecio sp. family Compositae. The dark pentagonal pattern seen in the photograph is a Type 1 configuration. One can test such dark regions for gas by applying high amplitude sound, which can cause the gas to be expelled. After such treatment the channels, now fluid-filled, appear more transparent. Fig. 1B shows the same cellular junctions as Fig. 1A after the expulsion of the intercellular gas.

Figure 1C shows a Type 2 array found in a portion of a living leaf of the aquatic plant Elodea canadensis. It is in Elodea that Johnsson and Lindvall[8] reported viscoelastic changes produced by ultrasound at (average ?) intensity levels of only 40 mW/cm^2.

That plant roots are richly provided with Type 2 gas-filled channels is shown in Figs 1D and 2A for the broad bean Vicia faba; we have found the same to be true for Indian corn, Zea mays. In Fig. 1D, a transverse section from the elongation region of the root tip, the intercellular tubes appear in their triangular cross section at the junctions of three cells. In the longitudinal section of Fig. 2A, one can discern dark streaks parallel to the axis of the root in the meristimatic region; these are the triangular tubes of Fig. 1D in their long aspect. The distribution of gas in roots of Vicia faba is of special interest because of its extensive use in studies of ultrasonic bio-effects; a review has been published by Carstensen, Miller and Linke.[3]

Further examples of intercellular gas spaces appear in Figure 2B, a transverse section of highly vacuolate tissue from the petiole of squash (Type 2 channels), and Fig. 2C, another example from Vicia faba. For this latter photograph, a slice was taken from the cotyledon of a germinating seed (near the cotyledonary node) to display the extensive Type 1 gaseous channels with which this storage tissue is provided.

We have made similar hand sections of many tissues, from very young embryos to maturing plants, and we are struck by the ubiquity of gas as a separate phase in the cellular environment. That space for the gas should exist between the cells is reasonable from the geometry of cells in contact. The volume and shape of intercellular spaces is quite variable, dependent on cell sizes, shapes and contacts. Intercellular gas might be expected also from another point of view: Since plant tissues lack the circulatory system of animals the presence of an extensively ramifying network of gas-filled cavities is an adaptive device for ensuring an adequate (quickly diffusing) supply of oxygen and CO_2.

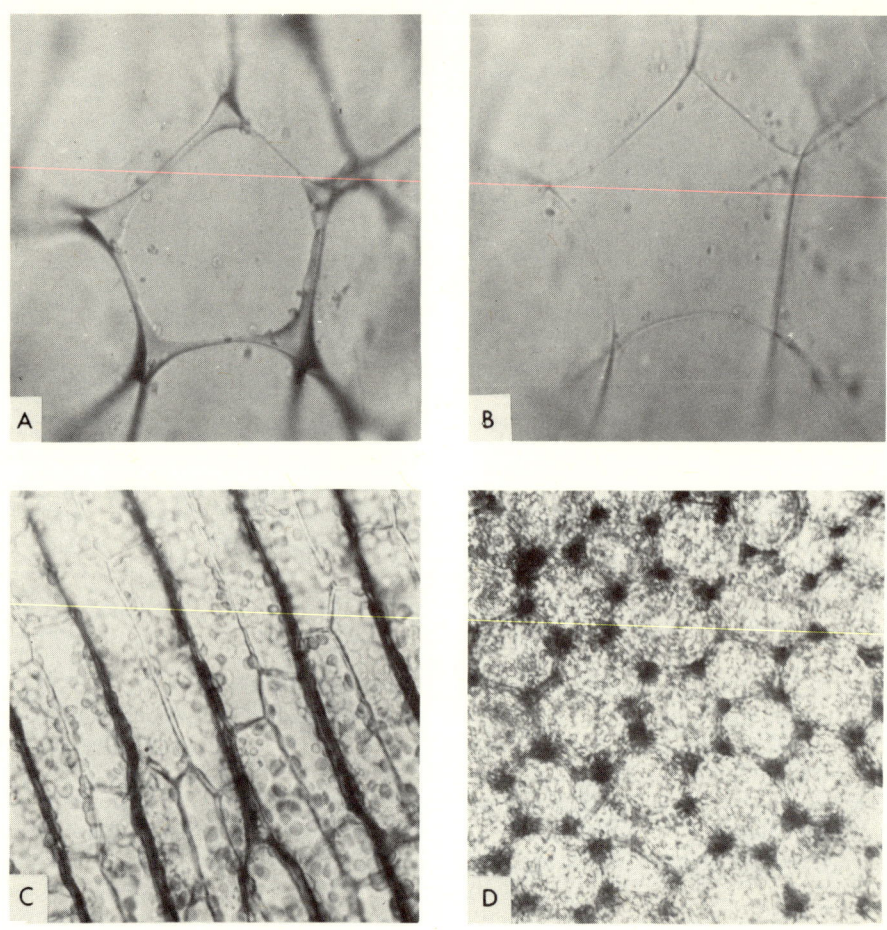

Fig. 1. A: Section of fleshy leaf of Senecio (sp.) showing intercellular space containing gas. Approx. 400X. B: Same after expulsion of gas by ultrasound. C: Leaf of Elodea showing long aspect of gas-filled channels. Approx. 500 X. D: Transverse section through cortex in elongation region of root tip in Vicia faba. Dark spots are gas-filled spaces at 3-cell junctions. 650 X.

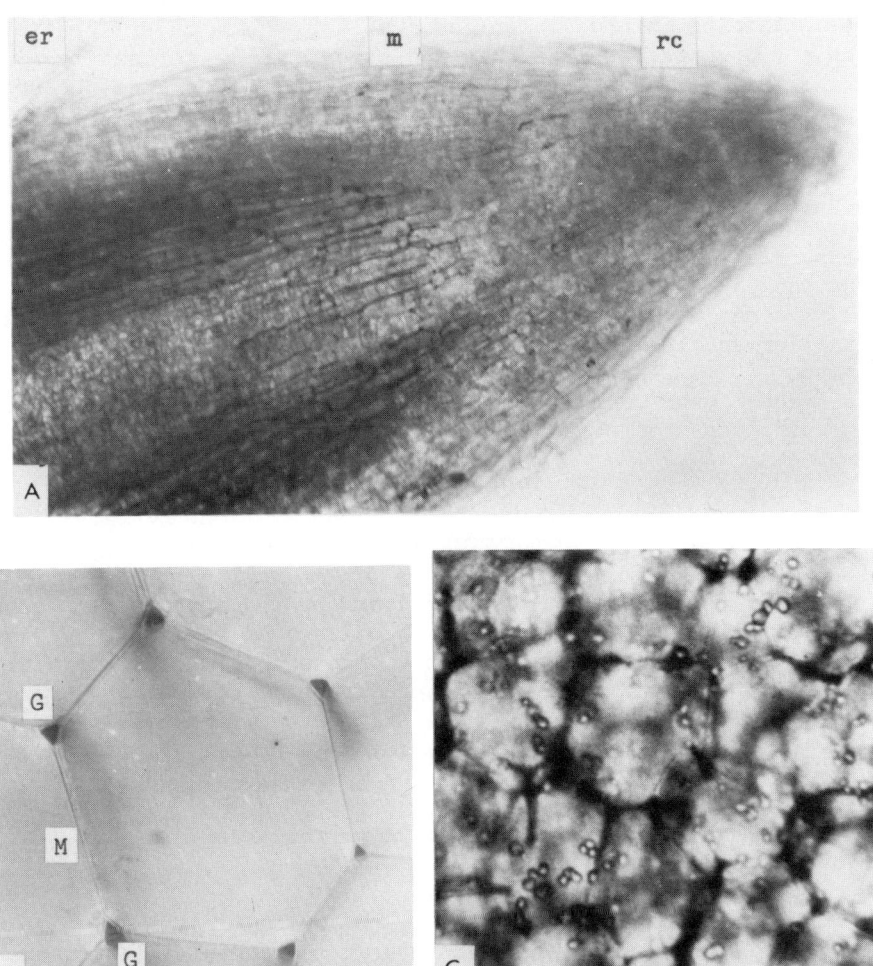

Fig. 2. A: Longitudinal section of Vicia faba root tip. The anatomical regions are; root cap, rc, and the meristem, m, which blends into the early elongation region, er. Approx. 100X.
B: Transverse section of highly vacuolate squash petiole, showing triangular gas-filled spaces at 3-cell junctions. Approx. 400X.
C: Section of cotyledon of germinating seed of Vicia faba, taken close to emerging seminal root. Seen are networks of gas-filled intercellular space (dark) and starch grains (resembling open circles). Approx. 150 X.

We proceed now to report on recent experiments in which we have made direct observations through a microscope on plant tissues containing intercellular gas, while they are under sonation. A variety of particle movements and structural perturbations are seen in the cells. At the lowest ultrasonic levels these occur primarily near the "triangular" gas-filled spaces at tri-cellular junctions, such as are seen particularly clearly in Fig. 2B. It is reasonable that these junctions should be sites of activity since the highly compressible gaseous body at a junction will respond to sound by executing volume pulsations. These pulsations necessarily cause localized vibrations in the walls of cells which bound the gas space. Localized wall vibrations, in turn, can lead to a range of intracellular perturbations, as has been shown in earlier studies in which cell walls are contacted by microvibrators[9,10]. In the next two sections we discuss work done (1) at a frequency of approximately 1 MHz with the ultrasound applied from below the sample and (2) at 85 kHz with ultrasound coming from the side.

RESULTS: 1 MHz

In the "megahertz" work we used an arrangement similar to one first described by Harvey and his associates[11]; the frequency was 985 kHz. In our arrangement the biological specimen is contained within a cylindrical volume of water supported between a quartz-disc transducer (which serves as a supporting microscope slide) and a quartz-disc cover (which may act as a receiver). Electroding is omitted from the center of the discs and conventional optical microscopy is used to observe the specimen. For this work, the cylindrical volume was 1.28 mm thick and had a radius of 2.225 mm.

The acoustic field generated in the cylindrical volume has been determined when filled with water. Interferometric measurements of the displacement boundary values at the transducer and at the cover, in conjunction with an approximate analytical solution of the wave equation, provide a detailed description of the pressure field. (Additional interferometric measurements, via an acousto-optical interaction, of the average pressure in the field as a function of the radial coordinate resolve an ambiguity in sign associated with the boundary values and confirm the analytical results.) In our approximation, the field is a cylindrical standing wave, with two pressure nulls in the radial direction and none in the vertical direction. Using the analytical solution calculations were also made of the time-averaged energy density E at various points in the field. A detailed description of this apparatus and its calibration is to be published later.

We have carried out observations on several of the different kinds of plant tissues represented in Figs. 1 and 2. Visible movements, distortions and other events were generated in the tissues by ultrasonation. Some of these resemble effects reported by previous investigators[9,10,11]; we can now give quantitative data on acoustical conditions which will produce them. Unfortunately, the acoustic field in the treatment space is not simple; it has the character of a nonuniform standing wave and cannot be specified by a single parameter which is constant throughout the space. Instead we provide information on four characteristic quantities, each with its own significance: (1) P_m, the maximum pressure amplitude in the space; (2) the intensity I_m as it would be in a traveling plane wave in which the pressure amplitude is P_m; (3) $c\bar{E}$, the average value in the treatment space of the product cE, where E is the time-averaged energy density referred to earlier and c is the velocity of sound; and (4) cE_m, the maximum value of cE in this space. We believe P_m is the important quantity when pulsation of gas-filled spaces is responsible for the observed events; under these circumstances I_m is also significant, since the same events should occur in a traveling plane wave of that intensity. Like I_m, the quantities $c\bar{E}$ and cE_m have the units of intensity; they may sometimes be superior to I_m as indices of "effective intensity". The values of P_m and I_m are given below as they exist when the treatment space is filled with water; they may be modified somewhat when a tissue sample is present. It was found that $c\bar{E}$ and cE_m are given approximately by

$$c\bar{E} = 0.069\ I_m\ ;\quad cE_m = 0.50\ I_m\ .$$

The response of the different tissues with intercellular gas spaces was remarkably uniform, although tissues with small gas spaces (characteristic dimension about 10 microns) were particularly sensitive. This enhanced sensitivity may be related to the well known resonance phenomena of bubbles. (At 1 MHz the diameter of a free resonant air bubble in water is about 7.5 microns). At the lowest levels, the sound was pulsed on and off at 1 sec intervals so that acoustically generated intracellular motions could be distinguished from normal cyclosis. At P_m = 0.32 atm (I_m = 35 mW/cm^2) slight perturbations are occasionally observed, but not below this level. The average level at which perturbations are first observed is approximately P_m = 1 atm (I_m = 350 mW/cm^2). At these low levels, effects are limited to displacement and/or rotation of a chloroplast or plastid during the pulse, and its return to its original position during the interpulse. Occasionally acoustic streaming eddies can be seen inside the vacuole. At these levels the movements are observed primarily near the intercellular gas spaces, and especially in that part of the sound field where the pressure amplitude is maximum (e.g., near the location of P_m).

At levels near P_m = 3.2 atm (I_m = 3.5 W/cm^2) a variety of effects occur. Chloroplasts tend to aggregate near the intercellular gas spaces, but do not return their original positions when the sound is turned off. Individual chloroplasts, and even the aggregated masses often rotate, still enclosed within the parietal layer. Streaming within the vacuole is more vigorous, and chloroplasts may be dislodged and taken up in the vacuolar streaming pattern; they execute orbits about the interior of the cell, with the most rapid motion adjacent to the intercellular gas.

Irradiation at P_m = 10 atm (I_m = 35 W/cm^2) produces an intensification of effects. Free mixing of cytoplasm and vacuolar contents occurs with rapid streaming involving the entire cell. Round masses of cytoplasm, including chloroplasts, sometimes separate from the cell wall and rotate freely. Cell nuclei, when visible as in Vicia faba roots, are often seen to rotate freely. In tissue slices the gas tends to leave the intercellular spaces, often quite rapidly, and occasionally forms very active spherical bubbles within or near the (now water-filled) intercellular cavities. Essentially all the gas may be expelled from the intercellular spaces at this level, and the velocity of streaming motions subsides after such expulsion.

At P_m = 25 atm (I_m = 220 W/cm^2) rapid disruption of cellular organization occurs. Free bubbles of near-resonance size may be seen appearing and disappearing even inside cells, with consequent homogenization of cell contents, including the apparent disintegration of chloroplasts and fragmentation of nuclei in root-tip cells of Vicia faba. This level is also the average threshold at which a subharmonic (493 kHz) signal can be received from the cover crystal, for tissue specimens containing air spaces, and also for ordinary tap water. Effects at or above this threshold level can be considered effects of transient cavitation; see Introduction.

Observations of specimens of plant cells devoid of the intercellular gas spaces (such as the alga Hydrodictyon) indicate that levels near P_m = 10 atm are required to produce effects similar to those seen at P_m = 1 atm in tissues with intercellular gas. In tissues with gas spaces, maximum activity occurred near regions of maximum pressure amplitude, while for the gas-free cells, intracellular activity was more uniformly distributed throughout the volume.

RESULTS: 85 kHz

In the work at 85 kHz a Mason horn, described previously[10,12], is used as source transducer. By means of a micromanipulator the horn, with its vibration axis horizontal, is positioned so that its vibrating tip, the effective source of ultrasound, is brought into acoustic contact with an edge of a tissue slice, this slice being mounted on the stage of a microscope. During sonication, visual observations were made on a portion of tissue whose distance from the sound source varied from 50 to 500 microns. Since the latter, the tip of a metal horn, is only about 45 microns in diameter, it is small compared to the sonic wavelength (about 17.5 mm in water at 85 kHz). Hence the sound field has a divergent character resembling the field of a monopole or dipole. While the tip amplitude is measured, and is typically in the micron range, the amplitude in the visual field is greatly reduced by divergence and, unfortunately, is not known accurately. Perturbations were readily produced in a variety of plant tissues and were similar in character to those observed in the megahertz studies.

With the amplitude held constant, perturbations were found to increase in extent with increasing time. In a series of experiments at increasing amplitude, events occurring after a fixed time interval were in approximately the following sequence: (i) reversible short displacements of chloroplasts; (ii) irreversible displacements of same; (iii) (irreversible) rotation of small bodies in the parietal cytoplasm; (iv) enlargement of the rotating masses; and (v) rotational and circulatory movement of the entire cell contents. At low amplitudes the motions occur only near gas-filled spaces at junctions such as G in Fig. 2B; at higher amplitudes they occur also at points, such as M in Fig. 2B, which are midway between consecutive junctions.

Of special interest are the orbits executed by small cytoplasmic particles at the higher amplitudes. As a particle approaches a wall it experiences an impulse, especially at gas spaces such as G or at intervening points such as M in Fig. 2B. This impulse apparently occurs in an acoustic boundary layer and reflects the character of the wall vibration.

DISCUSSION

When gas bodies exist between cells a sound field will produce pulsations of the gas, since its compressibility is more than 10^4 times that of aqueous media. These pulsations cause localized vibration of cell walls. In plant tissue there is an abundance of small stable intercellular gas-filled spaces. We find that near these spaces even at low ultrasonic levels visible events occur which take place only at much higher levels in the absence of gas. Threshold levels for these visible perturbations are in the same broad range as those reported for such bio-effects in plant tissue as viscoelastic changes in cytoplasm[8], chromosome damage[2,13,14], and growth retardation[1,15,16] in plants. It would seem likely that some of those bio-effects are related to our visual observations, and arise from the pulsation of gas-filled spaces.

Plants are useful as models, since they yield insight on conditions under which living systems are most vulnerable to ultrasound. Based on results with plants it is reasonable to form the following hypothesis for tissue of any kind: the threshold for bioeffects will be at its lowest if stable discrete gas bodies (especially of resonance size) exist in the tissue. If this hypothesis is valid it is imperative, for purposes of determining safe levels of medical ultrasound, to obtain information on any small stable gaseous bodies which may exist in human tissue. Some information is already available; for example, Gramiak, et al.[17], have obtained evidence which suggests the presence of gas microbubbles in human cardiac chambers. However, systematic studies of the distributions and significance of such microbubbles have apparently not been carried out.

REFERENCES

1. W. D. Gregory, M. W. Miller, E. L. Carstensen, F. L. Cataldo and M. M. Reddy, Non-thermal effects of 2 MHz ultrasound on the growth and cytology of Vicia faba roots, British Journal of Radiology 47, 122-129 (1974).

2. F. L. Cataldo, M. W. Miller, W. D. Gregory and E. L. Carstensen, A description of ultrasonically-induced chromosomal anomalies in Vicia faba, Radiation Botany 13, 211-213 (1973).

3. E. L. Carstensen, M. W. Miller and C. A. Linke, Biological effects of ultrasound, Journal of Biological Physics 4, 173-192 (1974).

4. F. A. Eames, E. L. Carstensen, M. W. Miller and May Li, Ultrasonic heating of Vicia faba roots, J. Acoust. Soc. Am. 57, 1192-1194 (1975).

5. W. L. Nyborg, D. L. Miller and A. Gershoy, Physical consequences of ultrasound in plant tissues and other bio-systems, Proceedings of Seventh Rochester International Conference on Environmental Toxicity 1974 (Plenum Publishing Company).

6. H. G. Flynn, Physics of cavitation, pp 57-172 in Physical Acoustics, Vol. 1B, Ed., W. P. Mason, Academic Press, New York 1964.

7. E. N. Harvey in Decompression Sickness, Ed., J. F. Fulton, W. B. Saunders, Philadelphia, 1951, Chap. IV.

8. A. Johnsson and A. Lindvall, Effects of low-intensity ultrasound on viscous properties of Helodea cells, Naturwissenschaften 56, 40 (1969).

9. H. J. Dyer and W. L. Nyborg, Ultrasonically induced movements in cells and cell models, IRE Trans. Med. Electron. ME-7, 163 (1960).

10. A. Gershoy and W. L. Nyborg, Perturbation of plant-cell contents by ultrasonic micro-irradiation, J. Acoust. Soc. Amer. 54, 1356-1367 (1973).

11. E. N. Harvey, E. B. Harvey and A. L. Loomis, Biol. Bull. 55, 459 (1928).

12. W. L. Wilson, F. J. Wiercynski, W. L. Nyborg, R. M. Schnitzler and F. J. Sichel, Deformation and motion produced in isolated living cells by localized ultrasonic vibration, J. Acoust. Soc. Amer. 40, 1363 (1966).

13. G. G. Selman, The effect of ultrasonics on mitosis, Experimental Cell Research 3, 656-674 (1952).

14. J. Slotova, Z. Karpfel and I. Hrazdira, Chromosome aberrations caused by the effect of ultrasound in the meristematic cells of Vicia faba, Biologia Plantarum 9, 49-55 (1967).

15. B. I. Bleaney and R. Oliver, The effect of irradiation of Vicia faba roots with 1.5 MHz ultrasound, British Journal of Radiology 45, 358-361 (1972).

16. E. R. Hering and B. J. Shepstone, The effect of irradiation of Vicia faba roots with 1.5 MHz ultrasound, British Journal of Radiology 45, 786-787 (1972).

17. R. Gramiak and P. M. Shah, Detection of intracardiac blood flow by pulsed echo-ranging ultrasound, Radiology 100, 415-418 (1971).

ACKNOWLEDGEMENT

This research was supported in part by the National Institutes of Health via Grant GM-08209

CLINICAL RESULTS OBTAINED WITH AN ULTRASONIC SPECTRAL ANALYSIS SYSTEM

F.L. Lizzi; M.A. Laviola; D.J. Coleman *
Riverside Research Institute, New York,
New York 10023; * Columbia University,
The E.S. Harkness Eye Institute, New York,
New York

Spectral analysis techniques promise to play an important role in determining tissue characteristics which can be used to identify classes of pathology that now present diagnostic problems in ophthalmology and other branches of medicine. These techniques can be used to determine such basic tissue properties as ultrasonic reflectivity and the frequency dependence of absorptivity. In addition, spectral analysis can provide statistically stable estimates of backscatter power spectra for use in delineating diagnostic "signatures".

This paper discusses the theoretical considerations underlying three types of applications where spectral analysis of reflected ultrasound can be especially useful. The first situation involves tissue structures with boundary segments that can be approximated as parallel planes. The ocular lens and certain cysts are examples of such structures. In this case, spectral analysis can provide measures of ultrasonic reflectivity and absorptivity as a function of frequency.

The second application involves tissues with a heterogeneous internal structure (e.g., malignant melanoma, angioma, and organized vitreous hemorrhage). Here, spectral analysis can be used to obtain estimates of backscatter power spectra that are essentially independent of transducer and system characteristics. By cross-range averaging, statistically stable estimates can be obtained to identify distinct tissue "signatures." Additionally, ratios of power spectra obtained at different tissue depths can be used to determine frequency dependent attenuation characteristics.

The third application involves acoustic shadowing measurements. Here, spectral analysis can be used to determine the frequency dependent attenuation characteristic of tissue elements by spectral measurements taken within posterior tissue regions.

This paper describes the bases for each type of application. It also presents *in vivo* results obtained from a clinical ultrasound system used for ophthalmological examinations at the Harkness Eye Institute. The spectral analysis system used for the clinical measurements provided a frequency coverage from 7 to 14 MHz depending on the transducer employed. Spectral resolution was typically 500 KHz providing 14 resolution cells in the output spectra. Spectral averaging along parallel transducer orientation was provided to study heterogeneous tissues, the number of individual spectra included in this average was variable. In most cases, less than 100 averages provided sufficient statistical smoothing.

Additional discussion relating to the spectrum analysis system and *in vivo* clinical results can be found in the references.

References

1. Smith, M.E., Franzen, L.A., Lizzi, F.L., Coleman, D.J., "Power Spectral Resonance Analysis in the Evaluation of Vitreous Pathology," Ultrasound in Medicine 2. Edited by D.N. White and R.W. Barnes. Plenum Press, New York, pp. 255-256 1976

2. Lizzi, F.L., and Laviola, M.A. "Ultrasonic Spectral Analysis for Tissue Characterization". Ultrasound in Medicine 2. Edited by D.N. White and R.W. Barnes. Plenum Press, New York. pp. 419-431 1976

3. Lizzi, F.L., and Laviola, M.A. "Power Spectrum Measurements of Ultrasonic Backscatter from Ocular Tissues." Ultrasonic Symposium Proceedings of the I.E.E.E. Group on Sonics and Ultrasonics, 1975.

Acknowledgement

The authors wish to acknowledge the very important

contributions made by Leslie St. Louis, Louise Franzen and Mary Smith.

This investigation was supported by Public Health Service grants EY-01212-02 and EY-01218-02 from the National Eye Institute.

INTERACTION OF ULTRASOUND WITH TISSUES

Edwin L. Carstensen

Department of Electrical Engineering

University of Rochester, Rochester, N.Y. 14627

As the applications of ultrasound are extended in diagnosis, therapy and surgery it is essential that we obtain a thorough knowledge of the biological effects of this radiation. These studies have become one of the most interesting subjects of applied research today. On the one hand, sound energy is absorbed and affects tissue by the heat produced. In addition, there is now a large body of evidence that ultrasound can affect biological material by specific, nonthermal mechanisms. As examples, purely thermal processes can explain focal ultrasonic lesion production in brain tissue at intensity levels below 200 W/cm^2. This is shown by considering acoustic absorption, heat diffusion, and the thermal sensitivity of brain tissue. On the other hand, nonthermal mechanisms are clearly needed to explain reduction in growth rate, mitotic index and chromosomal aberrations which are observed in plant roots irradiated by ultrasound. In spite of extensive applications of ultrasound in diagnosis, therapy and even surgery, there are still many problems to be solved in the basic physics of sound propagation in tissues. Sound absorption occurs primarily at the macromolecular level. There is evidence to indicate that this absorption can be profoundly modified by macromolecular interaction. The specific physical or chemical relaxation mechanisms responsible for the absorption are unknown. The macroscopic inhomogeneities in tissue affect sound propagation and can lead to artifacts in certain methods of measurement of tissue absorption. The problem of localized heating at interfaces and the question of linearity require investigation.

ULTRASONIC HEATING AT TISSUE INTERFACES

Leon A. Frizzell* and Edwin L. Carstensen

University of Rochester

Electrical Engineering Department, Rochester, N. Y.

A number of investigators have observed localized heating by ultrasound near impedance discontinuities within tissues. It was hypothesized that mode conversion to shear waves at impedance discontinuities and subsequent absorption of these waves in a very small distance was the explanation for this heating. To test this hypothesis preliminary measurements of the shear acoustic properties of soft tissues at low megahertz frequencies were made. At these frequencies soft tissues are viscosity dominated, but the viscosities are orders of magnitude below those reported at lower frequencies. The low viscosities result in low velocities and extremely high absorption coefficients for shear waves in tissue. A mathematical model for mode conversion at a plane interface between two viscoelastic media was developed. Longitudinal and shear properties of tissue were then used to calculate the amount of mode conversion at tissue-air and tissue-water interfaces. It was found that negligible energy was converted to the shear mode.

Other possible explanations were then investigated, including surface waves, non-linear effects and superposition of the incident and reflected beams. The pattern of lesion development in beef liver tissue as a function of intensity was used to determine the ultrasonic intensity pattern in air and in water backed samples. It was found that consideration of changing beam profile, absorption and superposition of incident and reflected beams could explain the heating pattern observed at a tissue-air interface.

*Present address: Bioacoustic Research Lab, University of Illinois, Urbana, Illinois 61801

ULTRASONIC DETERMINATION OF TISSUE MACROSTRUCTURE BY FREQUENCY SWEEPING

R. C. Waag; R. Gramiak; R. Lerner

Departments of Electrical Engineering and Radiology
University of Rochester, Rochester, New York

Ultrasound may be used to determine the acoustic structure of tissue on a scale corresponding to the wavelengths employed. The underlying concept is the relation between the spacing of tissue elements, ultrasonic wavelength, and scattered signal. There is selective reinforcement or cancellation of certain frequencies depending on the relation of wavelength and reflector spacing. A Fourier analysis of the received signal as a function of frequency reveals the variation in acoustic impedance which corresponds to structure. By employing a swept-frequency ultrasonic signal, data similar to that obtained by angle scanning at a fixed frequency in x-ray diffraction is obtainable. Frequency scanning appears more readily applicable for diagnostic purposes in patients. The theory is illustrated by two specific reflector configurations. One is for regular periodic structures in which point reflectors are represented as rapid changes in impedance and yield well-known Bragg diffraction effects. The other is for a random variation in acoustic impedance in which the structure information is obtained as an impedance correlation function. The frequency scanning results are identical with those for angle scanning when the medium is statistically regular or isotropic. Instrumentation capable of measuring scattered signal intensity as a function of frequency and range has been assembled. Test data obtained with this apparatus demonstrates interference effects from thin slabs and frequency dependent scattering from randomly distributed organic molecules of different sizes. Differences in scattering have been observed from an ultrasonically created lesion in beef heart muscle. Pilot studies of liver specimens have revealed marked differences in intensity-frequency distributions of individual disease processes. Cirrhosis of the liver and infiltration with myologenous leukemia have both differed from normal liver. These results are encouraging since they demonstrate the capability to study disease conditions that are expected to show obvious as well as relatively subtle tissue abnormalities.

THROUGH TRANSMISSION PATTERNS IN SOLID TUMORS

N. Hassani, R. Bard [1] and L. von Micsky [2]

Bio-acoustical Laboratory Queens Hospital Center
Jamaica, New York (1)
Director, Ultrasound Department St. Luke's Hospital
New York, New York

Through transmission is the sound energy that passes through a structure and is then recorded by the receiving transducer. If the receiving transducer is also the sending transducer, an echo producing medium must be immediately distal to the structure to qualitatively document the acoustical beam intensity. Through transmission is inversely proportional to the attenuating properties of the medium. It is registered on the oscilloscope as the number of echoes and their amplitude at the distal interface of the region insonated.

In order to evaluate the transmission characteristics of a structure, the posterior border must be identified. The distal border is visualized at low sensitivity settings when the medium is highly transsonic. This occurs in fluid filled structures and parenchymatous glands such as the liver and spleen. When the medium is poorly transsonic, great attenuation of the sound beam occurs and the sensitivity must be increased to amplify distal echoes. This is noted in acoustically homogeneous tumors such as leiomyoma uteri. This echo free region is differentiated from a cyst by the poorly delineated posterior wall indicating a lack of through transmission.

Through transmission does not occur when scanning over bone or air, since these interfaces highly reflect sound waves. The net effect is a lack of penetration of the ultrasonic beam. During scanning, an acoustical shadow of absent echoes is noted when scanning through bone or air. If the incident sonic energy is sufficient multiple axial reflection artifacts may occur.

The series included the following groups of solid tumors: thyroid adenoma-sixty four, thirty with internal degeneration; pancreatic carcinoma-fifty four, three with internal degeneration; renal cell carcinoma-seventy nine, thirty one with internal degeneration; leiomyoma uteri-two hundred thirty, twelve with internal degeneration. All tumors were sonographically interrogated with commercial A-mode, B-scan, real time and gray scale systems prior to histological analysis.

Tumors with internal degeneration permitted better through transmission than masses of the same histological type that were architecturally intact. Production of fluid filled necrotic spaces within a tumor increases the beam transmission and appears on the oscilloscope as a lesion with multiple posterior echoes. At low sensitivity, the anterior and posterior borders of a degenerating tumor may be outlined and the high posterior echo density may simulate a simple cyst. This error is avoided during attenuation studies which reveal a characteristic echogenic mass as gain is increased. Indeed, certain tumors have a biological tendency to degenerate (thyroid adenomas and renal cell carcinomas) and the demonstration of increased through transmission in a previously poorly transmitting tumor documents internal degeneration.

In summary, there appear to be two qualitative echographic patterns that may prove useful in evaluating degenerating tumors: a) change of an echo free tumor to an echogenic mass over a period of time and b) presence of high through transmission density in a solid echogenic tumor.

STUDIES ON ACOUSTICAL ATTENUATION, ABSORPTION AND SCATTERING FOR

DIAGNOSIS OF TISSUE PATHOLOGY

P. P. Lele; N. Senapati; A. I. Murphy

Laboratory for Medical Ultrasonics
Massachusetts Institute of Technology
Cambridge, Massachusetts 02139

Frequency dependent acoustical attenuation has previously been shown to correlate well with the state of viability of skeletal and cardiac muscle, viz. normal, ischemic, infarcted or necrotic. The study has been extended to normal and pathological specimens of other mammalian tissues and their acoustic attenuation "signatures" have been obtained. Scattering of ultrasound from the exposed surfaces as well as within the specimens, was measured at different ultrasonic frequencies and different orientations of the specimens, to assess its contribution to acoustic attenuation. Absorption coefficients were also measured. The specimens were examined histologically to correlate the structure with the acoustic measurements. These data will be presented and their usefulness in differential diagnosis will be discussed.

Supported in part by U.S.P.H.S. Grant FD00680 and Contract N.H.L.I. 72- 2017.

THE EFFECTS OF ACOUSTIC STREAMING ON NERVE CONDUCTION

P. P. Lele; R. Mecca

Laboratory for Medical Ultrasonics
Massachusetts Institute of Technology
Cambridge, Massachusetts 02139

Under certain experimental conditions, acoustic streaming from a resonant bubble in an ultrasonic field has been shown to have highly destructive effects on biological systems. In order to assess the effect of streaming on the physiological activity of nerve tissue, and to investigate the possibility of using streaming as a method of selectively blocking nerve function, frog sciatic nerves were exposed to streaming from single, captured resonant bubbles in 83, 49.4 and 39 kilohertz sound fields, for varying time intervals. Identical control experiments were run with no bubble in the field. The nerves were electrically stimulated before and after exposure, and changes in the spike heights of the five component elevations of the action potential were monitored, as was the temperature of the nerve surface at the point of exposure. The results obtained will be presented and discussed.

ANIMAL STUDIES OF CATARACTS PRODUCED BY HIGH-INTENSITY
ULTRASONIC ENERGY

F.L.Lizzi,Eng.Sc.D.;A.J.Packer*,B.S.;D.J.
Coleman*, M.D.
Riverside Research Institute,80 West End Ave.,
New York, N.Y. 10023; *Columbia University,
The E.S.Harkness Eye Institute, New York, N.Y.

The ability of high-intensity ultrasound to produce cataracts has been known for many years. This study was carried out to delineate the cataractogenic effects of high frequency ultrasound at intensities well above clinically employed levels. The ultimate aim of this research is to delineate the limits of "safe" high-frequency, short-duration irradiation of human ocular tissues so that future, advanced diagnostic systems can be designed within more accurately prescribed limits of safety.

Cataract production was studied in a series of <u>in-vivo</u> experiments using anesthetized rabbits whose proptosed eyes were exposed to carefully determined amounts of ultrasonic energy through a coupling medium held at constant temperature. Following irradiation the rabbit eyes were examined for short term cataractogenic effects. Irradiated eyes were examined via slit lamp photography to document the size, shape, and location of cataracts. Small scale structural changes were studied with light- and electron-microscopy. A series of animals was also monitored for long term changes.

The irradiation conditions encompassed several frequencies within the range from 1.4 to 20 MHz obtained by operating a focused transducer at odd harmonics of its resonant frequency. Typically, 9.8 MHz (seventh harmonic) operation yielded a focal spot size of 0.4 mm and average intensities as high as 500 watts/cm^2 could be achieved. At such high intensities, cataracts were produced within time intervals on the order of 0.1 sec. Intensity-time duration "threshold" data was obtained for exposures between 0.05 seconds and 10 seconds. Pulsed application of the same amounts of total energy was also studied.

Generally, cataracts produced at threshold levels appeared as thread-like opacities in an otherwise clear lens. These "threshold" cataracts gave the same gross appearance for all time durations that were employed. If irradiation was continued past initial cataract formation, the cataract grew very rapidly and could eventually occupy the entire lens thickness. These growth characteristics were studied by slit-lamp photography of a series of cataracts produced at a single intensity level applied for various time intervals.

The physical mechanisms involved in any ultrasonic tissue alterations should be identified for the most meaningful extrapolation of animal data to human diagnostic or therapeutic systems. Therefore, the quantitative data on both toxic irradiation conditions and corresponding measures of macroscopic and microscopic structural changes are being employed to further elucidate mechanisms, such as thermal phenomena, responsible for ultrasonic cataract production. These investigations also employed other types of measurements, such as _in vivo_ absorptivity determinations, to provide much-needed data on relevant tissue properties.

THE EFFECT OF CONTINUOUS WAVE ULTRASONIC THERAPY ON MYOCARDIAL

INFARCTION IN THE DOG

T. D. Franklin, Jr., J. T. Fallon*, R. C. Eggleton and
F. J. Fry
Indianapolis Center for Advanced Research, Indiana University School of Medicine, Indianapolis, Indiana 46202
*Department of Pathology, Massachusetts General Hospital,
Boston, Massachusetts 02114

Previous studies have indicated that ultrasonic therapy has some beneficial effects on wound healing specifically with increased vascularity and decreased fibrosis formation. To investigate potential benefits in myocardial healing after ischemic and infarcted events, 24 dogs were studied after coronary artery ligation. Mongrel dogs weighing from 20 to 30 kg. were anesthetized with sodium pentobarbital (30 mg/kg) and a left thoracotomy was performed at the fifth intercostal space. A portion of the fifth rib was removed and the pericardium incised. The heart was suspended by suturing the pericardium to the thoracic wall at five or six points to form a cradle. The pericardium so attached retained the lung from the anterior surface of the heart and thus provided a very good window for the post-operative ultrasonic treatment. The left anterior descending coronary artery or one or two of its anterior branches were ligated depending on the distribution pattern. The dogs were divided into three groups of eight animals each. Group A was studied for <u>four</u> weeks post-operatively, Group B for <u>three</u> weeks and Group C for <u>two</u> weeks. Each group contained four dogs that were treated with the ultrasound and four control dogs that received placebo massage with no ultrasound therapy. Treatment with ultrasound was commenced between six and eighteen hours after surgery using a continuous wave ultrasonic source. The frequency used was 1MHz, the average intensity was 1.5 watts/cm^2, and the treatments were performed for ten minutes three times a day on weekdays and twice a day on weekends. Control dogs were handled the same as treated ones, except that the ultrasonic generator was turned off. The transducer was coupled to the shaved chest wall with a water-soluble gel. The total power output of the ultrasound unit was checked weekly on a radiation pressure measurement device to verify stability. Electrocardiograms were taken before coronary artery ligations and post-operatively on days 1, 2, 3, 4, 7, 14, 21 and 28. Blood samples for total LDH and LDH isoenzymes were obtained pre-operatively and then post-operatively at days 1, 2, 3, 7, 14, 21 and 28. At the termination of the treatment period, the animals were anesthetized and the heart was removed and perfused with an enzyme specific solution which stained the viable tissue a deep blue and left the infarcted area (dehydrogenase depleted) unstained. After formalin fixation the heart was sectioned transversely at 1 cm intervals from apex to base. Blocks for histological study were selected and stained with H and E and Masson's tetrachrome.

A rise in the myocardial fraction of the serum LDH isoenzymes gave indications of myocardial damage and verified the infarctions. The untreated controls peaked higher than the isoenzyme levels of the treated animals. On several animals with pronounced premature ventricular contractions, the ultrasound treatments seemed to elicit some anti-arrhythmic response and restored the sinus rhythm. A blind histological examination was performed and the infarcted areas treated with ultrasound demonstrated (1) a decrease in the dense collagenous scar tissue, (2) more vascularization and (3) more viable myocardial cells around the small arteries and arterioles (perivascular sparing). This preliminary study has indicated significant effects which are difficult to quantify from histological findings. Studies are underway to evaluate functional aspects more quantitatively.

EFFECTS OF EXPOSURE OF THE NINE-DAY RAT EMBRYO TO ULTRASOUND

M. R. Sikov; B. P. Hildebrand; J. D. Stearns

Biology and Applied Physics & Instrumentation Departments
Battelle, Pacific Northwest Laboratories
Richland, Washington 99352

Review of the literature indicates that ultrasound may have deleterious effects on development but that these would occur at some indeterminate level above that used clinically. We will describe our ongoing studies which are providing quantitative data on the relationships between the intensity of exposure of the rat embryo and the effects produced. These include three series of experiments using 3.2 and 0.71 continuous wave and 2.0 MHz pulsed ultrasound to simulate doppler, therapeutic, and echographic conditions respectively.

In each case, individual embryos at 9 days of gestation are exposed for 5 to 15 minutes to randomly assigned intensities of ultrasound. The focused beams are coupled directly to the pregnant uterus, which is exteriorized through a mid-line incision. We have performed detailed calibrations to describe the intensity and shape of the beams and so may express exposure as the intensity incident on the uterus. The effects of insonation are evaluated after 20 days of gestation by detailed teratologic examination.

The studies with 3.2 MHz continuous wave ultrasound have been completed, resulting in typical sigmoid curves relating mortality to intensity. The curves for 5 and 15 minute exposures were not significantly different, providing a pooled LD_{50} of 17.6 W/cm^2 and an "apparent threshold" of about 3 W/cm^2. Neither the weight nor length of the surviving fetuses was affected. A limited number of malformations were observed; these were found only in fetuses insonated at intensities of 10.5 W/cm^2 and greater.

The studies at 0.71 MHz are not yet completed but there are sufficient data for preliminary analyses. The shapes and quantitative aspects of the mortality curves appear to be similar to those at the higher frequency although there is a tendency toward greater effect with 15 than with 5 minute exposures. The maximum average intensity employed in an ongoing series with 2.0 MHz pulsed ultrasound approximates the "apparent threshold" found with continuous wave exposure. Insonation at this level does not appear to affect prenatal mortality but the incidence of fetuses with abnormal morphology, particularly of the heart, is elevated. The frequency appears to be a function of the intensity over the range of peak intensities from 30 to 400 W/cm^2. We are currently attempting to establish threshold levels for this effect and to identify the mechanisms by which it is produced.

(These studies were supported by NIH research grant number R01 GM20661 from the Institute of General Medical Sciences.)

ULTRASONICALLY INDUCED FETAL WEIGHT REDUCTION IN MICE

W. D. O'Brien, Jr.
Division of Biological Effects, Bureau of Radiological
Health, Food and Drug Administration, Rockville, MD

The use of ultrasound in the clinical practice of medicine continues to increase. And yet an adequate assessment of the risk associated with such exposures is not available (O'Brien et al., 1972). In an effort to develop experimental data which would be useful in the assessment of risk, pregnant mice have been exposed to ultrasound at the eighth day of gestation. This is the period of development which corresponds to neurogenesis and early organogenesis. The neural grove is open throughout its length and midgut is wide open. Embryologically, this period corresponds to approximately the 20th day of human gestation (Rugh, 1968).

CF1 mice are time-mated by generally placing 2 males with 8 females for a 2 hour period. After the males are removed, evidence of successful mating is determined by examining for the presence of a vaginal plug.

At the eighth day of gestation, the mice are weighed and anesthetized with veterinarian sodium pentobarbitol diluted to 10% with 0.9% sodium chloride administered intraperitoneally according to weight. The total abdominal surface is shaved and the ears are punched to code the animal. The mouse is positioned on axis in the exposure field at a distance of 24 cm from a 3.18 cm diameter, 1 MHz transducer with 0.9% sodium chloride as the transmission medium. All reported ultrasonic intensities (accuracy $\pm 20\%$) represent the spatially averaged intensity at the site of the mouse but without the animal in place, which is determined by dividing the total ultrasonic power by the transducer surface area. Beam plots of the ultrasonic field at 24 cm from the transducer yield a 3 dB beam width of 1.3 cm and a ratio of on-axis intensity to spatially averaged intensity of 2.8. See O'Brien et al (1974) for further equipment, dosimetry and animal handling details.

The fetuses were removed by laparotomy at the eighteenth day of gestation, which is one to two days prior to birth. The experiment was performed double blind, that is, both the irradiation and examination were performed without the knowledge of the exposure condition.

A total of 2866 fetuses from 273 litters were examined. The following table shows the average fetal weight and number of fetuses for each of the seven exposure conditions.

EXPOSURE INTENSITY (W/cm^2)	EXPOSURE TIME (Sec)	NUMBER OF FETUSES	AVERAGE WEIGHT (GM)	PERCENT CHANCE (RE: SHAM)
0 (SHAM)	300	837	1.15	--
0.5	300	411	1.08	- 6.1
0.7	300	263	1.04	- 9.6
2.0	20	441	1.07	- 7.0
3.0	20	210	1.05	- 8.7
3.0	10	498	1.07	- 7.0
5.5	10	206	0.94	-18.3

The nonparametric Kruskal-Wallis statistical test showed that the average fetal weight reduction, shown in the table is significant at the 0.1% level ($P \alpha \leq 0.001$).

O'Brien, W.D., Jr., C.L. Christman and S. Yarrow, (1974). Ultrasonic Bioeffect Exposure System. In 1974 Ultrasonics Symposium Proceedings (ed by J. deKlerk) pp. 57-64, IEEE Cat. # 74 CHO 896-1 SU, New York.

Rugh, R., (1968). The Mouse. Burgess Publishing Co.

O'Brien, W.D., Jr., M.L. Shore, R.K. Fred and W.M. Leach, (1972). On the Assessment of Risk to Ultrasound. In 1972 Ultrasonics Symposium Proceedings (ed by J. deKlerk) pp. 486-490, IEEE Cat.# 72 CHO 708-8 SU, New York.

ULTRASONIC TOXICITY STUDY OF THE MOUSE REPRODUCTIVE SYSTEM AND THE PREGNANT UTERUS+

F. J. Fry, F. Dunn*, J. Brady*, W. D. Erdmann, P. Strang, Rozsa Kohn*, I. Baird and J. Cobb*
Indianapolis Center for Advanced Research, Indiana University School of Medicine, Indianapolis, Indiana 46202
*Bioacoustics Research Laboratory, Dept. of Electrical Engineering, University of Illinois, Urbana, Illinois 61801

This research is concerned with ultrasonic irradiation of the male mouse testes, the non-pregnant female mouse ovaries and the pregnant mouse uterus. A transcutaneous approach is used for the male testes and the pregnant uterus while a skin incision is made to permit accurate placement of the focused sound field over the ovaries. The animals are irradiated under Metofane anesthesia and are suspended in a 37°C temperature controlled degassed mammalian Ringer's solution. One aspect involves ultrasonic irradiation of 1MHz fundamental sound frequency delivered in short bursts (several μs to 125 μs) at a 1000Hz repetition frequency. These delivery regimes are meant to approximate those presently used in clinical diagnostic medicine. Spatial peak intensities and average intensities generated in this delivery mode are selected at maximum values to produce readily identifiable bioeffects. Animals are then irradiated in a graded reducing set of ultrasonic dosage regimes from this maximum. A continuous wave (c.w.) delivery format is also being used so that an intercomparison between c.w. and clinical relevant pulse regimes can be compared with regard to specific bioeffects. Bioeffects are recorded of a histological (light microscope level of specific organ and tissue sites), functional and gross structural (fetal teratology and gross tissue changes) nature. Irradiated males are tested for their ability to impregnate known quality females and the delivered litters are assayed. Irradiated non-pregnant females are tested for conception and litter delivery by mating with known quality males. Fetal status is assessed for Caesarian section delivered litters from animals irradiated over the uterine horns at day 8 or 9 post-conception as evaluated by plugging.

In order to achieve the necessary sound intensities (spatial peak intensities of 1000-1500 watts/cm^2 and time average intensities 30-150 watts/cm^2) to elicit grossly observable bioeffects in the short burst regimes, a focused ultrasonic beam is used. Multiple sound beam positions are used to cover the desired irradiation site. Each beam position involves an irradiation period of 20 seconds. For the c.w. regime, fewer beam positions are needed to cover a specific site because of the relative ease in obtaining the necessary ultrasonic intensities for irradiation with a beam of larger lateral dimensions than that used for the short burst regime.

Dosage conditions have been determined for the production of a late cage death syndrome (animals apparently recovered from the irradiation sequence, but die at periods from 12 hours to 2 weeks post-irradiation). This condition occurs for time average sound intensities in the short burst regimes in the range of intensities mentioned above. In this range of intensities for the short burst regimes, animals (male and female) which survive are functionally capable from a reproductive viewpoint. There is a high incidence of reduced fetal weight (0.6gm-1.0gm for individual fetuses compared to 1.2gm for fetuses from control animals) and size in the progeny of irradiated males and non-pregnant females, and a small reduction in numbers of fetuses in the litter (10% reduction) at these very high intensities. Irradiated pregnant females show some increase in resorption sites with little increase of gross structural fetal teratology.

The c.w. regimes show similar phenomena at lower intensities (10 watts/cm^2). There appears to be a higher incidence of fetal teratology in the c.w. regime for the pregnant female series.

The numbers of irradiated and control animals at present (approximately 1000) has just now begun to permit a statistical evaluation of the data which will be available in the next several months.

+This research supported by National Institutes of Health Grant No. R01-FD00665-03.

EARLY POSTPARTUM MORTALITY FOLLOWING ULTRASOUND RADIATION

Karen A. Curto
Division of Biological Effects, Bureau of Radiological
Health, Food and Drug Administraion, 5600 Fishers Lane
HFX-120, Rockville, MD 20852

The use of ultrasound for diagnostic and therapeutic applications is increasing.[1] Cautions based on lack of knowledge of the biological consequences of exposure and the need for further research have been expressed.[2] As part of a study of the behavioral effects of prenatal exposure, time-mated CF1 mice were sonicated in utero on the 13th day of gestation (the period of late organogenesis). The exposure system and procedure are described elsewhere by O'Brien et al.[3] Briefly the procedure involved anesthetizing the pregnant female mouse, positioning the abdominal area on-axis 24 cm from the surface of the transducer in a normal saline bath maintained at 30° C. The transducer produced an exposure of 1 MHz CW ultrasound with an effective radiating area of 7.9 square cm. Exposure times were 3 minutes and the levels (accuracy ± 30%) were sham, 0.125 W/cm^2 (low), 0.25 W/cm^2 (medium), and 0.5 W/cm^2 (high) spatially averaged over the effective radiating area of the transducer in the free exposure field condition. Choice of power levels was based on earlier findings in our laboratory which suggested that these levels were low enough not to interfere with the mother's ability to raise the pups to 21 days post partum or weaning.

All litters were randomly reduced in size to six pups shortly after birth. Reduction was done to insure adequate nourishment for all pups. A record of death of pups, female's failure to deliver or cannabalism was maintained for each litter up to day 21. A significant effect occurred for survival rate. The percent of offspring dying before the twenty-first day post partum were: sham 4.2%, low 14.4%, medium 13%, and high 26.7%. Percents were based on a total of 450 pups where numbers before death were sham 120, low 132, medium 108, and high 90. These totals exclude loss of pups due to mother's death, failure to deliver a litter, or visible cannabalism. Chi-square tests show that each group is significantly different from the sham at the 1% level ($P\alpha \leq .01$).

References

[1] J. Marx, Diagnostic Medicine: The Coming Ultrasonic Boom, Science 18 October, 1974.

[2] W. L. Nyborg, Letters, Science, 14 December, 1974.

[3] O'Brien, W. D., Christman, C. L., and S. Yarrow. Ultrasonic Biological Effect System, In Ultrasonics Symposium Proceedings 1974, IEEE, #74CHO 896 1SU, New York, p. 57-63.

PHYSICAL BASIS AND NECESSITY FOR GREY-LEVEL PHANTOM DEVELOPMENT

Terrance Matzuk, Ph.D., P.E. and M. Leon Skolnick, M.D.

Carnegie-Mellon University and University of Pittsburgh

Pittsburgh, Pennsylvania 15213

    Acoustical phantoms having several layer interfaces in simple geometric configurations and having controlled reflection coefficients at interfaces are proposed as grey-level phantoms. Such phantoms are useful for providing known ultrasonic reflection amplitudes at definite time intervals. These known reflection interfaces can provide an absolute standard to calibrate the instrument settings of conventional B-scanning equipment. Once so calibrated, diagnostic equipment can offer improved differential diagnostic capability to distinguish cystic from solid lesions and to monitor the progress of radiographic tumor treatment. In essence, the primary utility of the grey-level phantom is to provide an absolute gain calibration that includes the effects of the transducer by initializing the instrumentation prior to each examination procedure. Materials selections for the phantoms are shown to have physical properties and interfacial reflection coefficients closely approximating those values already documented for human tissue interfaces.
    Acoustical reflection amplitude information from soft tissue interfaces are presented in terms of the acoustical impedance contrast values and in terms of acoustical absorption values. The range of impedance and absorption values for normal-to-normal and for normal-to-pathological histological interfaces is presented. The physical basis for interfacial acoustical behavior is analyzed in terms of the absorption coefficients, velocity of sound, and density of tissue structures.
    Tabulated acoustical data, representing preliminary studies on a variety of soft non-biological materials, is presented wherein the acoustical velocities, densities, and absorption values lie generally within the range of human soft tissue values. It is

shown that through careful selection of materials, reflection coefficients and absorption values closely approximating tissue interfacial reflections can be simulated in a stable and reproducible manner. Such material selections, suitably molded into acoustical "grey-level phantoms", develop controlled small reflection signals when pulsed by conventional hand-held ultrasonic transducer probes. These controlled reflections are adjusted to standard display heights on an A-mode presentation (e.g., by manipulation of time-varying gain (TVG) controls, etc.) so that immediately subsequent patient examination via B-scan procedures is always made on a known absolute gain setting relative to the phantom. Illustrations of actual phantom images on several commercially available B-scanners will be demonstrated.

AUTHOR INDEX

Abboud, F.M. 84,85
Abowitt, S.H. 188,223
Al-Banna, S.J. 363
Alfidi, R.J. 195
Allen, H.D. 57,59,63,69,75,107
Amsterdam, E. 89,99
Anderson, C.F. 221,235
Anderson, G.D. 225
Anderson, J.M. 119
Angel, J. 89,99
Arnon, S. 453
Assad-Morell, J.L. 87
Asher, W.M. 179
Asokan, S. 207
Avallone, L.T. 165

Baird, I. 533
Baker, D.W. 317
Bard, R. 521
Barnes, R.W. 281,329
Barriga, P. 229
Baum, G. 469
Ben-Ora, A. 131
Bennett, L.R. 175
Beretsky, I. 401,411
Bezjian, A.A. 227
Boder, G.B. 441
Bosher, L. 71
Botvinick, E. 91
Boughner, D.R. 21,31,297
Brady, J. 533
Brenner, J.I. 103
Brockenbrough, E.C. 324
Brody, W.R. 277
Bronson II, N.R. 471
Brown, D.D. 85
Brown, M.D. 213
Burger, R.J. 281

Cannon, D.R. 95
Capek, V. 145
Cappaert, W.E. 261,263
Carpenter, D.A. 173,333
Carretero, M.M. 227
Carson, P.L. 391,445
Carstensen, E.L. 517,518
Casarella, W.J. 109
Cassidy, J. 229
Centor, R. 71
Chandra, M.S. 85
Chandraratna, P. 37,97
Chang, S. 74,83
Chown, T. 237
Christian, C.D. 221
Chuang, V.P. 183
Clark, O.H. 265
Cobb, J. 533
Coggs, G.C. 265
Coleman, D.J. 255,257,259,513,
   525
Cook, L.N. 225
Cunningham, D.A. 31
Curran, J.E. 183
Curto, K.A. 535

Daigle, R.E. 317
DeMaria, A. 89,99
Diethrich, E.B. 188
Dillon, J.C. 61,74,83
Doust, B.D. 183
Dunn, F. 533

Edelstein, A. 309
Eggleton, R.C. 239,251,441,
   481,527
Ellis, J. 199,219
Erdmann, W.D. 481,533

Erikson, K.R. 445
Estevez, C.M. 81
Evans, Jr., T.C. 321

Fallon, J.T. 527
Farrell, G. 401,411
Feigenbaum, H. 61,74,81,83
Felix, W.R. 309
Fester, A. 97
Findleton, L. 199,219
Fixler, D.E. 49
Fleischer, A.C. 213
Fox, H.E. 203
Frank, K.E. 261,263
Franklin, Jr., T.D. 239,251,521
Franzen, L.A. 255,257
Friedewald, Jr., V.E. 188,223
Friedman, G. 55
Frizzell, L.A. 512
Fry, F.J. 239,251,475,477,481, 527,533
Frye, R.L. 77
Fujii, J. 101
Funk, D.C. 85

Garrett, W. 341
Gau, G.T. 77
Gershoy, A. 501
Gerzberg, L. 273
Ghahramani, A.R. 105
Gibson, R. 309
Giles, H.R. 221,235
Girod, D.A. 61
Giuliani, E.R. 77,87
Glees, J.P. 173
Glenny, R. 191
Goldberg, B.B. 69,157,177
Goldberg, S.J. 57,59,63,69,75, 107
Goldman, L. 265
Goodman, A. 71
Gonzalez, L. 195
Gonzalez, Jr., R.R. 285
Gottlieb, S. 105
Graham, L.S. 175
Gramiak, R. 1,13,513
Green, P.S. 319,321
Green, W.M. 109
Greenspan, F.S. 265

Gresham, E. 239
Griffin, L. 225
Griffith, J.M. 75,107,277
Groch, M. 105
Gross, C.M. 1

Haaga, J. 195
Haak, Jr., E.D. 351
Haber, K. 179
Hagler, D.J. 65,87
Hancke, S. 451
Harrison, C.E. 321
Hassani, N. 521
Heimburger, R.F. 239,251
Heine, M.W. 235
Hendee, W.R. 391
Henry, W.L. 75,107
Hildebrand, B.P. 529
Hildner, F. 97
Hileman, R.E. 483
Hohler, C.W. 203
Holland, W.E. 71
Holm, H.H. 187,459,461
Holzemer, J.F. 319
Horgan, J.H. 71
Hottinger, C. 273
Hunt, S. 73
Hurwitz, R.A. 61

Ibrahim, F. 188,223

Jack, R.L. 257
Jacobsen, B. 231
Jensen, F. 187,231,459,461
Johnson, G.L. 93
Johnson, M.L. 55,465
Jones, J.P. 475
Justin, J. 309

Kak, A.C. 477
Kallos, N. 105
Kaplan, S. 93
Kato, K. 101
Kemp, V.E. 71
Kerber, R.E. 84,85
Kessler, L.W. 441
Kinard, S.A. 223
King, D.L. 109,363
Kisslo, J.A. 55,95,465

AUTHOR INDEX

Kohn, R. 533
Korfhagen, J. 93
Kossoff, G. 333
Kristensen, J.K. 187,459,461
Kurbarych, S.F. 225

Laird, W.P. 49
Larach, D.R. 363
Larsen, J.F. 231
Laughead, M.K. 223
Laviola, M.A. 427,513
Lee, T.G. 119
Lele, P.P. 523,524
Lerner, R. 519
Li, J.W. 324
Lichtenstein, B. 401,411
Lindgren, W.A. 485
Littman, B.B. 97
Lizzi, F.L. 255,427,513,525
London, E. 73
Lower, R.R. 71

McLeod, F.D. 325,327

Machleder, H.I. 487
Maklad, N.R. 183
Malindzak, Jr., G.S. 351
Manning, J. 1,13
Marich, J.W. 321
Markiewicz, W. 73
Marks, L. 191
Marshall, J.L. 271
Mason, D. 89,99
Matzuk, T. 485,537
Mayer, V. 269,271
Mecca, R. 524
Meindl, J.D. 273
Meyer, R.A. 93
Miale, Jr., A. 105
Miller, C.W. 325,327
Miller, D.L. 501
Miller, E.V. 329
Miller, P.G. 329
Miller, R. 99
Montesinos, C. 253
Muller, H.R. 285
Muller, J. 251
Murphy, A.I. 523

Nanda, N.C. 1,13
Nealeigh, R.C. 325,327
Neumann, A. 99
Nigam, A.K. 267
Nolan, J.P. 21,31
Norman, A. 487
Northeved, A. 459
Nyborg, W.L. 501

O'Brien, Jr. W.D. 531
Ohta, A. 101
Olinger, C.P. 267
Olson, R. 317
Oughton, T.W. 391
Ovitt, T. 69

Packer, A.J. 525
Paulus, H. 487
Payvandi, M.N. 84
Pedersen, J.F. 231,459
Peoples, W. 59
Pepper, H.W. 453
Perlmutter, G.S. 177
Persaud, J.A. 297
Petrovick, M.L. 351
Phillips, B.J. 188,273
Phillips, D.J. 373
Pickering, N.C. 465
Pieroni, D.R. 67
Po, J.B. 175,191,233
Poe, N.D. 175
Popp, R. 73
Porrath, S. 165
Premsagar, D. 207

Queenan, J.T. 225

Radovanovich, G. 333
Ramsey, S.D. 319
Rashid, A. 37,97
Rechnitzer, P. 21
Reid, J.M. 324
Ritter, D.G. 65,87
Robinson, D.E. 333
Roland, J.M. 67
Roseboro, T.A. 487
Rosenberg, D.B. 179,221,235
Roy, P. 77

Royal, D.R. 189
Russell, H.E. 281

Sahn, D.J. 57,59,63,69,75,107
Sample, W.F. 175,191,233
Sander, N. 131
Sanders, R.C. 185
Sanghvi, N.T. 477,481
Sarto, G. 229
Schattenberg, T.T. 77
Schiller, N.B. 91
Schy, N. 57
Senapati, N. 523
Seward, J.B. 65,79,87
Sigel, B. 309
Sikov, M.R. 529
Simmons, V. 317
Skolnick, M.L. 189,467,537
Smith, I.A. 173
Smith, L.R. 479
Smith, M.E. 255,257
Smith, S.W. 373
Smith, T.B. 383
Spencer, M.P. 324
Spigos, D.G. 145
Stearns, J.D. 529
Stern, R. 487
Stewart, H.F. 445
Stewart, J. 61
Stewart, S. 13
Stoner, J. 73
Strang, P. 533
Suarez, J.R. 319

Taenzer, J.C. 319
Takahashi, N. 101
Tajik, A.J. 65,77,79,87
Taylor, K.J.W. 173,182
Taylor, W.W. 473
Tenner, M.S. 253
Thurstone, F.L. 373,463,465
Toletino, A. 97

Valdes-Cruz, L.M. 67
Varghese, P.J. 67
Viles, P. 1
Vinson, F.S. 441
VonMicsky, L. 523
Von Ramm, O.T. 55,95,373,463,465

Waag, R.C. 519
Wardell, A. 271
Watanabe, H. 101,193
Watanabe, T. 101
Waugh, R.A. 103
Weyman, A.E. 61,74,81,83
Wilds, P.L. 213
Williams, E.S. 81
Williams, J. 309
Williams, J.B. 383
Wittmann, B. 237
Winder, A. 411
Wixson, S.E. 479
Wodraska, G. 253
Wood, J. 57,59
Wojcik, R. 57

Ziehm, D. 199,219

SUBJECT INDEX

Abdominal scanning 461,465,467
Abdominal scanning, Simethicone in 197
Acoustic holography 473
Acoustic microscopy 481
AIUM test object 445
Amniocentesis 229
Aneurysm, Aortic 157,188,461
Aneurysm, Ventricular 83
Aorta, Abdominal 157,188,189
Aortic arch 69
Aortic blood flow 297,325,327
Aortic stenosis 61,74,91
Aortic valve 1,37,61,91
Arrays, Transducer 55,219
Arterial imaging 319,321,327
Arteries, Upper abdominal 189
Arteriosus Truncus 87
Artery, Carotid 267,281,285,322
Artery, Frontal 281
Artery, Ophthalmic 281
Aspiration, Percutaneous 187
Atheroma 324
Athletes, Cardiac dimensions of 57,21
Atrial dimension 57
Atrial, Intra-, baffle 13
Atrial flutter 3
Atrial septal defects 1,13,67,87
Atrial septum 1
Atrioventricular canal defect 4
Autoimmune diseases 487

Biliary tract disease 177
Blood cells sensitivity to ultrasound 487

Blood flow, Cerebral 281,285
Blood flow measurement 273,277, 281,285,297,325,327
Brain disease 239,251,253,343
Breast diseases 345,469
Breathing, Foetal 203
Bundle branch block 101

Calibration 445,537
Cardiac dimensions 57,97,351 479
Cardiac disease, Congenital 69, 75
Cardiac imaging, Real time 55, 59,74,75,81,83,95,363
Cardiac blood flow 317
Cardiac output 89,351
Cardiac tamponade 91
Carotid artery 267,281,285,322
Carpal tunnel 269
Cataracts, Production by ultrasound of 525
Cavitation, Biological effects of 501
Choroid tumours 257
Ciliary body tumours 257
Circumferential fiber shortening, Velocity of ventricular 21
Colour display 469,471
Computer processing 363,427, 479,481
Computerized axial tomography, Abdominal 195
Congenital heart disease 69,75

When the subject indexed appears throughout a whole paper it is indexed only for the first page of the paper.

Coronary artery 21,31,97
Coronary sinus 5

Deconvolution techniques 401, 411,475,477
Dextraposition of great vessels 13
Diabetic vitreoretinopathy 263
Directional Doppler flow studies 281,297
Doppler systems 273,277,281, 285,297,309,317,324,327,329
Doppler systems, Directional 281,297
Doppler systems, Pulsed 273, 277,309,317,325
Drugs, Effect on embryo heart of 441

Ebstein's malformation 75
Echocardiography, Medium for "Stand-off" scanning technique in 107
Echoencephalography 239,251, 253,343,373
Ejection times, Ventricular 21
Embryo heart 441
Endocardial cushion defects 8
Endocarditis, Bacterial 77
Exercise and myocardial contractility 31
Fallot, Tetralogy of 69,87,93
Flow disturbances 281,285, 297,309
Flowmeters 273,277,297
Foetal abnormalities 221,223, 231
Foetal age 221,223
Foetal breathing 203
Foetal heart 207,223
Foetal injection 231
Foetal life 199,207
Foramen ovale, Patent 3
Frontal artery, Directiona- flow in 281

Gas, Intercellular in plants 501
Gray-scale technique 145,157, 173,175,177,179,182,191,213, 221,233,235,237,251,267,269, 333,341
Gynecological tumours 213,227, 233,235

Hepatic disease 173,175,177, 342,347,520
Holography, Acoustical 473
Hydrocephalus 343
Hyperemia, Reactive 329
Hypertension 49

Imaging, Real time 55,59,199, 203,219,267,319,321,363, 373,383,459,463,465,471, 473,481
Impedance, Blood flow 285
Impediography 401,411,475,477
Infarcted tissue, Effect of ultrasound upon 527
Inter-atrial septum 1
Inotropic contraction, Myocardial 21,35
Intrauterine contraceptive devices 237
Isometric exercise and myocardial function 31

Kidneys 109,183,185,187,342, 346
Kidney transplants 119,131,145
Knees 269,271

Liver disease 173,175,177,342, 347,520
Liver metastases 173
Lymphocytic destruction 487

Marfan's Syndrome 84
Maturity, Foetal see Foetal age
Microscopy, Acoustic 441
Mitral insufficiency 37,303
Mitral leaflet, Motion 55
Mitral stenosis 71,303

SUBJECT INDEX

Mitral valve 1,37,55,59,71,73, 84
Mitral valve motion 59
Mitral valve prolapse 59,73
Mortality, Postpartum 533,537
Multiscan echocardiography 55, 59,74,75,81,83
Myocardial contraction 21,31, 351
Myocardial infarction 31,89, 99,527

Nerve conduction, Effect of ultrasound on 524

Obstetrics 199,203,207,219,221, 223,225,227,229,231,345,348
OCTOSON 333,341
Ocular biometry 261
Ocular disease 255,257,261,263
Ophthalmic artery, Directional flow in 281
Orbital disease 259
Orthopaedics 269,271

Pancreatic disease 179,189
Patella 271
Pelvic inflammatory disease 233
Pericardial effusion 5,9,10,91
Photographic film for ultrasound systems 453
Placenta 221
Plants, Effect of ultrasound on 501
Plethysmography 329
Polycystic disease 336
Power spectral resonance analysis 255
Pregnancy, Complications of 199,219,227
Probe, Intravenous Doppler 327
Prostatic scanning 191,193
Pulmonary artery 69
Pulmonary obstructive disease 63
Pulmonary valve 63,87
Pulmonic stenosis 93

Radiation therapy, Planning of 165
Radiometer 485
Radiocardiographic probe placement 105
Raylography 401,411,475,477
Real time imaging 55,59,199 203,219,267,319,321,363, 373,383,459,463,465,471, 473,481
Renal diseases 109,183,185 187,342,346
Renal transplants 119,131,145
Respiration and left ventricular dimensions 103
Resistance to flow in carotid system 285

Scanning systems 333,363,373, 459,463,467,469,471
Scanning systems, Doppler 319, 321,324
Scattering by tissue 373,513, 519,523
Septal defect, Atrial 67,87
Septal defect, Ventricular 63, 65,67,79,93
Septum, Atrial 1
Septum, Interventricular, thickness 57
Shunts, Cardiac 67,69,87
Simethicone in abdominal scanning 197
Skull 373,475
Sodium nitroprusside in heart failure 99
Spectral frequency analysis, Doppler 309
Spectral resonance analysis 255,427,513
Spleen, Enlargement of 182
Standardisation 445,537
Stenosis, Aortic 61,74,93
Stenosis, Mitral 71
Stenosis, Pulmonic 93
Suprasternal notch echocardiography 69

Tamponade, Cardiac 91
Test object, AIUM 421
Tetralogy of Fallot, 69,87,93
Teratology, Foetal 529,533
THAUMASCAN 95,463,465
Thrombo-embolic disease in pregnancy 231
Thyroid disease 265
Tissue characterization 513, 519,521,523,537
Tomography, Doppler 319,321, 324
Toxicity of ultrasound 487,501, 517,518,524,525,529,531,533, 535
Transaxial tomography 391
Transducer arrays 55,219
Transducers 483
Transmission techniques 391
Transplants, Renal 119,131,145,
Tricuspid valve 1,79
Truncus arteriosus 87
Tumours, see under organ involved

Valve, Aortic 1,37,61,74,93
Valve, Mitral 1,55,59,71,73,84
Valve, Pulmonary 63
Valve, Tricuspid 1,79

Ventricle, Common 65,79
Ventricle, Lateral 253,337,343
Ventricle, Left, dimensions 21, 31,49,57,92,97,99,103,479
Ventricle, Left function 21, 31,49,93,97,99,101,103,479
Ventricle, Left, volume 21,31, 49,95,103,351,479
Ventricle, Right, compression 91
Ventricle, Right, volume 89
Ventricular aneurysm, Left 83
Ventricular circumferential fiber shortening, Velocity of 21
Ventricular diverticulum 81
Ventricular ejection 21,97,351
Ventricular septal defect 63, 65,79,93
Ventricular septum 7,67,85,97, 101
Ventricular septum thickness 49
Ventricular wall thickness 49,57
Vessels, Transposition of 13
Vitreous disease 255

Wolff-Parkinson-White Syndrome 85